AF615667

LIVER DISEASES

AN ATLAS OF HISTOPATHOLOGY

ABOUT THE AUTHOR

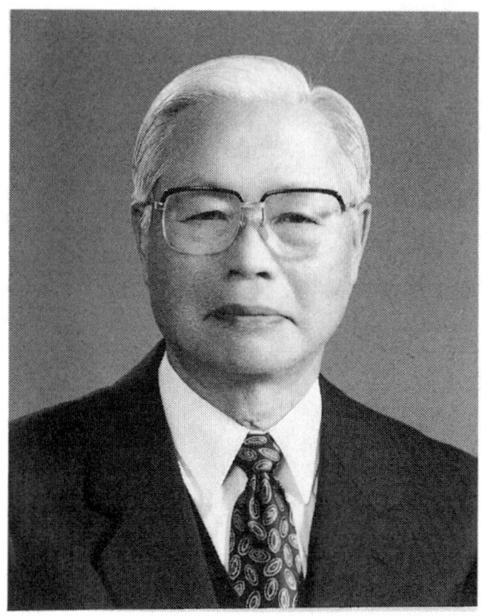

Dr. Whan Kook Chung was born in Nonsan-Goon, Choongchungnam-Do, Korea. He studied to be a doctor of medicine at Kyungpook National University Medical School in Taegu and did his internship and first year residency at the Seoul National University Hospital in Seoul. He also holds a Ph.D. from the Seoul National University.

After 13 years of medical experience he left the army as Colonel, Commander of Medical General Laboratory, and joined the staff of the Catholic University Medical College in Seoul. There he has held positions of increasing responsibility, including Department Head of Internal Medicine, Director of the Clinical Research Institute and Director of St. Mary's Hospital, which is part of the Catholic Medical Center.

Dr. Chung has had extensive academic activity in the research and study of the liver and has received numerous honors and awards. He is currently President of the Asian-Pacific Association for the Study of the Liver, Director of WHO Collaborating Center for Research on Viral Hepatitis, and Councillor of International Association for the Study of the Liver.

Dr. Chung is the author of four other books and more than 150 papers. He is the father of five children and resides with his wife in Seoul, with whom he has been married for fifty years.

LIVER DISEASES

AN ATLAS OF HISTOPATHOLOGY

WHAN KOOK CHUNG, M.D., PH.D.

Professor Emeritus
Department of Internal Medicine,
Catholic University Medical College,
Seoul, Korea

Foreword by F. Schaffner, M.D.

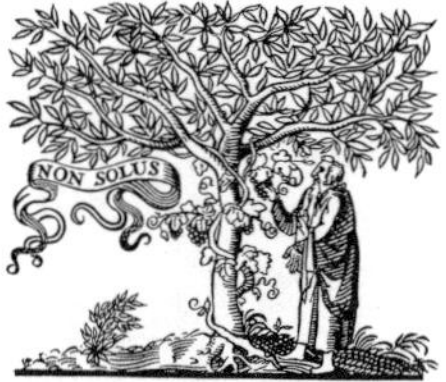

ELSEVIER
AMSTERDAM • LONDON • NEW YORK • TOKYO 1993

ELSEVIER SCIENCE PUBLISHERS B.V.
Sara Burgerhartstraat 25
P.O. Box 211
1000 AE Amsterdam, The Netherlands

Produced by: Dopazo & Company
Design and typesetting: Folio Graphic Company, Inc., New York
Color separations: TSI Graphics, Inc., New Jersey

Library of Congress Cataloging-in-Publication Data

Chung, Whan Kook.
Liver diseases: an atlas of histopathology/Whan Kook Chung; foreword by F. Schaffner.
p. cm.
Includes bibliographical references and index.
ISBN 0-444-81542-2
1. Liver—Histopathology—Atlases. I. Title.
[DNLM: 1. Liver Diseases—pathology. 2. Liver—pathology—atlases. WI 700 C5592L 1993]
RC846.9.C55 1993
616.3'6207—dc20
DNLM/DLC
for Library of Congress 93-11641
CIP

PRINTED IN THE U.S.A.

CONTENTS

LIST OF COLOR PLATES

LIST OF TABLES

ACKNOWLEDGEMENTS

I wish to express my sincere gratitude to my family, relatives and friends, especially the staff members of the Department of Internal Medicine, Catholic University Medical College, Seoul, and Dr. and Mrs. C.Y. Oh, M.D., The Mount Sinai Hospital, New York, all of whom have in many ways preserved me from the crises of life, helped me to live until this day and have encouraged me to complete the publication of this book.

The following persons deserve special thanks for their assistance or contribution in preparing the manuscript: B. M. Ahn, M.D., Instructor of Medicine, Catholic University Medical College (CUMC); I. S. Chung, M.D., Associate Professor of Medicine, CUMC; K. W. Chung, M.D., Professor of Medicine, CUMC; K. D. Han, M.D., Assistant Professor of Medicine, CUMC; J. W. Jeong, M.D., Former Assistant Professor of Medicine, CUMC; Y. B. Koh, M.D., Professor of Surgery, CUMC; B. S. Kim, M.D., Professor of Medicine, CUMC; J. K. Kim, M.D., Instructor of Medicine, CUMC; K. S. Kim, M.D., Former ROKA Captain, Capital Army Hospital; A. K. Lee, M.D., Former Assistant Professor of Medicine, CUMC; C. D. Lee, M.D., Assistant Professor of Medicine, CUMC; J. K. Lee, M.D., Director of Dongkwang General Hospital, Ulsan; Y. S. Lee, M.D., Instructor of Medicine, CUMC; Rev. Liam McCarron, CUMC; J. K. Moon, Ph.D., Professor Emeritus, CUMC; S. K. Moon, M.D., Professor of Pathology and Director of Fatima General Hospital, Taegu; S. I. Shim, M.D., Professor of Clinical Pathology, CUMC; H. S. Sun, M.D., Professor of Medicine, CUMC; J. Y. Yoo, M.D., Professor of Medicine, Halim University.

I am indebted to J. B. Chung, M.D., Professor of Medicine, Yonsei University; T. J. Chung, M.D., Professor of Medicine, Han yang University; J. K. Kim, M.D., Professor of Pediatrics, Inha University; C. H. Lee, M.D., Professor of Medicine, Korea University and J. M. Yang, M.D., Clinical Fellow of Medicine, CUMC, for providing materials. I am particularly grateful to Misses H. K. Kim, J. J. Nam, I. K. Kwoun, M. S. Park, H. H. Lee, Mr. S. C. Oh, S. J. Sohn and many other technicians for their administrative and technical assistance.

FOREWORD

Physicians interested in the pathology of liver diseases came from all over the world to hear and see what the late Hans Popper could show and teach them about this now rapidly expanding field of hepatology. One of these was Whan Kook Chung from Seoul, Korea. As a medical officer in the Republic of Korea Army, he had seen many cases of hepatitis and had been collecting liver biopsy specimens from these patients. He came to New York to learn how to best study and classify the variations in the clinical and pathological pictures he had observed. The wealth of this material also piqued Dr. Popper's interest and the months that they spent together in Dr. Popper's office on the fourth floor of the Atran Building of The Mount Sinai Hospital pouring over Dr. Chung's slides laid the foundation for Dr. Chung's life work in the study of liver diseases. Some of his colleagues followed him to New York so that they, too, could have the same teaching that was proving to be so helpful to Dr. Chung. Several of them are now contributors to this book.

I first met Dr. Chung at Mount Sinai soon after I had arrived from Chicago, following Dr. Popper with the idea that I would try to be his clinical arm. Dr. Chung and I both learned from our teacher and, at the same time, we all became friends. The learning experience did not stop when Dr. Chung returned home because the stream of Korean colleagues brought back new information and we all continued to meet at various places in the world to exchange ideas, observations and data. Furthermore, Dr. Popper reviewed slides that came from Korea until he fell ill a few years ago. Dr. Chung was a good pupil and in reading his manuscript I could imagine I was hearing Dr. Popper describing the various slides.

My friendship with Dr. Chung grew even greater during my visit to Korea 20 years ago at which time I had the rare and delightful opportunity to visit his home and meet his wife and children. This memorable experience for a Westerner was the highlight of the trip. Dr. Chung's warmth and charm were complemented by his delightfully wry sense of humor. In Seoul, I saw some of the patients that Dr. Chung describes in this book and looked at many of the follow-up liver biopsies that he had obtained.

From the point of view of information alone, this book is unique in two ways. First, it contains a wealth of detail about hepatitis, not only in numbers of cases but also in the long-term follow-ups that are provided. Secondly, this book contains descriptions of conditions that we in the Western world have seen little or none of, like typhoid fever, falciparum malaria and clonorchiasis, as they involve the liver. This book also tells us about a country, Korea, as it grew into a major industrial nation, about a man, Whan Kook Chung, as he grew into a leading educator and physician and about a lifetime of study devoted to many facets of diseases in one organ, the liver. I trust the reader will enjoy perusing these pages as much as I have when I read through the manuscript. Looking through the pictures was also a treat. Many illustrate what is quite familiar to us but many also are previously unseen views of unfamiliar diseases I know only from textbooks.

Dr. Chung has presented us with a monument to the liver, to Korea and to himself. I can only hope that this work will have several sequels.

FENTON SCHAFFNER, M.D.
George Baehr Professor of Medicine
and Professor of Pathology
Mount Sinai School of Medicine
New York, New York

PREFACE

Liver needle biopsy procedure was first introduced to Korea in the early 1950's. In the beginning, a small number of physicians who were interested in liver diseases carried out sporadic liver biopsies for the purpose of clinical diagnosis and research. From then on, however, the procedure has become so popular as to make a significant contribution to the diagnosis and treatment of patients with liver diseases, and this valuable method is now being employed in most large hospitals in Korea.

Between 1956 and 1991, I personally performed a total of 5,142 liver biopsies on Korean patients with various liver maladies, including hepatic lesions related to local epidemic diseases. On occasions, in order to find out the histologic course and outcome, I carried out serial multiple biopsies on a considerably large number of selected cases.

Through the study that I carried out during that period, I was able to establish the histologic entity and evolution of some liver diseases which had not been recognized previously.

Looking back upon the past, perhaps I was over-enthusiastic about liver biopsy in some cases. Luckily, however, among the patients on whom I conducted liver biopsy, there have been no cases that developed fatal complications.

As mentioned above, at a certain period of history in Korea, there was quite a large number of patients with hepatic lesions, but the number of such cases has now dwindled remarkably. This is a good indication that, as time passes, socio-economic development, change in behavioral patterns and mutual exchange of culture and technology within the global village will eventually result in the termination of geographic alienation and isolation and, as a result, some types of diseases once rampant in Korea, including the diseases described in this book, may be hard to find in future.

The primary significance of this book is, I admit, not so much in its availability as a histologic textbook but in the value it may retain for many years to come as a documentation of the histologic features of liver diseases found among the Korean people at one stage of the world's development.

Since the tissue slides used in this publication have been collected over a long period of time, it has been impossible to clearly reprint some of the photographs. However, they have been included as valuable records of my study.

I hope that clinicians and pathologists, especially hepatologists, and all those interested in this field of medicine, will find in this publication a useful reference and an enjoyable companion for a lasting period.

Seoul, Korea

WHAN KOOK CHUNG

LIST OF CONTRIBUTORS

BYUNG MIN AHN
Instructor, Department of Internal Medicine, Catholic University Medical College, Seoul, Korea.

IN SIK CHUNG
Associate Professor, Department of Internal Medicine, Catholic University Medical College, Seoul, Korea.

KYU WON CHUNG
Professor, Department of Internal Medicine, Catholic University Medical College, Seoul, Korea.

JIN WU JEONG
Former Assistant Professor, Catholic University Medical College, Seoul, Korea.

BOO SUNG KIM
Professor, Department of Internal Medicine, Catholic University Medical College, Seoul, Korea.

YONG BOK KOH
Professor, Department of General Surgery, Catholic University Medical College, Seoul, Korea.

JAE KWANG KIM
Instructor, Department of Internal Medicine, Catholic University Medical College, Seoul, Korea.

KIL SOO KIM
Former Captain, ROK Army.

AHN KI LEE
Former Assistant Professor, Catholic University Medical College, Seoul, Korea.

CHANG DON LEE
Associate Professor, Department of Internal Medicine, Catholic University Medical College, Seoul, Korea.

CHANG HONG LEE
Professor, Department of Internal Medicine, Korea University Hospital, Seoul, Korea.

JIN KWAN LEE
Director, Dongkwang General Hospital, Ulsan, Korea.

SAE KWANG MOON
Director, Fatima General Hospital, Taegu, Korea.

HEE SIK SUN
Professor, Department of Internal Medicine, Catholic University Medical College, Seoul, Korea.

JAE YOUNG YOO
Professor, Department of Internal Medicine, Halim University Medical College, Seoul, Korea.

LIVER DISEASES

AN ATLAS OF HISTOPATHOLOGY

1 NATURAL HISTORY OF ACUTE ICTERIC VIRAL HEPATITIS

Whan Kook Chung, M.D., Ph.D.,
Sae Kwang Moon, M.D., Ph.D.
Jin Kwan Lee, M.D., Ph.D., and
Kil Soo Kim, M.D.

Following the Korean War (1950–1953), an endemic prevalence of acute viral hepatitis (AVH) occurred in Korea. After the war, in the latter half of the 1950's and the first half of the 1960's, we worked as army surgeons in the ROK Army and encountered many AVH cases among the soldiers.

Initially we assumed that most cases of AVH recovered speedily, but sometimes chronic liver disease developed. However, this assumption has not been accepted universally.

Adult patients in Western countries show speedy recovery from type B AVH and only 10% of these remain chronic carriers(1). In Korea, however, the majority of cases remain carriers even after recovery.

The reason is, presumably, that in Western countries the primary infection occurs mostly in adulthood but, in Korea, the primary infection takes place in childhood (see Chapter 4). The infected patients maintain health until, in adult life, some factors spark acute episodic flare-ups, causing the latent state to develop to overt AVH.

The pathogenesis of the acute bout of AVH in healthy chronic hepatitis B virus (HBV) carriers remains problematic. It may be the result of exacerbation of hepatitis B, presumably associated with increased viral replication which may reappear after the preceding period of absence of viral replication. These patients seem to remain carriers even after recovery. In Korea, in such cases, clinical as well as histologic findings at the time of flare-up frequently present

AVH patterns. However, such cases of AVH often progress to chronic liver disease. Consequently, the natural course of AVH observed in Korea is thought to be different from that found in Western countries.

For the purpose of studying and establishing the natural histologic evolution of AVH in Korea, 183 young Korean male soldiers with biopsy-proven acute icteric viral hepatitis were selected from among jaundiced patients who were admitted to an Army hospital from 1956 to 1966. Of these, 143 patients were tested serially with needle biopsies during the period from the early acute phase to the convalescent stage (2). Of the 143 patients, 92 were available for long-term follow-up ranging from four months to 10 years after the initial attack (Table 1-1). Its etiology could not be established but, in a recent study, the majority (95%) of these AVH cases were of type B(3), prevalent among soldiers of the same age and sex in the same area where the previous study had been performed.

Histologic Features in the Initial Biopsy Specimens

The 183 patients were selected on the basis of detection of AVH by liver biopsy (Table 1-1). In all of the 183 patients, liver biopsy specimens demonstrated the features accepted as characteristics of viral hepatitis (4,5).

The majority of the cases were of a spotty necrotic type (prototype). Cholestasis and confluent (bridging or multilobular) necrosis were occasionally observed in addition to spotty parenchymal necrosis. Fulminant and fatal hepatitis with massive parenchymal necrosis was seen in one case (Fig. 1, see page 33).

Histologic Evolution as Evidenced by Serial Biopsies

Histologic features of the 143 of the 183 patients were evident around the end of the third month, after the onset of jaundice permitted a division of the patients into four groups (Table 1-1). The remaining 40 patients (Group V) were not available for follow-up biopsy in the third month.

Group I: Healed. Forty-four patients showed no abnormal features at the end of the third month.

Group II: Nonspecific reactive hepatitis. Seventy-five patients showed only Kupffer cell mobilization, some single cell necrosis and mild portal infiltration at the third month. All but three of the patients of this group were available for a follow-up biopsy study over a period of four months to 10 years (average 1.2 years) after the onset of jaundice. In the majority, the follow-up biopsy findings continued to exhibit nonspecific reactive hepatitis.

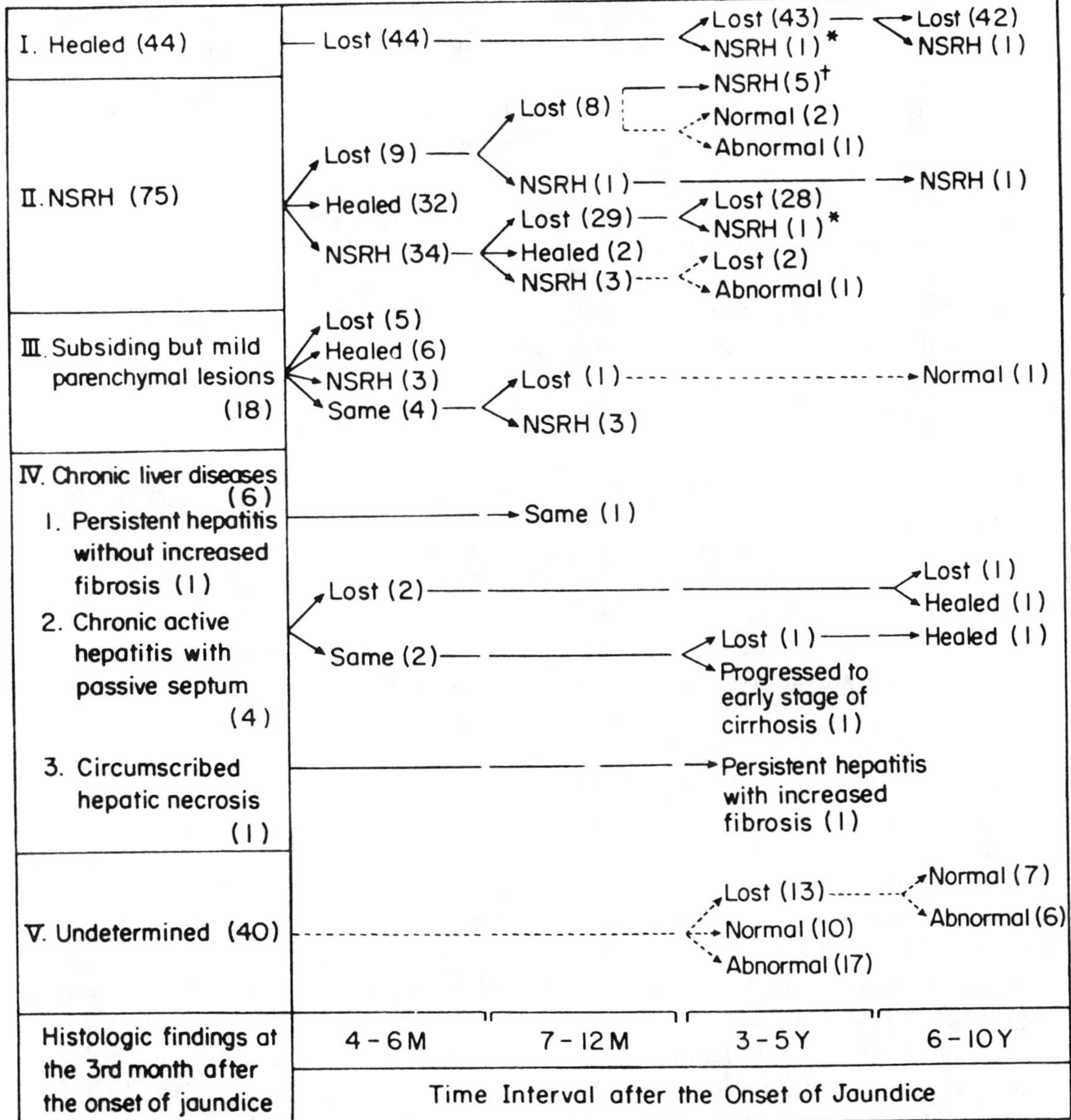

Table 1-1. Histologic and Clinical Evolution of 143 Cases of Acute (Icteric) Viral Hepatitis

Key: numbers in parentheses are the number of cases; unbroken lines denote histologic follow-up associated with clinical and laboratory observations; broken lines denote clinical follow-up; NSRH, nonspecific reactive hepatitis; † only an excess of lipofuscin pigments; *only an excess of lipofuscin pigments in four out of five cases. (Reproduced from Chung WK, Moon SK, Kim KS, et al., Korean J Internal Medicine 18:428–446, 1975, with permission)

Group III: Subsided but showed mild parenchymal lesions. This group comprised 18 patients. The appearance of hepatocytes varied only slightly. Acidophilic bodies were seen. Single-cell necrosis and Kupffer cell mobilization were also found, but in a lesser degree of intensity than in the initial biopsy specimens. Mild chronic portal inflammation was also noted. Some of the other features noted in the first biopsy specimens were absent.

Of these, 13 patients were followed for four to six months (average of five months) after the onset of jaundice: six patients revealed the disappearance of the abnormal histologic alteration, three improved to the grade of nonspecific reactive hepatitis, and four had still mild parenchymal lesions justifying the designation of persisting mild active hepatitis.

Illustrative Case Report

Case 474: A 23-year-old man was admitted to a hospital because of a high serum aspartate aminotransferase (SAST) found in a mass SAST survey originally designed to detect pre-icteric cases of viral hepatitis among the endemic population. The patient had been well until he began to have anorexia, indigestion and fatigue 15 days before hospitalization. He denied any history of jaundice, drug ingestion or related symptomatology of liver disease. Icterus was evident and the liver tip was palpable under the right costal margin. The serum bilirubin was 18.4 mg, the serum protein 6.8 gm (the albumin 2.7 gm, the globulin 4.1 gm) per 100 ml, the SAST was 1750 units, and the serum alanine aminotransferase (SALT) was 1420 units/100 ml.

Liver biopsy was performed on the second day of hospitalization, 16 days after the onset of jaundice. The biopsy specimen demonstrated spotty necrotic type AVH (Fig. 2, see page 33).

Two months after the onset of symptoms, the SAST and SALT gradually decreased to 260 and 159 units, respectively, while the serum bilirubin level persistently rose. Rebiopsy was performed. The biopsy specimen exhibited the glycogen storage phase usually seen in the healing stage. Variation of hepatic cells in size and staining qualities of nuclei and cytoplasm throughout the lobule, swelling and ballooning of hepatic cells, activated reticuloendothelial cells with bile pigment—these features were evident but showed a lesser degree of intensity than those in the first biopsy specimen. Most of the reticulum framework was well preserved except for a little condensation in part (Fig. 3, see page 33).

Three months after the first biopsy, a third biopsy was done. The histologic features were the same in principle, although hepatic cell variation was less conspicuous.

Consecutive biochemical tests afterwards revealed a gradual subsidence to a near normal level six months after the first biopsy. The last biopsy was performed six months after the first and the biopsy specimen showed a normal architecture, occasionally with two-cell thick plates and chronic inflammatory cell infiltration in the portal area without destruction of limiting plates. Almost complete healing occurred and no chronic progression developed.

Group IV: Chronic hepatitis. Serial biopsies of six patients in the third month revealed the features of persistent hepatitis in one, chronic active hepatitis with passive septal fibrosis in four and circumscribed hepatic necrosis (CHN) in one.

The patient with persistent hepatitis exhibited constant features without clinical, biochemical or histologic evidence of progression to cirrhosis until one year after the acute attack. Three of the four patients with chronic active hepatitis of a septal type were available for a long-term follow-up. Of these, two appeared to have attained complete healing without cirrhosis. In the remaining one, the histologic lesion failed to recover and ultimately progressed to an early stage of cirrhosis during the period of a three-year follow-up. In the patient with circumscribed hepatic necrosis with postnecrotic cirrhosis, regression progressed to a state of inactive, incomplete septal fibrosis without any abnormal biochemical tests three years after the initial study.

Whether these patients, who showed chronic progression, contracted the primary infection in their earlier life or later is not clear. All of the patients had returned to work after recovery from the original attack and had enjoyed their lives without any significant difficulties when last seen.

Illustrative Case Reports

Case 1048: Persistent hepatitis. A 26-year-old man was admitted to a hospital because of headache, dark urine and jaundice.

The jaundice developed 10 days after the initial symptoms. There was no history of jaundice or drug ingestion. Physical examination revealed mild icterus and a tender palpable liver edge. The SAST was 450 units, the SALT 560 units and the total bilirubin was 5 mg per 100 ml.

Liver biopsy was done on the day following the admission, 10 days after the onset of jaundice. Typical features of a spotty necrotic type of AVH were noted.

In the fourth week after the admission, the jaundice cleared and his only complaint was fatigue. Biochemical tests were all normal except SAST. Liver biopsy showed the portal tract expanded and infiltrated by chronic inflammatory cells. The lobular architecture was preserved and there was no piecemeal necrosis. Occasional focal necrosis and mild Kupffer cell activation were noted. While the other biochemical tests showed normal values, the SAST level remained elevated even until one year later. A third biopsy showed neither progression nor regression of the lesion. The portal tracts were slightly expanded but no appreciable parenchymal changes were seen.

Case 1059: Chronic active hepatitis with passive septal fibrosis. A 24-year-old man was admitted to a hospital because of dark urine and jaundice. He had no history of jaundice or drug ingestion. Icterus was evident but the skin was free of spider nevi or palmar erythema. The total bilirubin was 7.7 mg and the total protein 6.7 gm (the albumin 4.2 gm and the globulin 2.5 gm) per 100 ml. Liver biopsy was done on the day following the admission, five weeks after the onset of jaundice. All features of classic AVH were noted.

In the seventh month after the first biopsy, the liver was no longer palpable but a mild elevation of serum aminotransferase activity was noted. A second liver biopsy was done, and the specimen showed a bridging type of parenchymal necroinflammation. The patient returned for reexamination three years later. He was symptom-free and working, but hepatosplenomegaly was noted again. The SAST was 146 units, the SALT 640 units, the total serum bilirubin 0.8 mg per 100 ml and the total protein 7.5 gm (the albumin 3.6 gm and the globulin 3.9 gm) per 100 ml. The third biopsy specimen revealed expanded portal tracts infiltrated by mononuclear cells, piecemeal necrosis and the beginning of nodule formation (Fig. 4, see page 33). The morphologic criteria of chronic active hepatitis with early cirrhosis were satisfied.

Case 141: Chronic active hepatitis with passive septal fibrosis. A 24-year-old man was admitted to a hospital because of dark urine and jaundice. He denied a history of jaundice, drug ingestion and related symptomatology of liver disease. On physical examination, icterus was evident but the skin was free of spider nevi or palmar erythema. The edge of the liver and the spleen were palpable. The total bilirubin was 10.2 mg per 100 ml. A biopsy was performed on the day following admission, seven weeks after the onset of jaundice. Acute viral hepatitis with spotty necrosis was noted.

Seven weeks after the initial study, the icterus and hepatosplenomegaly remained but they subsided considerably in degree. Mild pitting edema in both shins and questionable ascites were noted. A second biopsy was done and the histologic features revealed that the disease process had further advanced with passive collapse, fibrotic septa formation, nodular regeneration and piecemeal necrosis (Fig. 5, see page 33). It was predicted that this patient would develop cirrhosis.

He was discharged from the hospital 10 days after the second biopsy, and for 10 years thereafter had not been available for follow-up treatment or observation until he returned for reexamination. He stated that he had been obliged to go back to work soon after his return home and that he paid no particular attention to the regimen for the liver disease. Apart from the slightly palpable liver, no appreciable symptoms or signs were noted. The SAST was 27 units, the SALT 4 units, the total bilirubin 0.9 mg and the total protein 7.6 gm (the albumin 4.1 gm and the globulin 3.5 gm) per 100 ml. The biopsy specimen showed a normal architecture, with occasional two-cell-thick plates but hardly any variations in hepatic cells and in nuclear size (Fig. 6, see page 33). Complete healing occurred and no cirrhosis developed.

Case 1317: CHN. A 21-year-old man was admitted to a hospital because of dark urine and jaundice. The patient, who had been well, began to have anorexia, indigestion, fatigue and dark urine 10 days before admission. He denied any history of jaundice, drug ingestion or related symptomatology of liver disease. On physical examination, icterus was evident but the skin was free of spider nevi and palmar erythema. The liver and spleen were not palpable. The serum bilirubin was 15 mg and the serum protein was 8.5 gm (the albumin 4.7 gm, and the globulin 3.8 gm) per 100 ml. The SAST was 360 units, the SALT 340 units. A liver biopsy was performed on the third hospital day, two weeks after the onset of jaundice. The biopsy specimen demonstrated the histologic features of AVH.

Ten days later, the patient became delirious, but did not fall into a deep coma. The delirium persisted for three days, but gradually subsided. Development of ascites followed this episode. Another episode of similar mental deterioration appeared one month after the first occurrence. Although the serum levels of bilirubin, the SAST and the SALT persistently rose for two months after the onset of symptoms, the consecutive tests thereafter revealed a gradual subsidence to a near normal level five months after the onset of jaundice. Rebiopsy was performed 12 weeks after the first biopsy under the condition of complete subsidence of ascites and the presence of mild jaundice. The biopsy specimen exhibited CHN with postnecrotic cirrhosis (Fig. 7, see page 33). The hepatocytes were isolated in a rosette-like fashion by fibrotic tissue and, in the greater part of the remaining area of the specimen, the hepatocytes were replaced by broad fibrotic scar tissue with chronic inflammatory cell infiltration. The patient returned for reexamination three years after the initial study. Apart from ready fatigue, he felt relatively well and was able to perform his duties as a factory hand. The edge of the liver and spleen were questionably palpated. The biochemical tests were normal. A third biopsy was performed. On microscopic examination, a small amount of incomplete strands of septal fibrosis was noted but the most part of the specimen was fairly intact. When last seen 10 years after the third biopsy, no appreciable clinical or biochemical abnormalities were noted, even though the patient had been working hard for more than 10 years.

Summary

One hundred and eighty-three icteric patients with biopsy-proven acute viral hepatitis were selected for the study and subjected to serial studies of liver needle biopsy and clinical and laboratory examinations during the period from the early acute phase to the convalescent stage. Of 183, 92 patients were available for a long-term follow-up ranging from four months to 10 years after the original attack. Of 143 patients, who were available for serial histologic studies around the third month after the onset of jaundice, 119 patients (83%) showed recovery to normal or nonspecific reactive hepatitis within three months after the onset of jaundice. In 13% of the 143 patients, the histologic lesion continued to subside. Three months later, only a few acute parenchymal changes remained, and all recovered within a year after the original attack. In an additional six patients (4%), the transition of acute viral hepatitis into chronic liver disease during three months of acute illness was also observed by serial histologic study: one showed persistent hepatitis without fibrosis, four chronic active hepatitis with passive fibrotic septum and the remaining one revealed circumscribed hepatic necrosis with cirrhosis.

The patient with persistent hepatitis exhibited constant features without clinical, biochemical or histologic evidence of progression to cirrhosis until one year after the acute attack. Three of the four patients with chronic active hepatitis of a septal type were available for a long-term follow-up. Of these, two appeared to have complete healing without cirrhosis. In the remaining one, the histologic lesion failed to recover and ultimately progressed to an early stage of cirrhosis during the period of a three-year follow-up. In the patient of CHN with cirrhosis, regression progressed to show a state of inactive incomplete septal fibrosis without any abnormal biochemical tests three years after the initial study.

Abnormal clinical and laboratory features, without association of significant organic hepatic lesions, were observed in a sizable minority of patients who had recovered from acute viral hepatitis three to 10 years earlier. Such an abnormality by itself is not a reason for reinstituting bed rest or restricting activity.

Addendum

In Korea, 79% of post-transfusion hepatitis cases (6) and 5% of sporadic AVH cases were HBsAg-negative (3). Recently, we examined these HBsAg-negative samples for antibody to hepatitis C virus (anti-HCV) using the Abbott enzyme immunoassay method. Among 57 HBsAg-negative patients with post-transfusion hepatitis, 38 (66.7%) were positive for anti-HCV. Of the 85 HBsAg-negative patients with sporadic chronic hepatitis, 42 (49.4%) were positive for anti-HCV (7).

A case with type C AVH: A 61-year-old female was admitted to a hospital because of epigastric fullness and easy fatigability since seven days prior to admission. She had no history of jaundice or drug ingestion within six months prior to the onset of illness. She had no icteric sclerae but showed a tender palpable liver edge. Her SALT and SAST levels were elevated initially and persisted for one month, while the bilirubin levels were within normal limits during the period of observation. No markers for hepatitis A and B were detected and anti-HCV was positive. Liver biopsy was performed 10 days after the initial observation. In the liver biopsy, in addition to the general features of acute viral hepatitis, the picture was one of marked sinusoidal and portal zone cellular infiltration, somewhat resembling infectious mononucleosis (Fig. 8, see page 33). Fatty change was seen.

References

1. Ganem, D. Persistent infection of humans with hepatitis B virus; Mechanisms and consquences. Rev Infec Dis 4: 1026–1047, 1982.

2. Chung, W.K., Moon, S.K., Kim, K.S. and Lee, J.K. Long term follow-up studies of acute viral hepatitis. Korean J Int Med 18: 428–446, 1975.

3. Paik, N.J., Chung, T.J., Jung, K.W., Kim, B.S. and Chung, W.K. Non-A, non-B hepatitis in Korea. Korean J Gastroenterology 11: 75–79, 1979.

4. Dible, J.H., McMichael, I. and Sherlock, S. Pathology of the hepatitis; aspiration biopsy studies of epidemic, arsenotherapy and serum jaundice. Lancet 2: 402, 1948.

5. Smetana, H.F. The histologic diagnosis of viral hepatitis of needle biopsy. Gastroenterology 26: 612, 1954.

6. Chung, K.W., Chung, W.K., Chung, I.S., Sun, H.S., Kim, B.S. and Kim, S.M. Post-transfusion hepatitis in Korea. Bull Clin Res Inst, Catholic Medical Center 11: 1–6, 1983.

7. Chung, K.W., Sun, H.S., Chung, W.K., Shin, H.K., Park, C.K., Yoo, J.Y., DiBisceglie, A.M., Waggoner, J.J. and Hoofnagle, J.K. A preliminary report on the prevalence of type C hepatitis in Korea. Korean J Internal Med 38: 750–753, 1990.

{This is an extension and revision of the study previously done by us (2).}

Legends

Fig. 1. Fatal massive necrosis (Case 73).

A needle biopsy specimen obtained from a patient, who had no history of drug ingestion during the six months preceding hospitalization, seven days after the onset of illness. Minor, not complete, collapse of reticular framework is seen in the area where confluent necrosis occurs. Needle biopsy, reticulin, ×200.

Fig. 2. A case from Group III (self-limited with retarded recovery) (Case 474).

First biopsy specimen obtained 16 days after the onset of jaundice, showing a picture of acute viral hepatitis with spotty necrosis of parenchymal cell, variation of hepatic cells in size and staining qualities of nuclei and cytoplasm throughout the lobule, the swelling and ballooning of hepatic cells, acidophilic bodies in the tissue space, activated reticuloendothelial cells and conspicuous mononuclear inflammatory cell reaction of the portal tract. Needle biopsy, HE, ×100.

Fig. 3. Second biopsy specimen obtained two months after the onset of jaundice.

The lobular architecture is preserved. There is a slight condensation of reticulin between the centrilobular area and the portal tract. Needle biopsy, reticulin, ×100.

Fig. 4. A case exhibiting transition to chronic active hepatitis with passive septal fibrosis (Case 1059).

Third biopsy specimen three years after the first, showing persistent portal chronic inflammation, piecemeal necrosis and the beginning of nodule formation. Needle biopsy, trichrome, ×100.

Fig. 5. A case exhibiting a course of reversible cirrhotic change (Case 141).

(Reproduced from Chung, W.K., Moon, S.K., Kim, K.S. et al., Korean J Internal Medicine 18: 428–446, 1975, with permission)

Second biopsy specimen obtained seven weeks after the first, showing confluent necrosis (subacute hepatic necrosis) with close approximation of portal tracts and central veins with no intervening parenchyma. Needle biopsy, HE, ×100.

Fig. 6.

Last biopsy specimen obtained 10 years after the first, showing complete healing. Note the intact architecture and the normal hepatic cell arrangement with no abnormal reaction. Needle biopsy, HE, ×100.

Fig. 7. A case exhibiting transition to cirrhosis (Case 1317).

(Reproduced from Chung, W.K., Moon, S.K., Kim, K.S. et al. Korean J Internal Medicine 18: 428–446, 1975, with permission)

Second biopsy specimen obtained 12 weeks after the first one, showing isolation of hepatocytes in a rosette-like formation of fibrotic tissue (circumscribed hepatic necrosis). Needle biopsy, HE, ×400.

Fig. 8. Liver biopsy specimen obtained from a case with type C acute viral hepatitis 17 days after the onset of illness.

Note the marked sinusoidal cell infiltration and fat change in liver cells. Sinusoidal cells are composed of mononuclear cells and polymorphonuclear cells. Needle biopsy, HE, ×100.

2

LIVER BIOPSY FINDINGS IN 'HEALTHY' HEPATITIS B SURFACE ANTIGEN CARRIERS

Whan Kook Chung, M.D., Ph.D.

Infection with hepatitis B virus (HBV) can lead to a variety of outcomes. The majority of persons (60–70%) infected with this virus do not manifest any overt symptoms of illness. From a clinical viewpoint, chronic HBsAg carriers can be divided into two forms: 1) those with chronic liver disease, 2) those without.

The first group usually refers to those having chronic type B hepatitis and the second to those being in the "healthy" chronic HBsAg carrier state. The "healthy" carrier state is conventionally considered as a persistence of infection in the absence of "clinical" and significant "laboratory" abnormalities. However, neither term is satisfactory, nor is usually accepted.

The "healthy" carrier state often develops into chronic hepatitis, cirrhosis or hepatocellular carcinoma, or sometimes serves as the source of infection. With regard to the ultimate outcome, prognosis and infectivity, it is important to clarify the clinical, biochemical, immunologic and histologic entities of the "healthy" carrier state and to differentiate it from chronic type B hepatitis.

The presence or absence of symptoms is often used to distinguish between HBsAg carriers with potentially serious forms of chronic type B hepatitis and those without significant liver disease. Indeed, the majority of patients with HBV-related chronic liver disease have no symptoms or complain only of mild and intermediate degrees of fatigue or lack of energy (1). Thus, clinical symptoms should not be used to decide whether a HBsAg-positive patient has chronic type B hepatitis or is a "healthy" carrier.

Although serum aminotransferase activities often serve as standards to distinguish between chronic type B hepatitis and the "healthy" carrier state, they are not always reliable.

The test for HBeAg is presently the most practical and generally available means of assessing the state of viral activity. Most patients with HBeAg will have chronic type B hepatitis, while the "healthy" carriers have occasionally anti- HBe. However, there are many exceptions.

Liver biopsy findings have been the traditional standard by which to measure whether a patient has significant underlying disease or is a "healthy" carrier. The truly "healthy" carrier should have normal or minimally abnormal liver histology. The most common abnormality found in "healthy" carriers is the ground glass-appearing hepatocytes, a cell with abundant HBsAg in the cytoplasm. However, these cells are also seen in chronic type B hepatitis and even in acute hepatitis and drug hepatitis. Therefore, no single, simple means can define all aspects of chronic HBV infection.

The histologic pattern and natural history of the "healthy" carrier vary depending upon geographic location, race, age, sex and duration. In countries with low carrier rates, histologic changes usually do not, or only slightly progress, and sometimes they can even regress. However, in areas with high carrier rates, insidious progression to cirrhosis is seen, mostly in males. Many of the researcher's interests may be related to the age at acquisition and to the duration of the carrier state. In high incidence areas like Korea, the carrier state is usually acquired at birth or in early childhood (2), often without active liver disease, and appears to have a life-long nature and a potential to insidiously progress to cirrhosis and hepatocelluar carcinoma (HCC).

Healthy Carriers

In Korea, chronic anicteric hepatitis, chronic active hepatitis, cirrhosis and HCC are common. Observations here have shown HBsAg to be frequent usually in these conditions (3), suggesting that serious liver disease may develop in some chronic carriers. For this reason, and because there is little detailed information on the hepatic histology of the HBsAg carrier state in Korea, liver biopsies were undertaken to assess the nature, frequency and severity of liver disease in apparently "healthy" HBsAg chronic carriers in a volunteer group of HBsAg-positive blood donors, provided by Dr. T. J. Chung, who was working at Capital Army Hospital, ROK Army, Seoul, and by a group of "healthy" HBsAg chronic carriers observed at St. Mary's Hospital, Catholic Medical Center, Seoul.

Sixty-eight "healthy" young Korean males, found to be persistent HBsAg carriers, were investigated by means of liver biopsy, serial liver function tests and serological studies for HBV immune markers. Twenty-eight carriers showed normal features in biopsy. Forty of the carriers had histologic abnormalities: one had parenchymal bridging necrosis, one chronic active hepatitis, 27 chronic persistent hepatitis, seven steatosis, one incomplete septal fibrosis, and one nonspecific reactive hepatitis. In addition, one case with granulomatous hepatitis (Fig. 9, see page 34), presumed to be tuberculosis, and one with marked periductal portal sclerosis were observed incidentally.

Histological Findings

Only two of the 68 cases of "healthy" carriers had progressive liver diseases, parenchymal bridging necrosis and chronic active hepatitis. However, "healthy" carriers are so common in Korea that even such a low prevalence of associated progressive liver disease might contribute to the high incidence of cirrhosis and HCC and be of considerable public health importance.

These patients may, on the basis of the histologic findings, be classified into two groups: the first group was presumed to retain the residual stage of acute viral hepatitis (AVH), while the second group was considered to maintain chronic sequelae of viral hepatitis. The histologic patterns of the first group included perivenular focal necrosis (Fig. 10, see page 34), large and ballooned hepatocytes aggregated in Rappaport Zone III, approximation of the central portal areas (Fig. 11, see page 34), the glycogen storage phase and restoration of the parenchyma showing multiple cell-thick plates.

The patterns of the second group comprised dense mononuclear cell infiltration restricted to the portal tract (Fig. 12, see page 34), regenerative nodules surrounded by septal fibrosis, bridging necrosis with chronic inflammatory cell infiltration, chronic periportal inflammation in association with progression and hepatocytes with ground glass-appearing cytoplasm (Figs. 13, 14, see page 34). From the above findings, these carriers are presumed to have a history of AVH.

Of many studies currently in progress, an increasing number of reports are related to the liver histology of these carriers (4), with wide discrepancies among these reports concerning the incidence, nature and severity of liver abnormalities found in these carriers. Therefore, the present study was undertaken to assess the nature, frequency and severity of liver disease in apparently "healthy" HBsAg chronic carriers.

In a Canadian study, 24 of 31 carriers showed chronic persistent hepatitis (5), whereas, in a Danish report (6), some 50% of the carriers had normal liver histology. Another report from Germany (7), on a large-scale study of 58 liver biopsies, revealed that 33% of the carriers had normal liver histology, 8.6% had chronic persistent hepatitis and the rest of the carriers showed various cytotoxic lesions. None of the carriers had chronic active hepatitis. Other reports (8,9) indicate a higher incidence of more severe chronic liver disease such as chronic active hepatitis and cirrhosis. The histologic patterns of "healthy" carriers vary depending upon geographic location.

The most common histologic abnormality found in "healthy" carriers has been considered to be the ground glass-appearing hepatocytes, a cell with increased smooth endoplasmic reticulum and a varying amount of glycogen. In my series, only one of the 68 cases showed scattered hepatocytes with ground glass-appearing cytoplasm in the normal liver. In a study done with cases that were partly dealt with in this study, orcein stain was positive in 50% of the carriers (10).

Therefore, we can suspect a carrier state of HBsAg, even when orcein-positive cells are detected in an otherwise normal liver in the absence of significant drug exposure.

Summary

Sixty-eight healthy young males, found to be persistent HBsAg carriers, were investigated by means of liver biopsy following serial liver function tests and immunological tests for hepatitis B virus.

Liver needle biopsy findings revealed that 28 cases (41%) were normal, 27 (40%) had chronic persistent hepatitis and seven (10%) had steatosis. Four showed chronic active hepatitis, bridging necrosis, incomplete septal fibrosis and nonspecific reactive hepatitis, respectively. Of the remaining two, one case of portal sclerosis and the other with granulomatous hepatitis, presumed to be tuberculosis, were observed incidentally.

Thus, it is presumed that apparently "healthy" HBsAg chronic carriers in Korea often have chronic hepatitis, usually persistent but rarely active. This finding indicates that liver biopsy still remains the most useful approach in the evaluation of these HBsAg carriers. The HBsAg carrier state seems to be well tolerated, but further long-term studies are needed to understand the natural history of this condition.

References

1. Hoofnagle, J.H. and Alter, H.J. Chronic viral hepatitis. In: Vyas, G.N., Dienstag, J.H. and Hoofnagle, J.H., eds. Viral Hepatitis and Liver Disease. Orlando: Grune & Stratton, pp. 97–113, 1984.

2. Chung, W.K., Yoo, J.Y., Sun, H.S., Lee, H.Y., Lee, I.J., Kim, S.M. and Prince, A.M. Prevention of perinatal transmission of hepatitis B virus: a comparison between the efficacy of passive and passive-active immunization in Korea. J Infect Dis 151: 280–286, 1985.

3. Chung, W.K. Chronic hepatitis in Korea. Edited by H. Popper and F. Schaffner. Progress in Liver Diseases, Vol VIII. New York: Grune & Stratton, pp. 469–484, 1986.

4. Villeneuve, J.P., Richer, G., Cote, J., Guevin, R., Marleau, D., Joly, J.G. and Viallet, A. Chronic carriers of hepatitis B antigen (HBsAg): histological biochemical and immunological findings in 31 voluntary blood donors. Digestive Diseases 21: 18–25, 1976.

5. Feinman, S.V., Cooter, N., Sinclair, J.C., Wrobel, D.M. and Berris, B. Clinical and epidemiological significance of the HBsAg (Australia antigen): Carrier state. Gastroenterology 68: 113–120, 1975.

6. Reinicke, V., Dybkjaer, E., Poulsen, H., Banke, O., Lylloff, K. and Nordenfelt, E. A study of Australia-antigen-positive blood donors and their recipients, with special reference to liver histology. N Engl J Med 296: 867–870, 1972.

7. Klinge, O., Kaboth, U. and Winckler, K. Feingewebliche befunde an der leber klinisch gesunder Australia-antigen-(HB-Ag) Trager. Virchows Arch A 361: 359–368, 1973.

8. Prince, A.M., Hargrove, R.L. and Jeffries, G.H. The role of serum hepatitis virus in chronic liver disease. Trans Assoc Am Physicians 82: 265–277, 1969.

9. Singleton, J.W., Fitch, R.A., Merrill, D.A., Kohler, P.F. and Rettberg, W.A.H. Liver disease in Australia-antigen-positive blood-donors. Lancet 2: 785–787, 1971.

10. Chung, T.J. The clinical, histological and electron microscopic observation: chronic carriers of hepatitis B antigen (HBsAg). Armed Forces Medical J (ROK Army) pp. 60–65, 1980.

Legends

Fig. 9. Incidental findings.

Granuloma with some central multinucleated giant cells and surrounding epithelioid cells and fibrosis. Needle biopsy, HE, ×100.

Fig. 10. Histologic findings presumably in the presence of the residual state of AVH.

Perivenular focal necrosis with mononuclear cell infiltration (arrow). Lymphocytes predominate in the infiltrate. Needle biopsy, HE, ×400.

Fig. 11.

Approximation of the central-portal area without intervening parenchyma. Needle biopsy, HE, ×100.

Fig. 12. Chronic sequelae of viral hepatitis.

There is significant mononuclear cell infiltration of the portal tract but a little piecemeal necrosis. Needle biopsy, HE, ×100.

Fig. 13.

Scattered hepatocytes with ground glass-appearing cytoplasm. Needle biopsy, HE, ×200.

Fig. 14.

Cluster of orcein stain-positive hepatocytes (left). Needle biopsy, orcein stain, ×200.

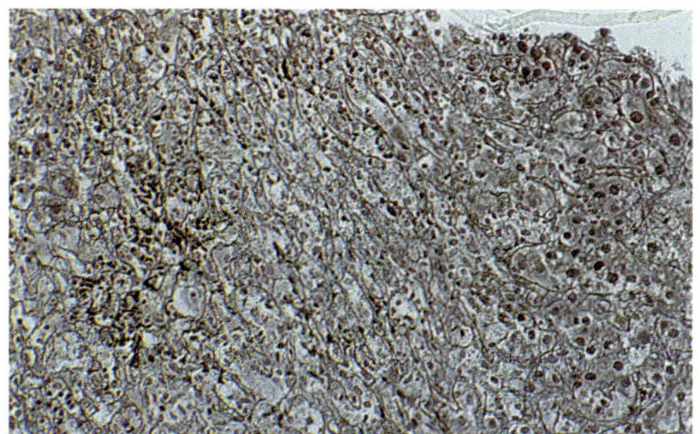

Fig. 1 See Legend page 25.

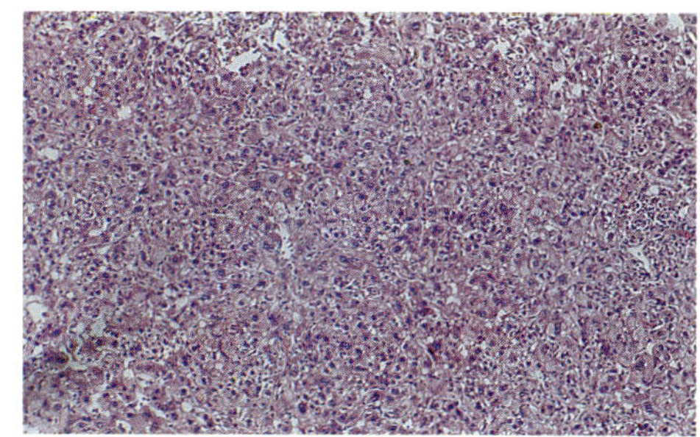

Fig. 2 See Legend page 25.

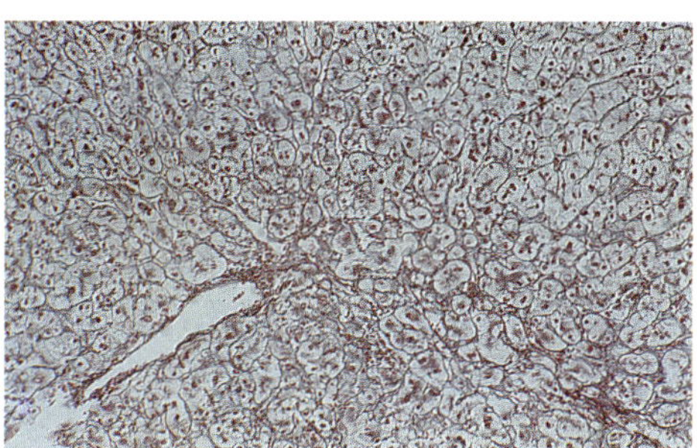

Fig. 3 See Legend page 26.

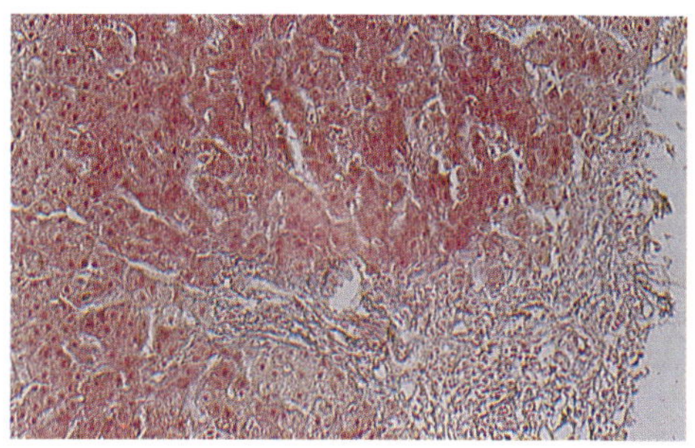

Fig. 4 See Legend page 26.

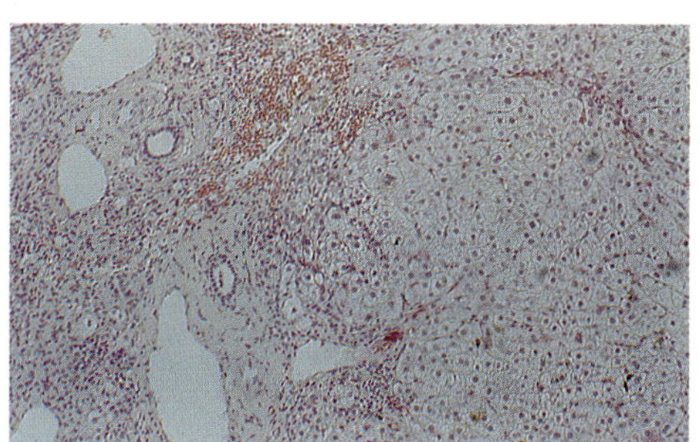

Fig. 5 See Legend page 26.

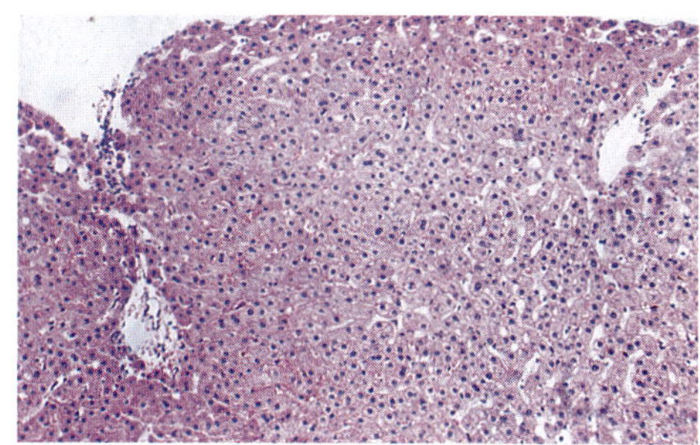

Fig. 6 See Legend page 26.

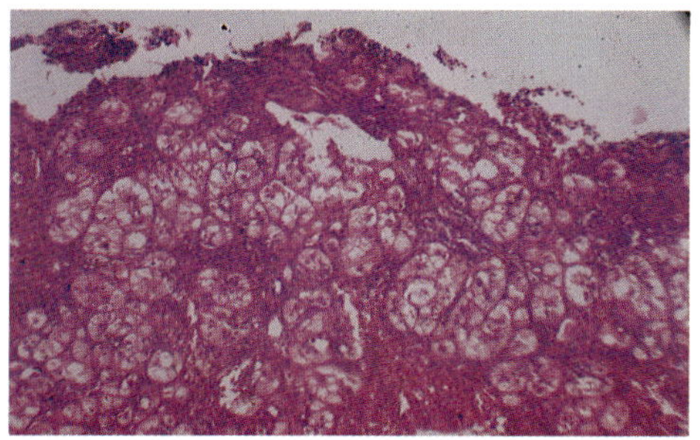

Fig. 7 See Legend page 26.

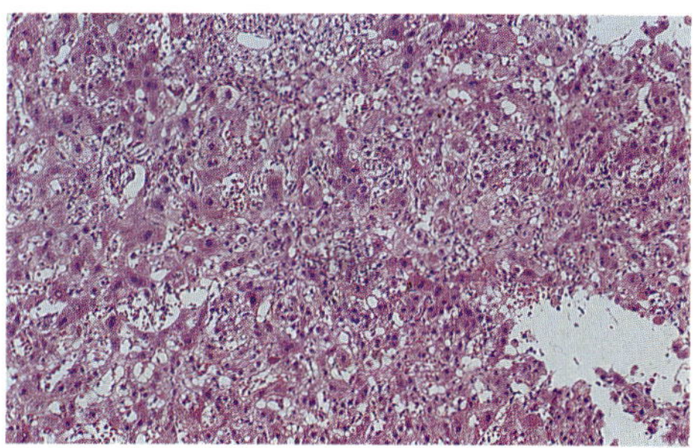

Fig. 8 See Legend page 26.

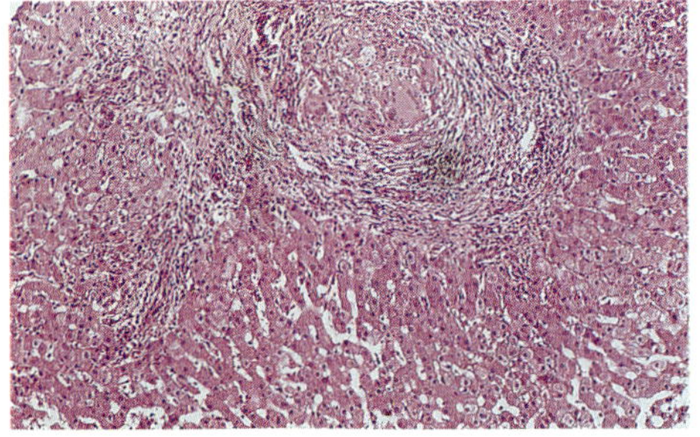

Fig. 9 See Legend page 31.

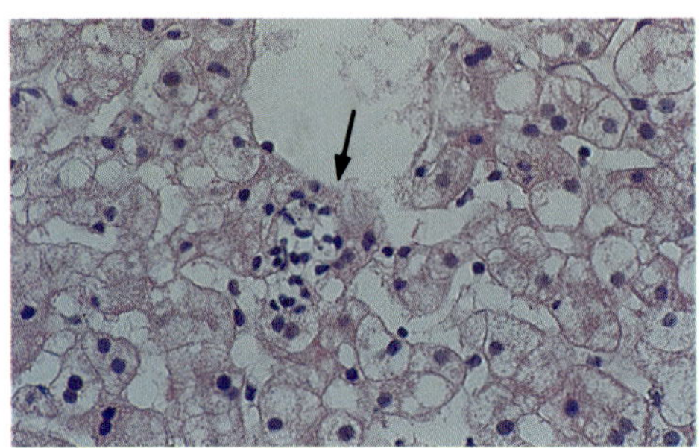

Fig. 10 See Legend page 31.

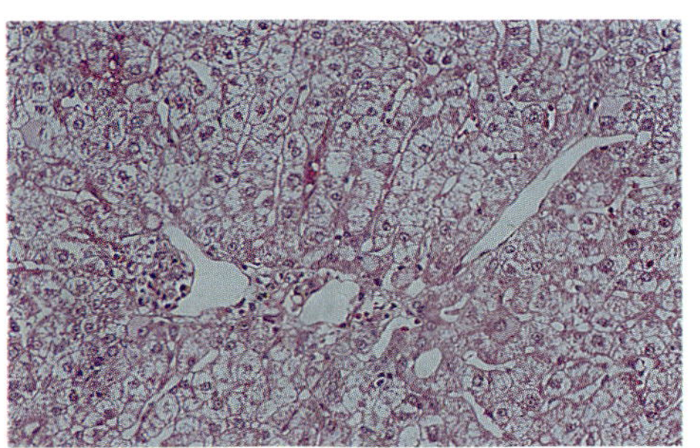

Fig. 11 See Legend page 31.

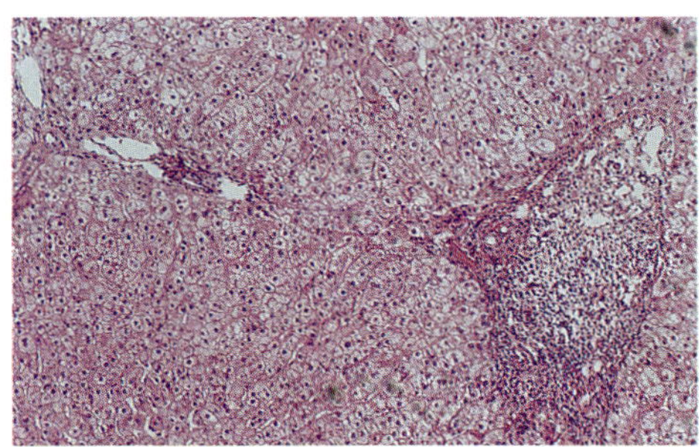

Fig. 12 See Legend page 31.

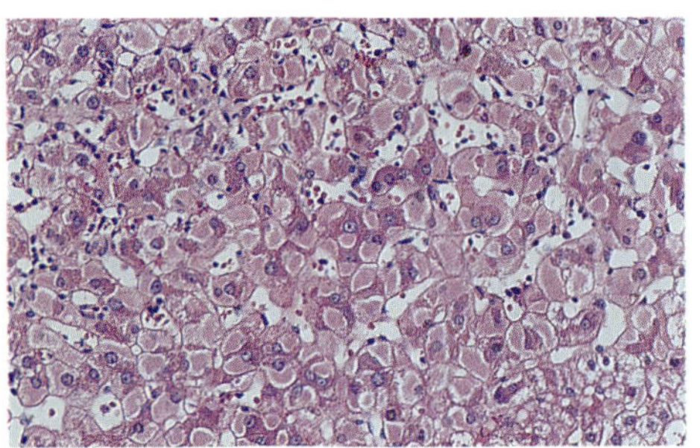

Fig. 13 See Legend page 31.

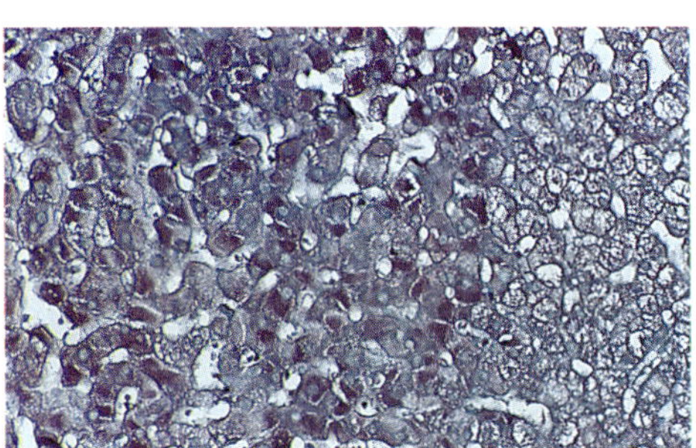

Fig. 14 See Legend page 31.

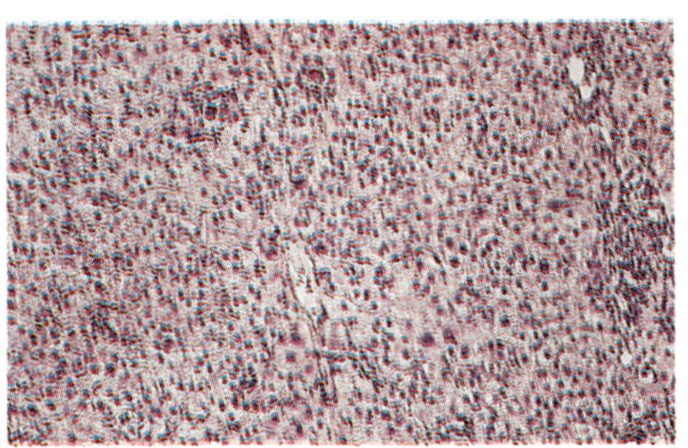

Fig. 15 See Legend page 48.

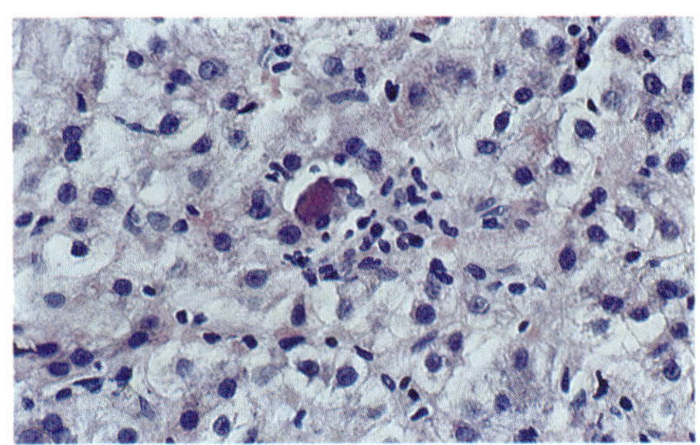

Fig. 16 See Legend page 48.

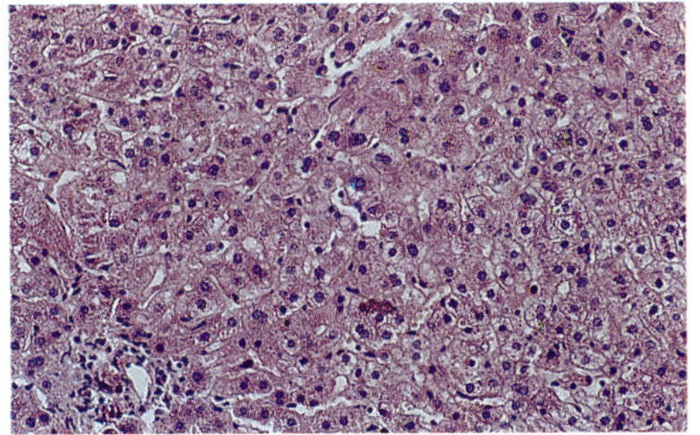

Fig. 17 See Legend page 48.

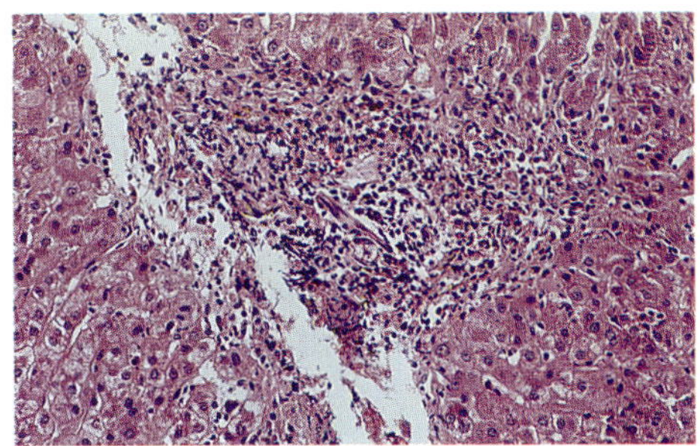

Fig. 18 See Legend page 48.

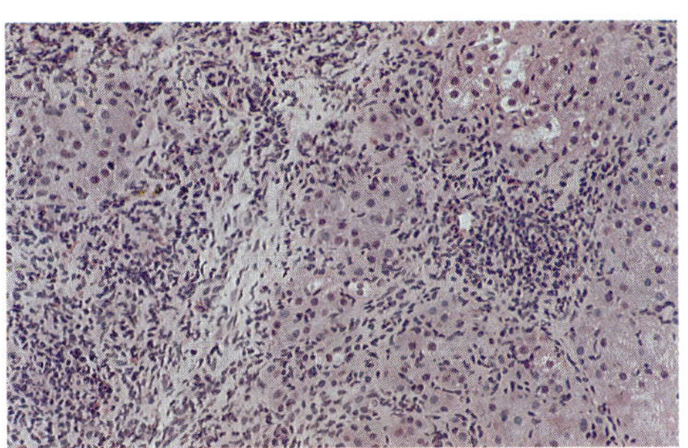

Fig. 19 See Legend page 48.

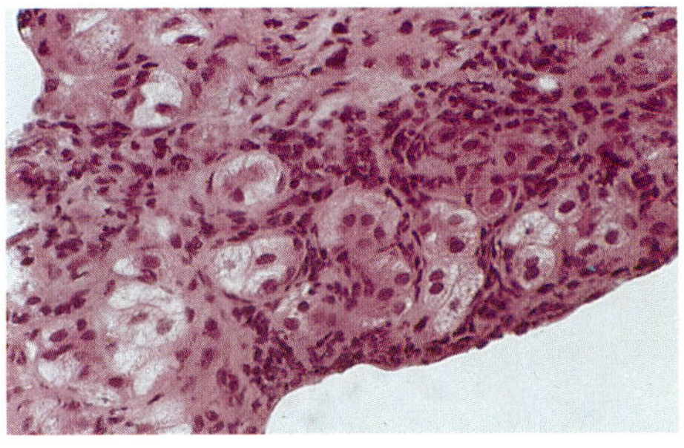

Fig. 20 See Legend page 48.

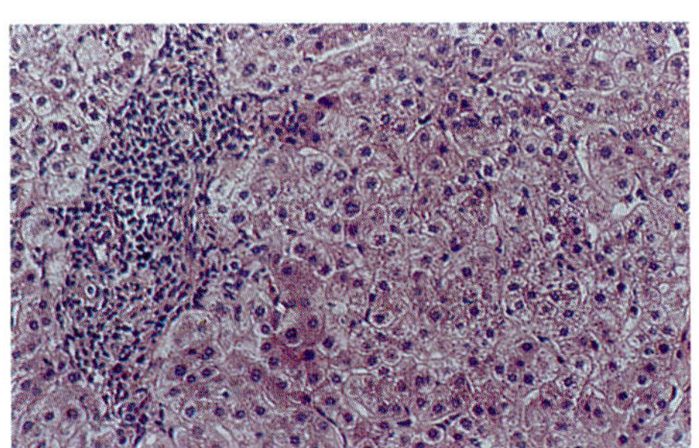

Fig. 21 See Legend page 48.

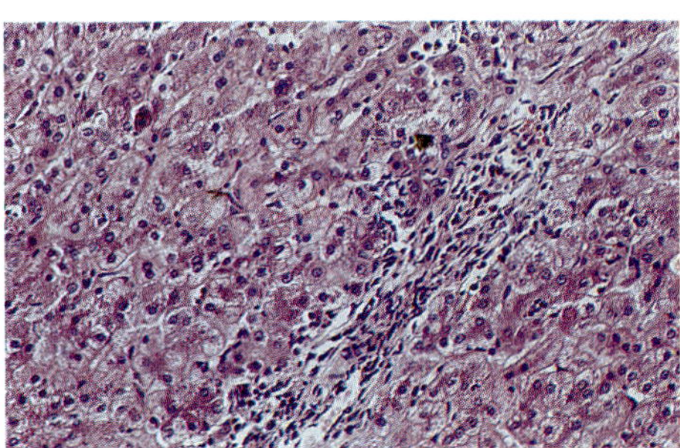

Fig. 22 See Legend page 48.

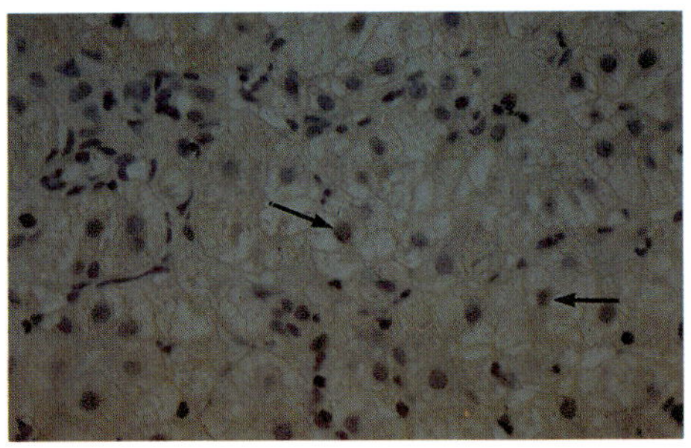

Fig. 23 See Legend page 57.

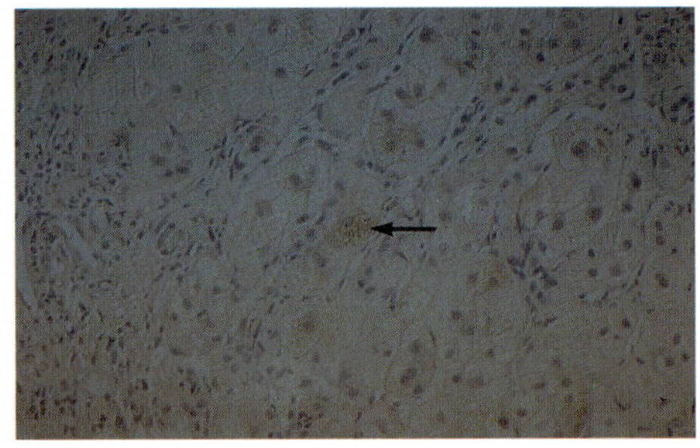

Fig. 24 See Legend page 57.

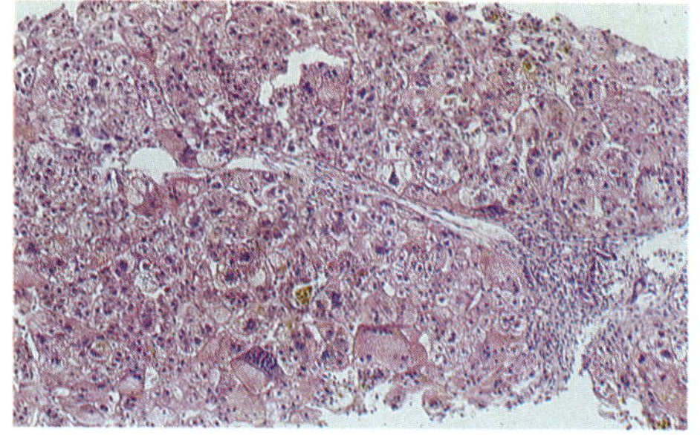

Fig. 25 See Legend page 57.

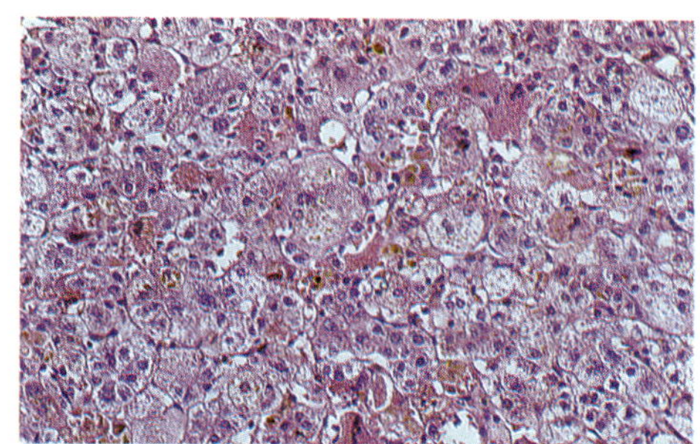

Fig. 26 See Legend page 57.

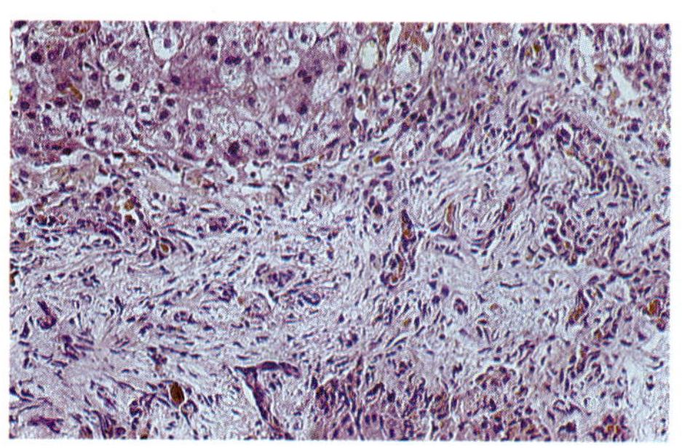

Fig. 27 See Legend page 57.

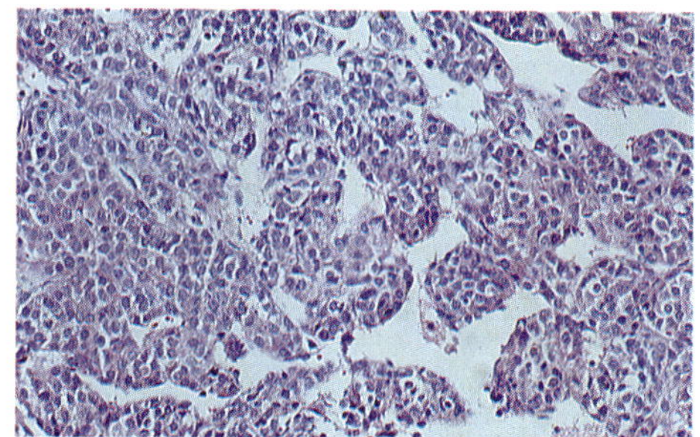

Fig. 28 See Legend page 57.

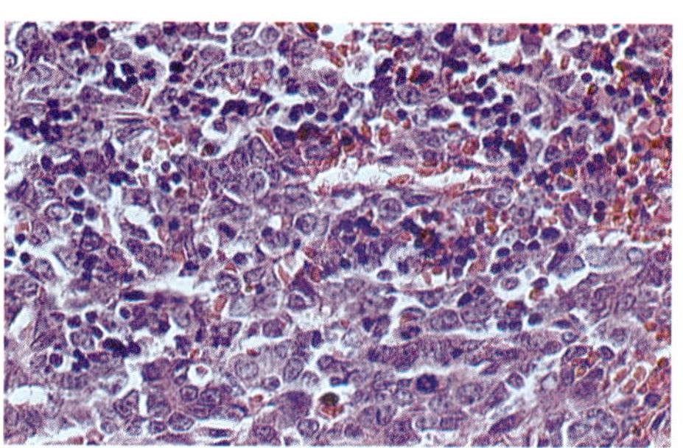

Fig. 29 See Legend page 57.

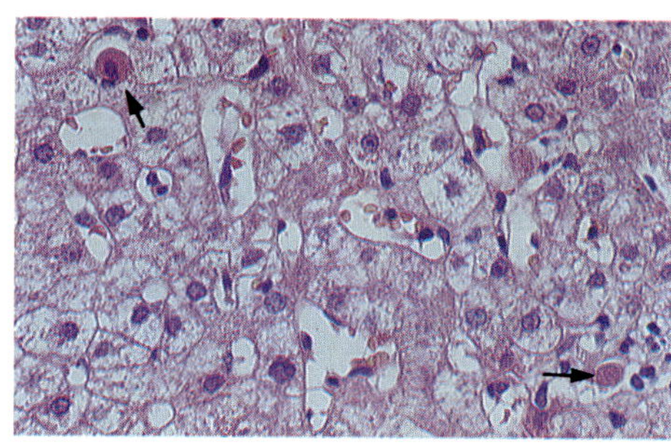

Fig. 30 See Legend page 57.

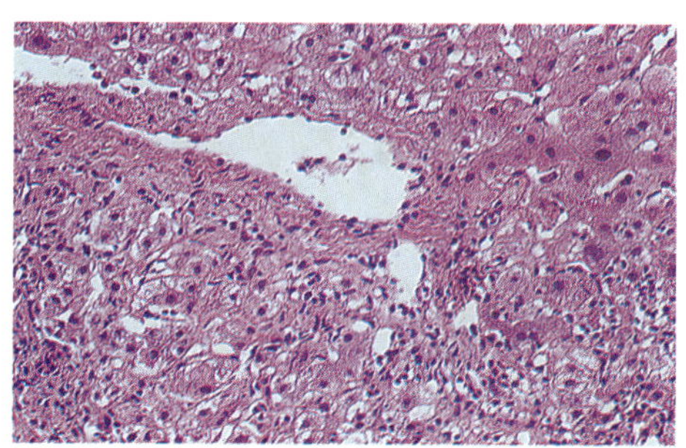

Fig. 31 See Legend page 57.

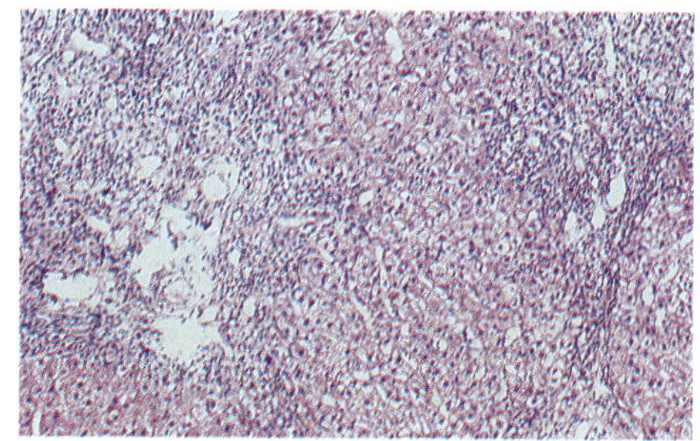

Fig. 32 See Legend page 58.

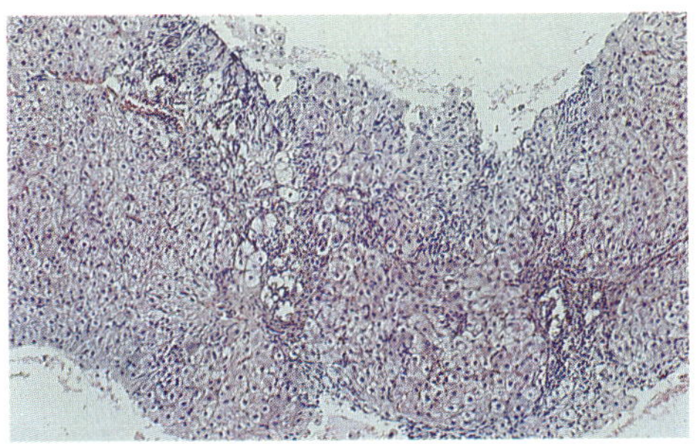

Fig. 33 See Legend page 58.

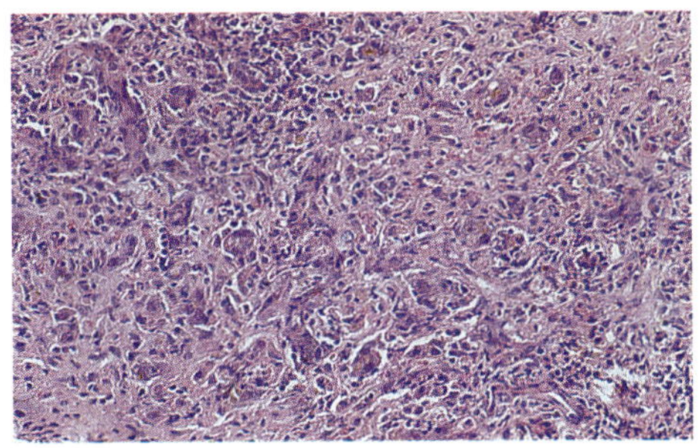

Fig. 34 See Legend page 58.

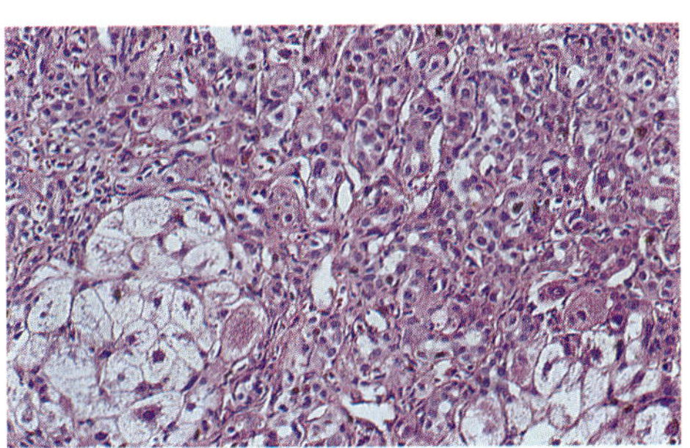

Fig. 35 See Legend page 58.

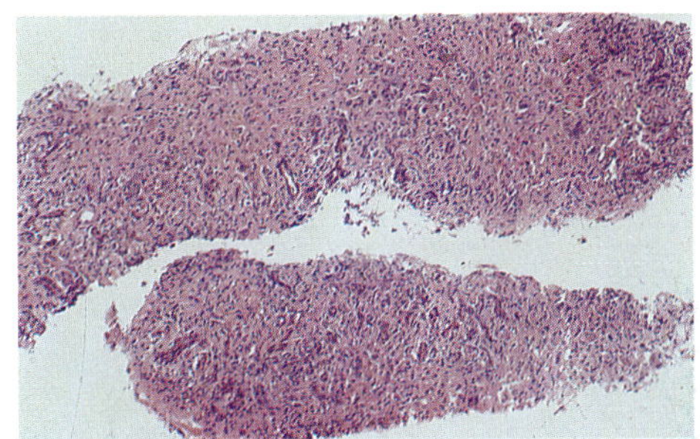

Fig. 36 See Legend page 58.

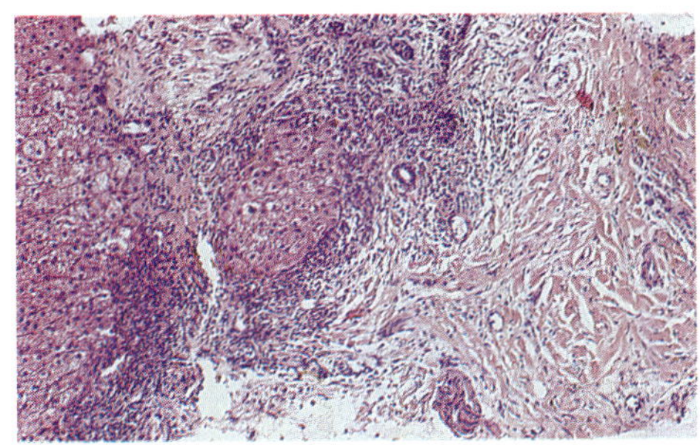

Fig. 37 See Legend page 58.

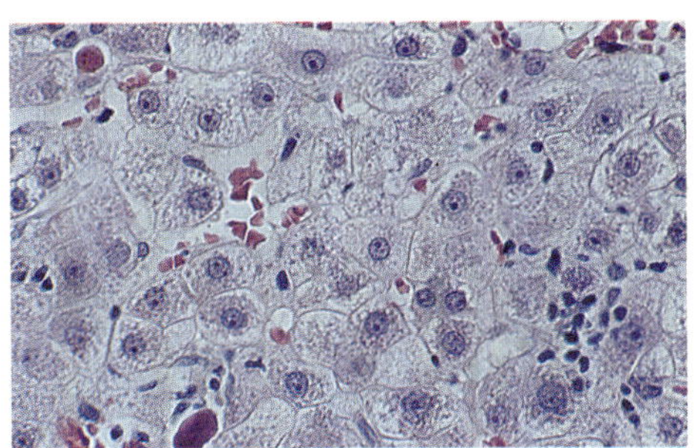

Fig. 38 See Legend page 58.

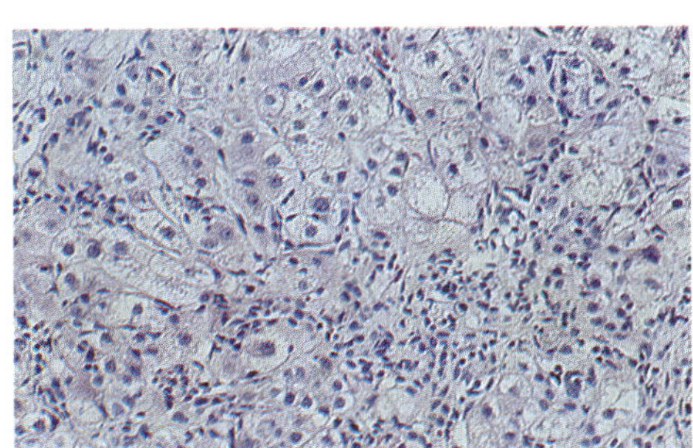

Fig. 39 See Legend page 58.

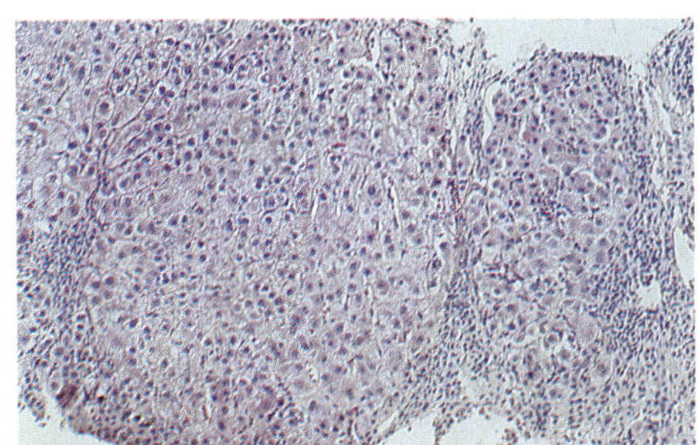

Fig. 40 See Legend page 58.

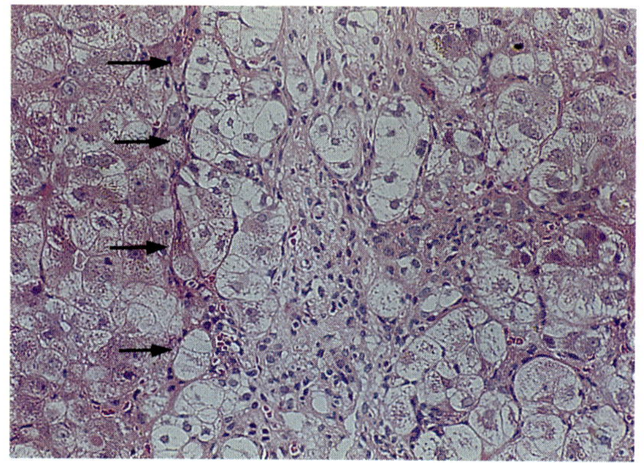

Fig. 41 See Legend page 68.

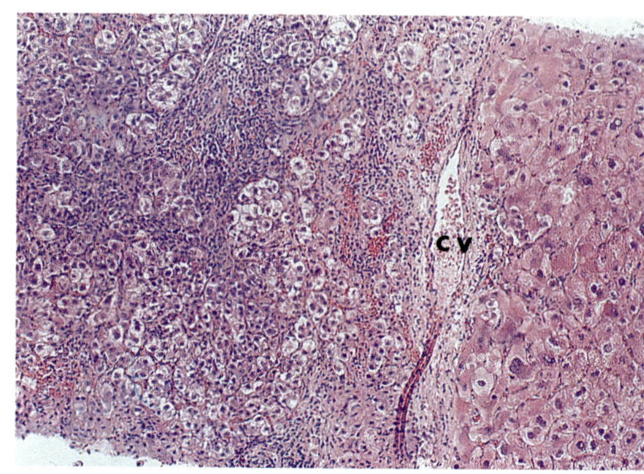

Fig. 42 See Legend page 68.

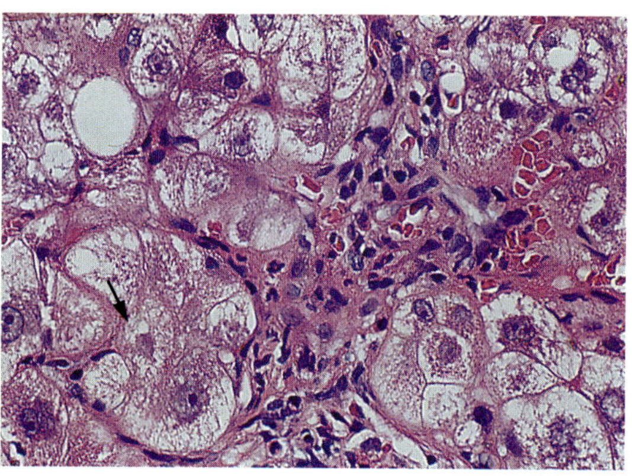

Fig. 43 See Legend page 68.

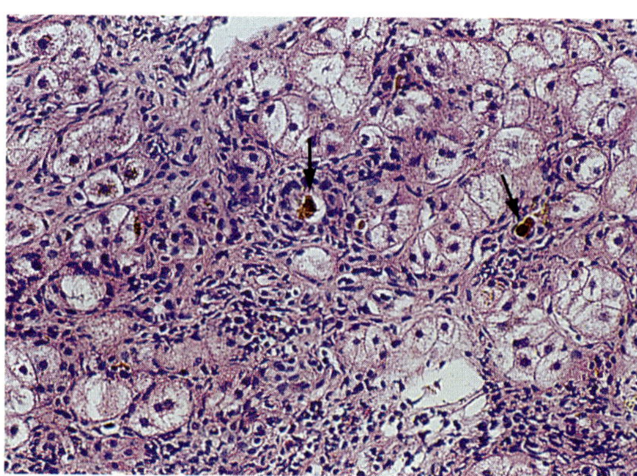

Fig. 44 See Legend page 68.

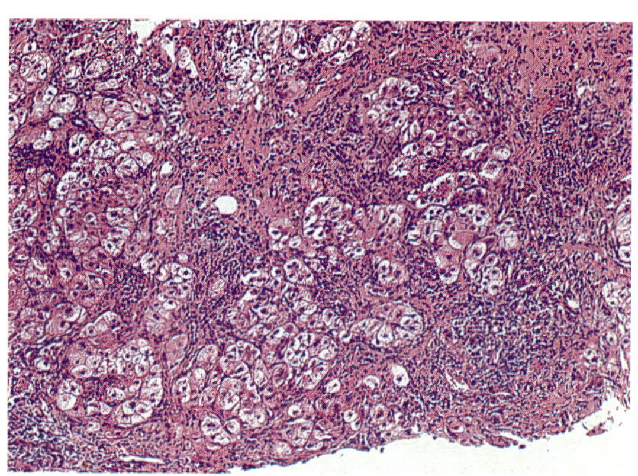

Fig. 45 See Legend page 68.

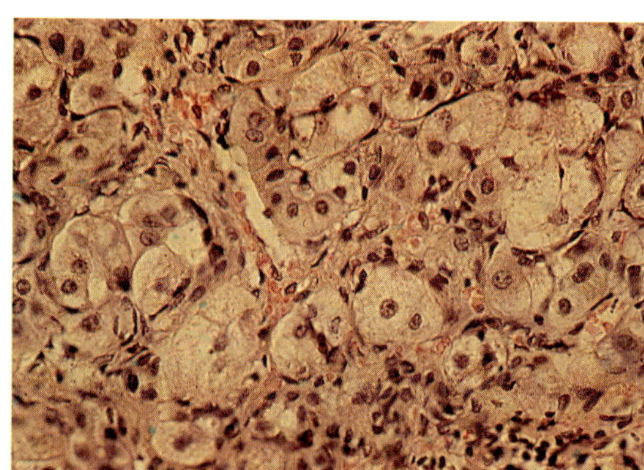

Fig. 46 See Legend page 68.

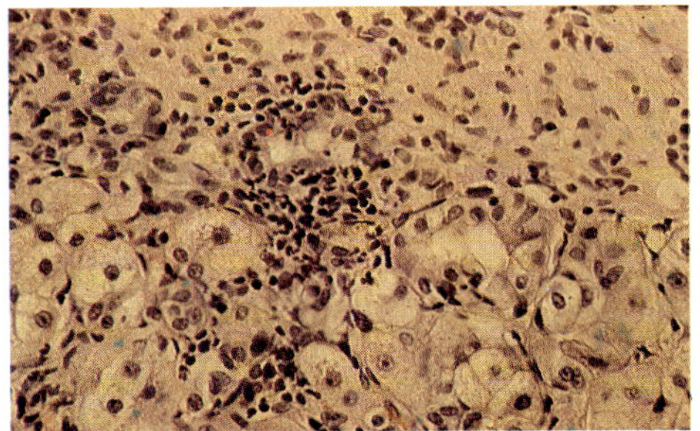

Fig. 47 See Legend page 68.

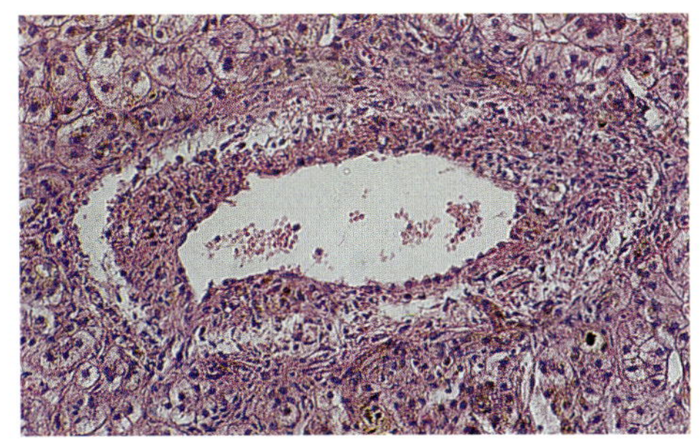

Fig. 48 See Legend page 68.

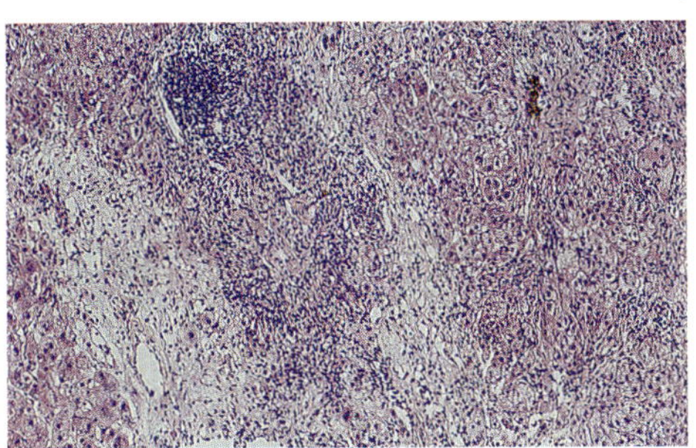

Fig. 49 See Legend page 68.

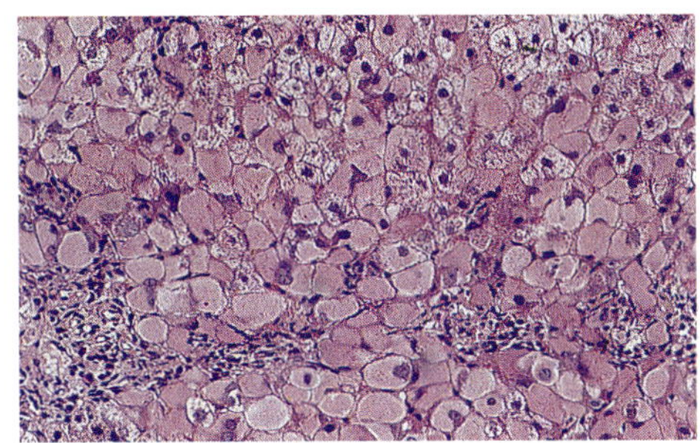

Fig. 50 See Legend page 69.

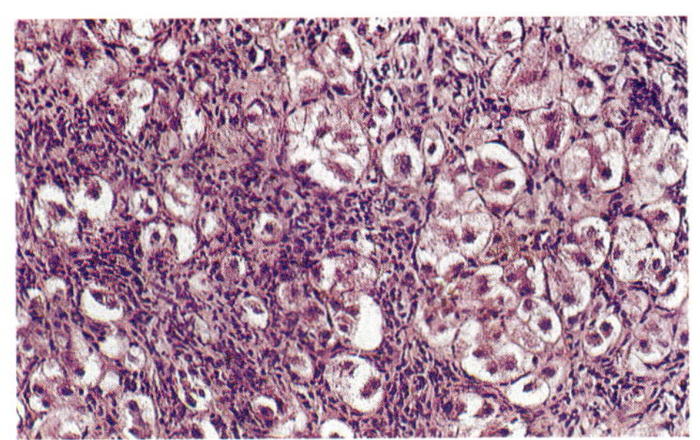

Fig. 51 See Legend page 69.

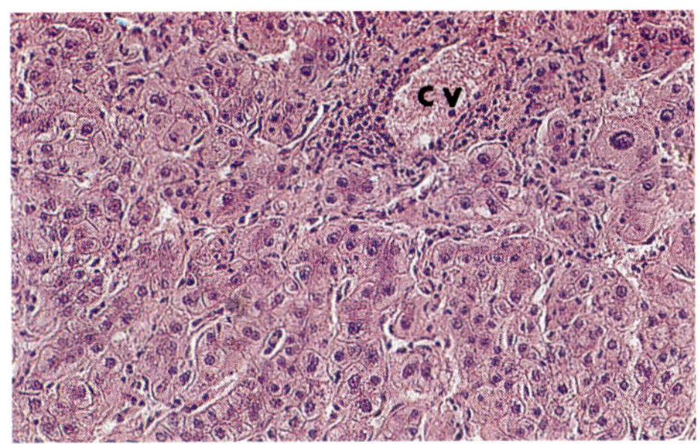

Fig. 52 See Legend page 69.

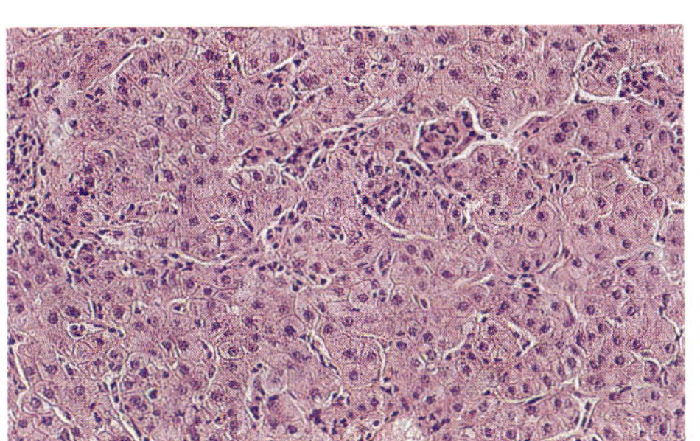

Fig. 53 See Legend page 69.

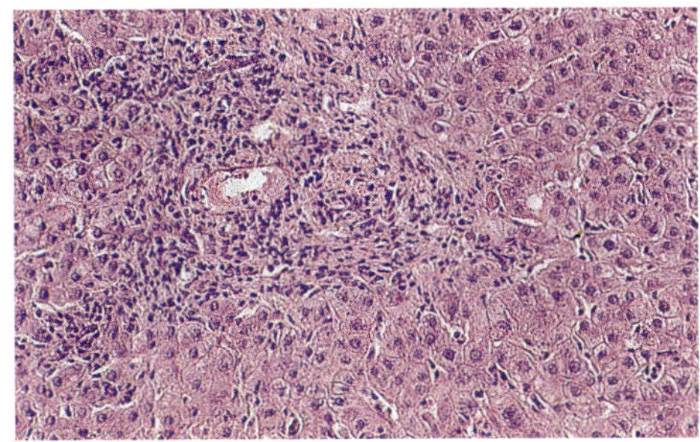

Fig. 54 See Legend page 69.

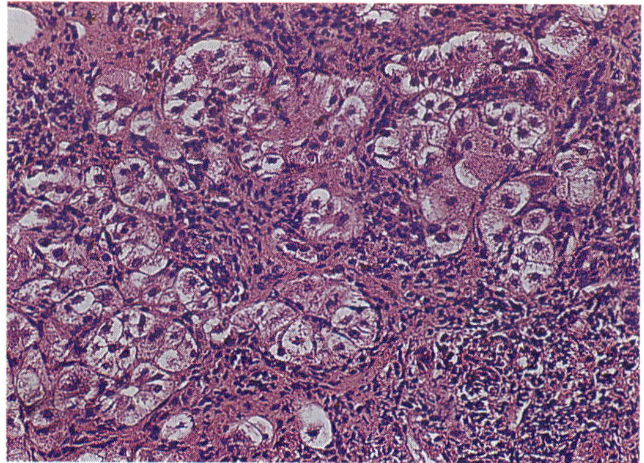

Fig. 55 See Legend page 69.

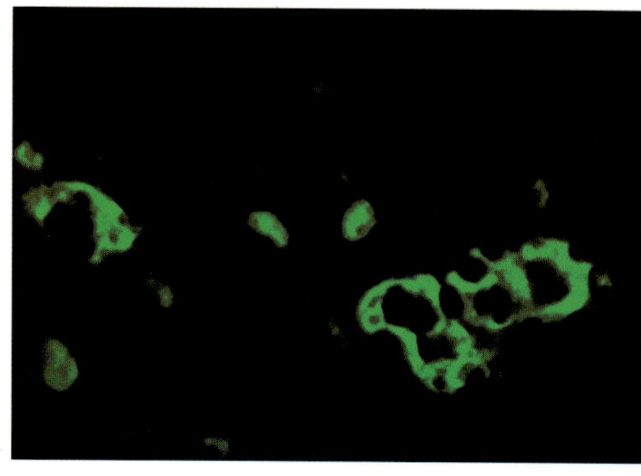

Fig. 56 See Legend page 87.

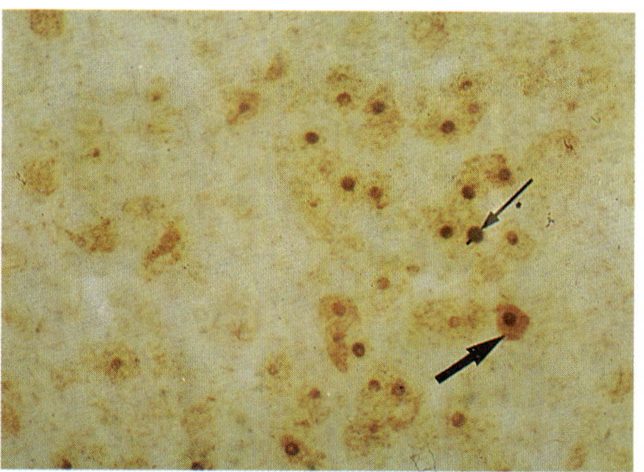

Fig. 57 See Legend page 88.

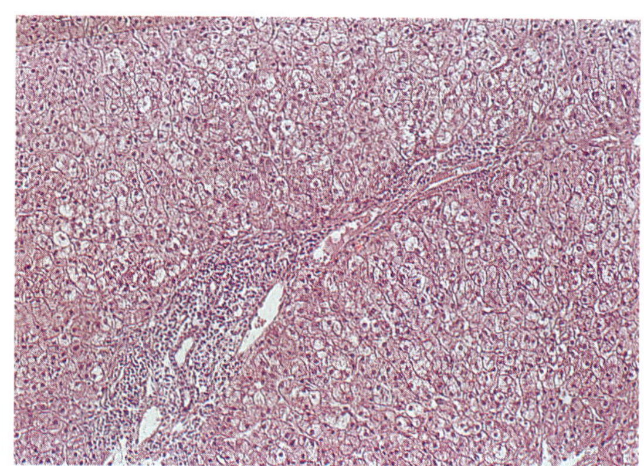

Fig. 58 See Legend page 88.

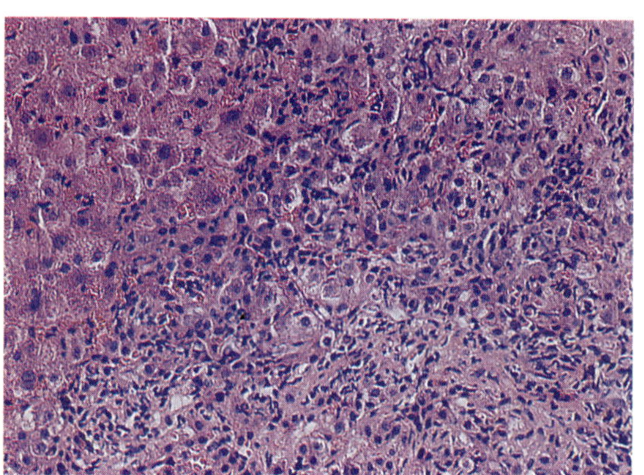

Fig. 59 See Legend page 88.

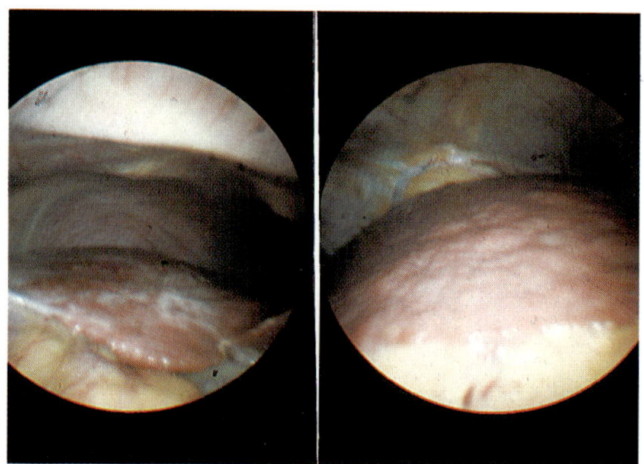

Fig. 60 See Legend page 88.

3 NATURAL HISTORY OF ANICTERIC HEPATITIS: MAJOR SOURCE OF CHRONIC LIVER DISEASES

Whan Kook Chung, M.D., Ph.D. and
Sae Kwang Moon, M.D., Ph.D.

During and after the Korean War, liver diseases—acute and chronic hepatitis, cirrhosis and hepatocellular carcinoma (HCC)—were prevalent in Korea. These liver diseases presented a grave health hazard to a population already suffering from the ravages of a long war.

At that time, relatively little was known of the scientific basis and etiology of viral hepatitis, particularly of chronic hepatitis. For the purpose of detecting these diseases at their early stage and clarifying their etiologies, we undertook a study designed to detect pre-icteric cases of viral hepatitis. To this end, we conducted a mass serum enzyme survey on around 2,000 subjects selected from among the population with endemic viral hepatitis. We discovered 32 cases with anicteric asymptomatic hepatitis on the basis of significantly abnormal serum activities of aspartate aminotransferase and alanine aminotransferase.

These patients were hospitalized for intensive study—clinical, laboratory and histopathologic. Their clinical and laboratory manifestations and the histologic changes, based on three liver biopsies of each patient during a three-month period of observation, have been described in our previous reports (1,2). In the study, persistent parenchymal lesions justifying the designation of chronic active hepatitis (CAH) were found in 75%.

Of the 32 cases, nine showed serum hepatitis antigen in the liver (3). This detection was followed by the discovery of Australia antigen by Blumberg. Sera from eight of the nine patients had HBsAg (4), emphasizing the significance of the carrier state in the etiology of the anicteric hepatitis in Korea. Of the 32 cases, some were presumed to have, in addition to hepatitis B, non-A, non-B type viral infection, which may have caused or contributed to chronic hepatitis. As a matter of fact, these studies constituted one of the first descriptions of chronic hepatitis at that time. This disease gradually and generally became recognized as the result of the availability of these liver biopsies as well as of the determination of the serum activities of the aminotransferases.

Chronic hepatitis and chronic hepatitis-related diseases, including cirrhosis and HCC, are major causes of death in Korea. Most cases of chronic liver diseases in Korea seem to have retained such an anicteric asymptomatic state for a long time. The onset of chronic hepatitis comes after six months of persistent manifestation of hepatitis. Consequently, a study of a short period, such as our prior study (2) which was done in only three months, is not sufficient to document the natural course of anicteric hepatitis.

Therefore, chronic hepatitis needs a long-term follow-up of at least six months to confirm the chronicity. In this study, we performed a fourth biopsy six months after the first, and made a serial histologic reanalysis of the specimens together with the former biopsy specimens. After the fourth biopsy, we conducted a clinical and/or histologic follow-up study of these patients for periods ranging from four years to 27 years (an average of 16.5 years).

Classification of cases on the basis of histologic pictures of the first biopsy

The histologic features of the initial biopsy specimens permitted a division of the cases into five groups.

Group 1. Diagnostic viral hepatitis (DVH)—hepatitis with all features of viral hepatitis (one case). The cytoplasm and nucleus of the hepatic cells varied from cell to cell throughout the lobule in volume and staining qualities. Many ballooned cells as well as a few multinucleated giant cells were noted, mainly in the centrolobular zone. In additon, acidophilic round bodies with or without pyknotic nuclei were in tissue spaces. Single cell necroses were prominent, as evidenced by the absence of some liver cells and replacement of inflammatory cells, usually lymphocytes, and a few macrophages containing PAS-positive granules. Kupffer cells were mobilized throughout, and contained a large amount of PAS-positive lipofuscin pigment. The walls of the tributaries of hepatic veins were thickened, homogeneous and frequently surrounded by mononuclear inflammatory cells. The portal tracts were enlarged and exhibited ductular proliferation and periductular infiltration with predominantly mononuclear inflammatory cells. A few segmented leucocytes were also present in the inflammatory exudates. The border between the portal tract and the parenchyma was not sharp because of the disappearance of individual hepatocytes from the limiting plate and accumulation of inflammatory cells (piecemeal necrosis). No bile pigment was visible and the bile canaliculi were not dilated.

Group 2. Suggestive viral hepatitis (SVH)—hepatitis with some features of viral hepatitis (13 cases). The appearance of hepatocytes varied only slightly in this group. Acidophilic bodies, however, were seen throughout. Spotty necrosis of liver cells was also found in all cases, but the intensity was not severe as in Group 1. In many instances, some of the other listed criteria were absent. In some cases, eosinophilic leucocytes were numerous in the portal tract. Plasma cells were sometimes found in the littoral position.

Group 3. Nonspecific reactive hepatitis (NSRH) (five cases). Only Kupffer cell activation, some single cell necroses, and a little portal infiltration were seen in the five cases of this group (Fig. 17, see page 35). These changes were considerably less marked than in Groups 1 and 2. Characteristic acidophilic bodies were not found and several of the other features noted in the first group were absent. This type of lesion, which usually occurs as a reaction of the liver in many diseases, has also been noted in the defervescent stage of viral hepatitis (see Chapter 1).

Group 4. Chronic persistent hepatitis (CPH) (11 cases) (Fig. 18, see page 35). Inflammatory infiltration, mainly by mononuclear cells often including plasma cells, was confined to the portal tract. It was occasionally enlarged with short fibrous septa extending into the parenchyma, but the lobular architecture remained intact and intralobular changes were usually slight. The limiting plates were usually well preserved but sometimes mild piecemeal necrosis was noted.

Group 5. Chronic active hepatitis (CAH) (two cases) (Fig. 19, see page 35). The portal tracts contained a conspicuous exudate of predominantly mononuclear cells intermixed with a few segmented leucocytes. They extended into the surrounding periportal parenchyma, from which liver cells had disappeared (piecemeal necrosis), and the connective tissue septa radiating from the portal tract to the parenchyma, frequently linking the portal tracts. The septa also reached the central zone. Lobular alterations were mild.

Clonorchis sinensis infestation was found in eight of the 32 cases. One of them had the picture of diagnostic viral hepatitis, four suggestive viral hepatitis, one persistent hepatitis and two nonspecific reactive hepatitis. The incidence of Clonorchis sinensis infestation in the material studied was not different from that in the population at large, and no evidence was found which indicated that the infestation caused the type of hepatitis under study, but it might have contributed to the chronicity.

Course as evidenced by serial biopsies (Table 3-1)

In the group with DVH (Group 1), no changes occurred at the second, the third or the fourth biopsy during the period of six months follow-up (Figs. 15, 16, see page 34). Thus, the persistence of the original parenchymal lesion permitted the diagnosis of chronic lobular hepatitis . In the fifth biopsy, which was possible four years after the first, the biopsy findings showed complete regression.

In some of the cases with SVH (Group 2), the findings appreciably varied during the observation. Seven of the 13 cases with SVH returned for the fourth biopsy six months after the first: two developed chronic active hepatitis and two chronic persistent hepatitis; one revealed persistence of the original parenchymal lesion, at least for the period of the six months, to such a degree as to permit the diagnosis of chronic imperfect lobular hepatitis; two showed improvement or persisting nonspecific features.

Four cases of the five with NSRH were available for the fourth biopsy in the sixth month. Of the four cases, (Fig. 17, see page 35) one showed CAH and the others still revealed nonspecific reactive hepatitis.

Seven of the 11 cases with CPH returned for the fourth biopsy six months after the first. Of the seven, one (Fig. 18, see page 35) showed CAH and the others retained the same state as they had at the first biopsy.

There were two cases with CAH at the time of the initial biopsy. Both patients developed CAH with cirrhosis in the sixth month (Figs. 19, 20, see page 35).

Overall, of the 21 cases that were observed for six months, 17 revealed persistence of the original lesion or additionally developed CAH or cirrhosis of a degree similar to chronic hepatitis, at least for a period of six months; five cases were aggravated to CAH—two from the SVH group, one from the NSRH group, and two from the CPH group; two with CAH developed cirrhosis; the remaining 10 cases maintained the original lesions. Only two of the 21 cases showed improvement. Thus, the lesion persisted in 90% of all the cases, justifying the term "chronic hepatitis", and progression to cirrhosis occurred in 10% of the cases studied during the period of six months.

Long-term follow-up study by means of clinical and biochemical methods

Final observations by means of clinical and biochemical methods were possible in the 17 cases for a period from four years to 27 years (an average of 16.5 years) after the initial biopsies (Table 3-1).

One patient was found to have developed decompensated cirrhosis four years after the initial observation (Fig. 21, see page 35), and another hepatocellular carcinoma 27 years after the first biopsy (Fig. 22, see page 35). Both cases belonged to the group of patients with chronic persistent hepatitis

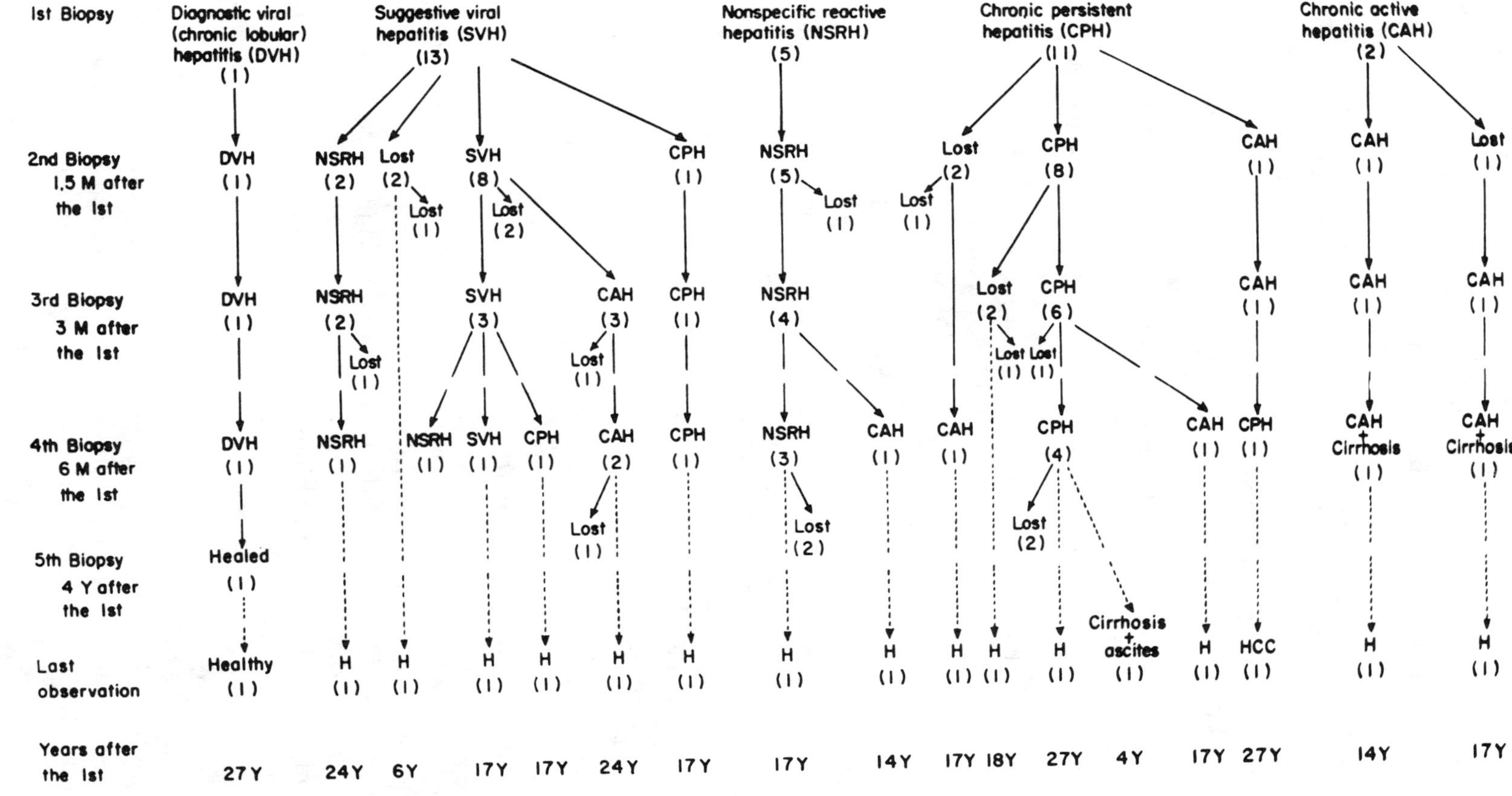

Table 3-1. Histologic and Clinical Evolution of 32 Cases with Anicteric Hepatitis
Key: unbroken rules, histologic follow up; broken rules, clinical follow up; ( ), number of cases studied; H, Healthy; HCC, hepatocellular caricinoma; M, months; Y, Years

(Table 3-1). All the remaining cases, including the two cases of CAH with cirrhosis at the time of the fourth biopsy were healthy.

Previous studies (1,2) indicate that the prevalence of anicteric hepatitis among young Korean adult males is around 2%. The lesion persisted in 90% of all cases, justifying the term "chronic hepatitis". Thus, the incidence of chronic hepatitis resulting from anicteric hepatitis in Korea is at least over 1.5% of the male population, indicating that the main type of chronic hepatitis prevalent in Korea is anicteric. The prevalence of anicteric hepatitis in Korea is related to social, economic and environmental conditions (5).

The benign, mild and inactive types of diseases such as SVH, NSRH and CPH were often exacerbated and developed into CAH. As a result, it is presumed that these types of diseases always have the potentiality of active progression.

CPH, in which inflammation is restricted to the portal tracts, is said to remain quiescent and inactive with only minor sequelae. However, a minority of patients with CPH appear to have developed CAH over a period of years (6). By contrast, CAH, in which continuous progression of periportal inflammation (piecemeal necrosis) to abolition of lobular architecture, is often associated with progression to cirrhosis. Through this study, we found that cases of CAH with cirrhosis showed no further progression during the period of the follow-up study, while some cases of CPH progressed to the acute episodic onset of ascites associated with cirrhosis, and other cases developed HCC.

Consequently, these results suggest that the popular belief that active chronic hepatitis B, particularly with piecemeal necrosis, very often progresses further, is not true.

Cases with CPH, which are frequently seen in asymptomatic "healthy" carriers (see Chapter 2) and anicteric hepatitis, are not always quiescent. Sometimes they have episodes of significant exacerbation in which histological aggravation is associated with conspicuous clinical and laboratory alterations, progressing to grave hepatic disorders.

To evaluate the state of the whole liver with chronic hepatitis is not easy by needle biopsy alone. Variability in sampling occurs because histologic changes of liver with chronic hepatitis are usually uneven. Consequently, it is incomplete to justify the histologic changing progress on the basis of a series of biopsies only. Nonetheless, liver biopsy remains the best way to identify progression or regression of chronic hepatitis.

Summary

In our prior studies (1), 32 clinically healthy Korean soldiers were selected on the basis of elevated activities of serum aspartate aminotransferase and subjected to repeated liver biopsies for a period of up to three months (2). On these subjects, the last (fourth) biopsy was conducted six months after the first, and histologic analysis was made of the specimens of the fourth biopsy comparing those of the first biopsy. Then, 17 of them were followed up for four to 27 years (an average of 16.5 years) after the fourth biopsy.

The initial biopsy revealed all the features of acute viral (diagnostic) hepatitis in one, most of the features of such (suggestive) hepatitis in 13 patients, those of nonspecific reactive hepatitis in five patients, those of chronic persistent hepatitis in 11 and those of chronic active hepatitis in two patients.

At the fourth biopsy, all of 21 cases, but two, had a persisting histologic lesion, justifying the designation of chronic hepatitis. Only two with suggestive viral hepatitis regressed to the state of nonspecific reactive hepatitis. The case with diagnostic viral hepatitis in the first biopsy showed the same features as those in the fourth biopsy. However, it regressed completely four years after the first biopsy. The findings from the serial biopsies showed that a total of five patients—two of the suggestive viral hepatitis group, one of the nonspecific reactive hepatitis group and two of the chronic persistent hepatitis group—developed chronic active hepatitis during the period of six months of histologic follow-up. Features of cirrhosis appeared in an additional two cases that had showed chronic active hepatitis in the first biopsy.

Of the seventeen cases who returned for clinical investigation after four to 27 years (an average of 16.5 years), one revealed decompensated cirrhosis and another showed hepatocellular carcinoma. Both of these cases were from the group of patients with chronic persistent hepatitis. The remaining cases, including the two cases of CAH with cirrhosis at fourth biopsy, were healthy.

Most of these cases were infected with hepatitis B virus but some were presumed to have non-A, non-B virus.

References

1. Chung, W.K., Moon S.K., Gershon, R.K., Prince, A.M., Park, Y.C. and Cho, Y.S. Anicteric hepatitis in Korea. I. clinical and laboratory studies. Arch Intern Med 113: 526–534, 1964.

2. Chung, W.K., Moon, S.K., Gershon, R.K., Prince, A.M. and Popper, H. Anicteric hepatitis in Korea. II. serial histologic studies. Arch Intern Med 113: 535–542, 1964.

3. Prince, A.M., Fuji, H. and Gershon, R.K. Immunohistochemical studies on the etiology of anicteric hepatitis in Korea. Am J Hygine 79: 365–381, 1964.

4. Prince, A.M. and Gershon, R.K. The etiology of chronic active hepatitis in Korea. Yale J Biol Med 52: 159–167, 1979.

5. Chung, K.W. Studies on latent hepatic lesions in Korea. J Catholic Med Coll 21: 71–84, 1971.

6. Chadwick, R.G., Galizzi, J. Jr., Heathcote, J., Lyssiotis, T., Cohen, B.J., Scheuer, P.J. & Sherlock, S. Chronic persistent hepatitis: hepatitis B virus markers and histological follow-up. Gut 20: 372–377. 1979.

Legends

Fig. 15. The fourth biopsy specimen obtained after six months.
Persisting spotty necrosis, pleomorphism, an acidophilic body, central vein reaction, and portal inflammation are seen. Needle biopsy, HE, ×100.

Fig. 16.
A higher magnification of an acidophilic body located in the tissue space where single cell necrosis occurred. HE, ×100.

Fig. 17. A case exhibiting transition from nonspecific reactive hepatitis to chronic active hepatitis (Case 243).
The first biopsy specimen showing mild portal infiltration, a little variation of hepatocytes. Note the liver cell plates are two-cell thick. Needle biopsy, HE, ×200.

Fig. 18. A case exhibiting transition from chronic persistent hepatitis to chronic active hepatitis (Case 249).
The first biopsy specimen showing the widening of the portal space. Chronic mononuclear inflammatory cell infiltrate is restricted to the portal tract. Needle biopsy, HE, x200.

Fig. 19. A case exhibiting transition from chronic active hepatitis to cirrhosis (Case 256).
The first biopsy specimen showing spotty necrosis, severe portal reaction, pronounced "piecemeal" necrosis, and a little scarring. Needle biopsy, HE, ×200.

Fig. 20.
The fourth biopsy specimen obtained six months later, showing isolation of hepatocytes surrounded by striking pericellular inflammatory fibrosis. Needle biopsy, HE, ×400.

Fig. 21. A case exhibiting transition from chronic persistent hepatitis to decompensated cirrhosis (Case 255).
The first biopsy specimen showing the widening of the portal tract with marked infiltration of chronic mononuclear cells and a little scar tissue. The border of the portal tract is intact. The parenchymal hepatocytes are highly regenerative. Needle biopsy, HE, ×200.

Fig. 22. A case exhibiting transition from chronic persistent hepatitis to hepatocellular carcinoma (Case 240).
The first biopsy specimen showing a mild variation of hepatocytes in size and staining quality and some acidophilic bodies, and chronic inflammation restricted to the portal tract. Needle biopsy, HE, ×200.

4 CHRONIC LIVER DISEASES IN CHILDHOOD

Whan Kook Chung, M.D., Ph.D.

Chronic liver diseases, including chronic hepatitis, cirrhosis and hepatocellular carcinoma (HCC), are common in Korea. The etiology is mainly related to hepatitis B virus (HBV) (see Chapter 7) (1). In Korea, the HBV carrier state is usually acquired at birth or in early childhood (2), often without active disease, and appears to have a life-long nature and a potential to progress insidiously to cirrhosis and HCC. However, there is little detailed information on hepatic histology of infants and young children in Korea.

In consideration of these facts, histologic studies were carried out by means of liver needle biopsy on 42 children, who were hospitalized for symptoms referable to the liver, in order to assess the nature, frequency and severity of the diseases.

Hepatomegaly was the most frequent clinical sign in patients with asymptomatic hepatitis (3). Twenty-nine cases with symptom-free hepatomegaly were selected and subjected to liver needle biopsy (some of the specimens were provided by Dr. C. K. Kim). For fuller understanding of the significance of hepatomegaly in children, the observations were compared with those of children who were hospitalized for symptoms referable to the liver. Furthermore, the observations of those biopsy specimens were compared with those obtained from 14 symptomless adults in whom the liver was palpated (4).

Acquisition of hepatitis B virus

The hepatitis B virus carrier state represents a major factor in the etiology of the chronic liver disease which is so common in Korean children. In Northwest Europe and North America, HBV infection in infancy and childhood is quite uncommon. By contrast, in Korea, up to 10% of all children become infected in the first year of life, predominantly in the perinatal period (5). Close contact with an HBeAg-positive mother is a particularly important predisposing factor. In a previous study of 20 infants born to HBeAg-positive mothers, 16 (80%) developed HBsAg during the first year of life (2). Most of these cases were infected within three months of age and maintained detectable antigenemia for a six-month or longer period and were thus presumed to have developed the chronic carrier state. While this carrier state is usually without active disease and appears to have a life-long nature, active hepatitis was rarely seen in its carrier state in the children observed by us.

A case report

A 34-month-old boy was admitted with abdominal distension and vomiting for two days. He had been normal at birth (normal spontaneous delivery, birth weight 4.2Kg).

On physical examination, he was alert and well-nourished. Slight icteric sclera was present. The liver was palpable to one finger breadth with firm mass below the right costal margin, but the spleen could not be felt. Laboratory investigations showed: total serum bilirubin 3.0 mg/100ml (conjugated bilirubin 2.2 mg/100ml), total serum protein 7.3 gm/100ml (albumin 3.9gm/100ml), serum alkaline phosphatase 15 King-Amstrong (KA) units, serum aspartate aminotransferase (SAST) 320 Karmen units, serum alanine aminotransferase (SALT) 280 Karmen units, and prothrombin time 100% of normal. Hepatitis B surface antigen (HBsAg) and hepatitis Be antigen (HBeAg) were positive in serum. One month later, he was discharged in good condition.

Six months later, he was readmitted with abdominal distension and anorexia. Physical examination disclosed hepatomegaly with a firm, smooth, nontender liver. Laboratory tests revealed SAST 270 Karmen units, SALT 390 Karmen units, total serum bilirubin 1.6 mg/100ml, serum alkaline phosphatase 38 KA units, and prothrombin time 74% of normal. HBsAg and HBeAg were positive. A percutaneous liver biopsy was performed on the fourth hospital day, and the biopsy specimen showed chronic active hepatitis.

His mother (33-years-old) had always been healthy. At the time of her son's illness, she was noted to be HBsAg-and HBeAg-positive. There was no past history suggestive of hepatitis. Physical examination disclosed hepatomegaly below the right costal margin.

Laboratory tests of sera revealed: SAST of 150 Karmen units, SALT 330 Karmen units, and total protein 7.7 gm/100ml (albumin 4.3 gm/100ml). Seven months later, she was readmitted with icteric sclera and anorexia. Percutaneous liver biopsy was performed on the fourth hospital day. The biopsy finding revealed chronic active hepatitis with early cirrhosis. In the biopsy specimens, from both the child and the mother, HBsAg and hepatitis B core antigen (HBcAg) were demonstrated in the cytoplasm and nucleus, by peroxidase-antiperoxidase technique (Figs. 23, 24, see page 35). His sister (5-years-old) was noted to be HBsAg- and HBeAg- positive. Physical examination and liver function tests were normal. His father had anti-HBs (Table 4-1) (This case was communicated by Dr. C. D. Lee).

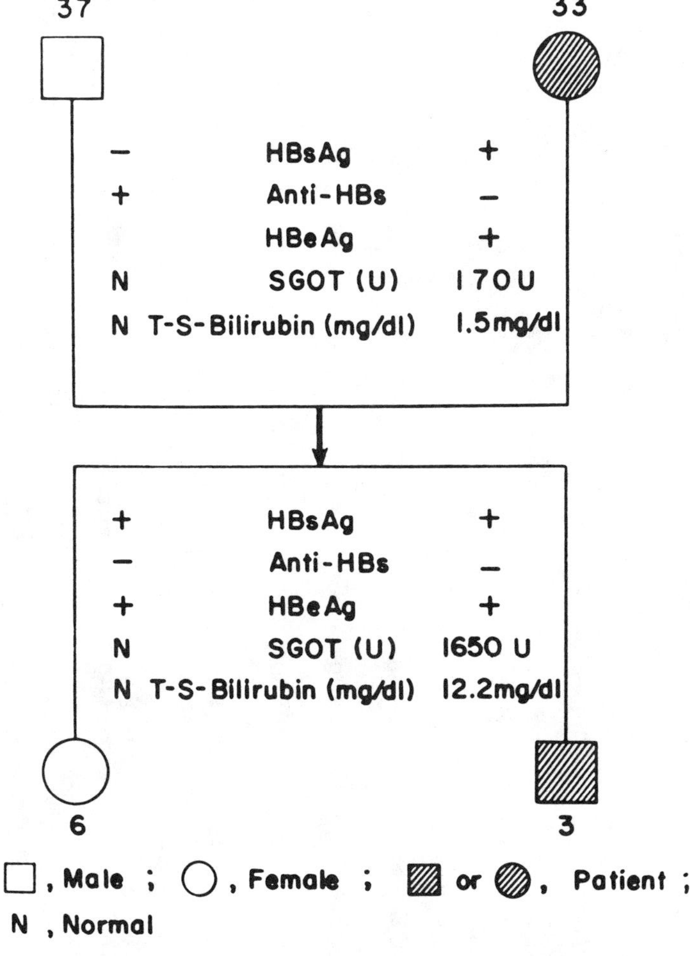

Table 4-1. Pedigree of a Hepatitis Family.

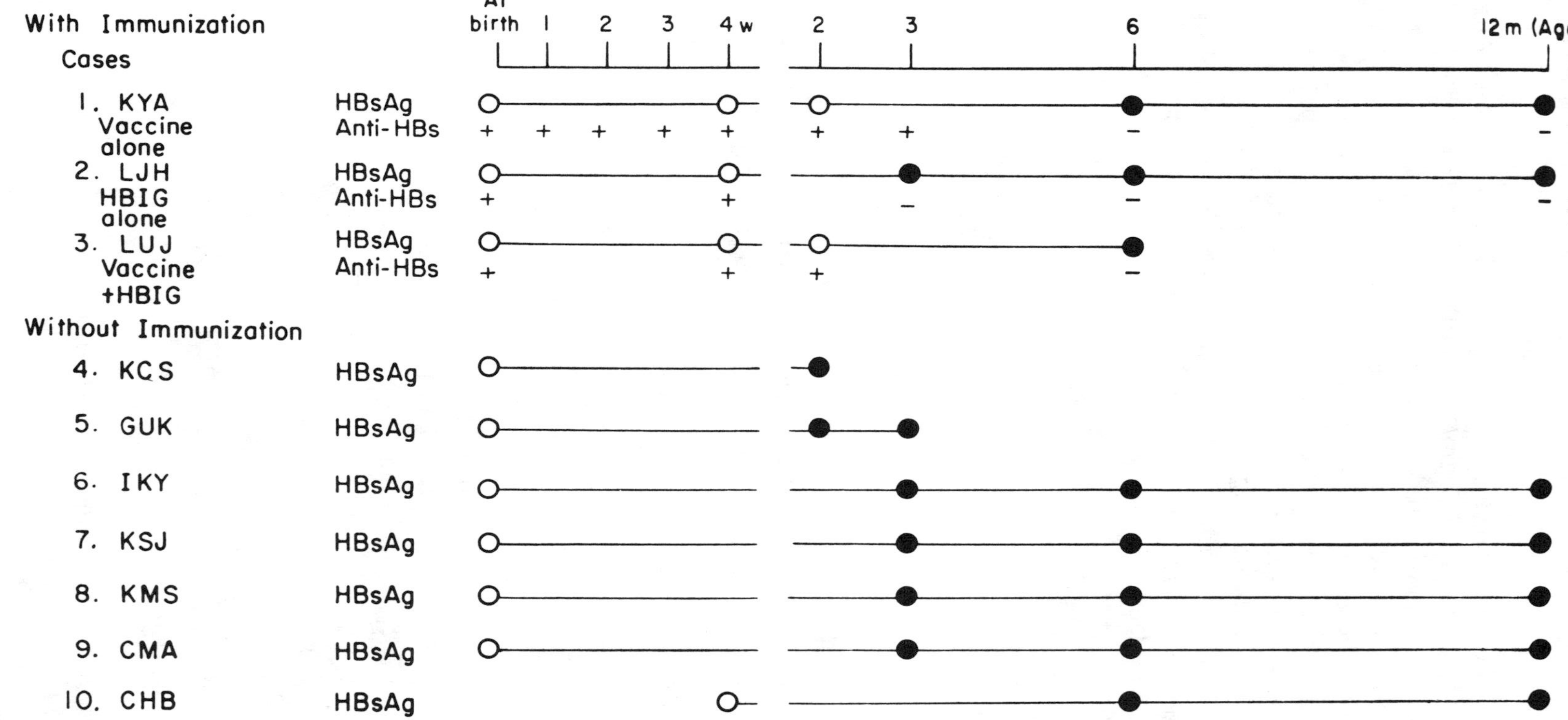

Table 4-2. Occurrence of HBsAg in Babies Born to HBeAg Positive Mothers

Key: Solid circle, HBsAg positive, determined by radioimmunoassay; Hollow circle, HBsAg negative, determined by radioimmunoassay, but surface and core gene of HBV-DNA positive, determined by polymerase chain reaction

Only four (5.8%) out of 69 HBsAg-negative newborn babies born to HBeAg-positive and anti-HBs-negative mothers had anti-HBs in their blood at birth. HBsAg appeared during the follow-up period in all the four babies, in spite of the fact that they already had prenatally acquired anti-HBs at birth and had received various types of immunization, passive, active or passive-active.

In three of the four babies, the sera, which were found to be HBsAg-negative at birth by radioimmunoassay, were confirmed to contain surface and core gene of HBV-DNA by polymerase chain reaction (Table 4-2).

Anti-HBs seems to be acquired prenatally and not transmitted from the mother but developed by the fetus itself. It acts not as a preventive but as an immune tolerogenic activity. However, it is not clear whether the intrauterine or perinatal infection with HBV genomic DNA can induce interruption of immunization.

Moreover, the babies born to HBeAg carrier mothers, infants who had no HBsAg at birth, but later developed HBsAg, maintained detectable antigenemia for a six-month or longer period. They were presumed to have developed a chronic carrier state. All seven HBsAg-negative samples of the newborns born to HBeAg positive mothers were found to contain the surface and core gene of HBV-DNA by polymerase chain reaction (Table 4–2). We, therefore, concluded that HBV-DNA was present in the form of genomic DNA in the sera at birth, prior to the occurrence of HBsAg.

This suggests that most of the babies born to HBeAg-positive mothers could have been infected already at birth with a genomic DNA in spite of the fact that HBsAg did not occur.

Symptomatic cases

Liver diseases presumed to be related to HBV infection are nonspecific reactive hepatitis, chronic persistent hepatitis, chronic active hepatitis and cirrhosis (Table. 4-3). However, in this study, HBsAg was found in two of four cases tested with persistent hepatitis, in all of three cases with chronic active hepatitis of a spotty necrotic type and in three of five cases with chronic active hepatitis of a periportal type. In cases with cirrhosis, six were tested for HBsAg, but the results were negative in five. Some of the cases with cirrhosis might have gone undetected or showed false negative results. However, metabolic or viral origins other than hepatitis B virus might have been involved. A fatty liver was observed in a patient with Froelich syndrome, and another was seen in a patient with malnutrition.

By contrast, giant cell hepatitis (Fig. 25, see page 36), more biliary atresia (Figs. 26, 27, see page 36) and hepatoblastoma were observed in earlier infancy or childhood than the other liver diseases. Three cases of hepatoblastoma were

TABLE 4–3.

Histologic Diagnosis of Biopsy-proven Symptomatic Liver Diseases in 42 Children (Age, < 15 years)

Histologic diagnosis	*No. cases*	*HBsAG (No. cases) Positive/Tested*	*Age Mean*	*Age (Range)*	*Sex M : F*
Nonspecific reactive hepatitis	2	0/0	6.5y	(3–12y)	2 : 0
Chronic persistent hepatitis	6	2/4	11.8y	(7–14y)	3 : 3
Chronic active hepatitis of spotty necrotic type	3	3/3	10.2y	(6–14y)	3 : 0
Chronic active hepatitis of periportal type	7	3/5	10.3y	(2–14y)	4 : 3
Cirrhosis	10	1/6	9.7y	(5–13y)	7 : 3
Diffuse fatty liver	2	0/2	12.0y	(11–13y)	2 : 0
Giant cell hepatitis	6	0/1	3.5m	(1m–7m)	6 : 0
Biliary atresia	3	0/2	3.7y	(13m–7y)	3 : 0
Hepatoblastoma	3	0/0	13.0m	(7m–24m)	2 : 1
Total	42		8.2y	(1m–14y)	32 : 10

Key: y, years; m, months; M, male; F, female

of an epithelial type. One was of an embryonal cell type and the other two were of a fetal cell type (Fig. 28, 29, see page 36).

Analysis of a variety of histologic features of hepatitis in the symptomatic cases permitted a separation into five structural patterns with only a few overlaps.

Group 1. Nonspecific reactive hepatitis (two cases).

These cases showed some of the same features as were found in Group 3, notably with acidophilic bodies absent (see Chapter 3).

Group 2. Chronic persistent hepatitis (six cases).

These cases revealed chronic inflammation restricted to the portal tracts (see Chapter 6).

Group 3. Chronic active hepatitis of a spotty necrotic type (three cases).

Most of the features, which were observed in instances accepted of viral hepatitis, were present. Scattered necrotic hepatic epithelial cells were replaced by small clusters of mononuclear cells, usually lymphocytes and occasionally a few macrophages containing PAS-positive granules. Round, deeply acidophilic bodies, with or without pyknotic nuclei, were frequent in tissue spaces (Fig. 30, see page 36). Neighboring hepatocytes varied in size and staining qualities of both cytoplasm and nucleus throughout the lobule. Activated sinusoidal cells scattered throughout the lobule contained a large quantity of PAS-positive lipofuscin as well as iron pigment. The walls of the central veins were occasionally thickened and homogenous and frequently harbored mononuclear cells (Fig. 31, see page 36).

The conspicuous portal inflammatory exudate consisted predominantly of mononuclear cells, such as lymphocytes, numerous plasma cells and histiocytes, some of which contained PAS-positive granules. Eosinophilic cells and a few segmented leukocytes were also present. Piecemeal necrosis was characterized by loss of single hepatocytes on the lobular periphery in close proximity to inflammatory cells. Connective tissue septa extended from the enlarged portal tracts into the lobular parenchyma.

Group 4. Chronic active hepatitis of a periportal type.

Seven of the 28 cases were included in this group in which periportal inflammation (piecemeal necrosis) is often associated with progression to cirrhosis. Of the seven cases, three were associated with progression to a cirrhotic pattern. This cirrhotic pattern seemed due to passively formed young septa following bridging necrosis rather than piecemeal necrosis (Figs. 32, 33, see pages 36, 37).

Group 5. Cirrhosis of undetermined origins (10 cases).

Ten patients developed cirrhosis without an intervening stage. Hepatocytes were surrounded by layers of reticulin and sometimes even hard collagen fibers which separate the hepatocytes to varrying degrees (Figs. 34, 35, see page 37). Inflammatory cells were predominantly macrophages, but lymphocytes were occasionally found. Sometimes bile duct epithelial cells were conspicuous (Fig. 35, see page 37). In some areas, hepatocytes disappeared and collapse of different extent was noted where the reticulin framework showed new formations of fibers, including hard collagen (Figs. 36, 37, see page 37). Usually these foci involved the periphery. These findings are consistent with chronic sequelae of subacute hepatic necrosis.

By contrast, the chronic liver diseases, including chronic persistent hepatitis, chronic active hepatitis of a spotty necrotic type, chronic active hepatitis of a periportal type and cirrhosis occurred at a time of near adult age and generally later than giant cell hepatitis, biliary atresia and hepatoblastoma.

Asymptomatic cases

For the purpose of elucidating hepatic lesions in cases with hepatomegaly without symptoms referable to the liver in children, 29 cases with hepatomegaly were selected and subjected to liver biopsy. Four of the patients with liver diseases evidenced by biopsy had a history of hepatitis or a clinical evidence of liver diseases (6). Of the 29 cases, chronic active hepatitis was found in one, chronic active hepatitis associated with cirrhosis in another, chronic persistent hepatitis in seven and nonspecific reactive hepatitis in eight. The other 10 cases were normal. In most cases, chronic persistent hepatitis and chronic active hepatitis associated with a cirrhotic pattern seemed to be at the stage of convalescence or sequelae of bridging necrosis.

The observations with those biopsy specimens were compared with specimens obtained from 14 symptomless adults in whom the liver was palpated (4). In 14 adult cases, chronic active hepatitis was found in four and chronic active hepatitis was associated with cirrhotic pattern in two (Figs. 38, 39, 40, see page 37). Incidences of chronic active hepatitis and chronic active hepatitis with cirrhosis were significantly fewer in symptom-free children with hepatomegaly than in adults. Thus, in Korea, the hepatitis B virus carrier state is presumed to be acquired at birth or in early childhood, often without active disease. It seems to have a life-long nature and a potential to progress insidiously to cirrhosis and hepatocellular carcinoma in adulthood.

Summary

The etiology of chronic active hepatitis in childhood seems to be related mainly to hepatitis B virus.

The hepatitis B carrier state, usually acquired at birth or in early childhood, often without active disease, seems to have a life-long nature and a potential to progress insidiously to cirrhosis and hepatocellular carcinoma in adulthood.

The etiology of the majority of cirrhosis in childhood has not been established but, in Korea, factors other than hepatitis B virus, such as metabolism and viruses, should be taken into consideration.

In most cases, the cirrhotic pattern in childhood seems due to passively formed reticulin collapse and fibrosis resulting from confluent necrosis or young septa following bridging necrosis rather than piecemeal necrosis.

References

1. Lee, A.K. and Chung W.K. Observations of HBsAg by radioimmunoassay in chronic liver diseases and hepatocellular carcinoma in Korea. J Catholic Medical College 30: 61–72, 1977.

2. Chung, W.K., Yoo, J.Y., Sun, H.S., Lee, H.Y., Lee, I.J., Kim, S.M. and Prince, A.M. Prevention of perinatal transmission of hepatitis B virus: A comparison between the efficacy of passive and passive-active immunization in Korea. J Infect Disease 151: 280–286, 1985.

3. Chung, W.K., Moon, S.K., Gershon, R.K., Prince, A.M., Park, Y.C. and Cho, Y.S. Anicteric hepatitis in Korea. I. Clinical and laboratory studies. Arch Intern Med 113: 526–534, 1964.

4. Chung, W.K., Moon, S.K. and Popper H. Anicteric hepatitis in Korea: comparative studies of asymptomatic and symptomatic series. Gastroenterology 48: 1–11, 1965.

5. Chung, D.K. and Chung, W.K. Vertical transmission of hepatitis B antigen. J Catholic Medical College 27: 257–267, 1974.

6. Kim, C.K. and Lee, D.B. Clinico-pathological evaluation of hepatomegaly in Korean children: Emphasized on hepatomegaly, unknown etiology. J Catholic Med College 18: 303–309, 1970.

Legends

Fig. 23. HBsAg and HBcAg in Hepatocytes.

HBcAg in the nucleus (arrows) of hepatocytes (mother). Needle biopsy, PAP method for HBcAg followed by hematoxylin stain, ×400.

Fig. 24.

HBsAg in cytoplasm (arrow) of hepatocytes (mother). Needle biopsy, PAP method for HBsAg followed by hematoxylin stain, ×400.

Fig. 25. Giant-cell (neonatal) hepatitis.

A seven-month-old male, HBsAg-. The parenchyma consists of multinucleated giant liver cells and is infiltrated by mononuclear cells. There is a portal tract in the right side of the field and a capillary bridging between the portal tract and the central vein. Needle biopsy, HE, ×200.

Fig. 26. Extrahepatic biliary atresia.

A one-year-old male. Some giant multinucleated hepatocytes, often bile-stained, are seen. Wedge biopsy, HE, ×400.

Fig. 27.

The same biopsy specimen illustrated in Fig. 26. Portal inflammation and fibrosis are confined to the portal tract. Proliferated bile ductules are distorted. HE, ×400.

Fig. 28. Biopsy specimens of epithelial cell-type hepatoblastoma.

A fetal-cell type. A two-year-old male, alpha-fetoprotein 726.5 ng/ml. A higher magnification of fetal cell type hepatoblastoma showing trabecular type growth. Note the uniformity of cells and the absence of mitotic figures. Wedge biopsy, HE, ×200.

Fig. 29.

Fetal cell type hepatoblastoma. An eight-month-old female. Note the marked hematopoietic activity. Most of the cells are of an erythroid series. Wedge biopsy, HE, ×400.

Fig. 30. Chronic active hepatitis of a spotty necrotic type.

A nine-year-old male, HBsAg+. Two round and deeply acidophilic bodies (arrows) with or without a pyknotic nucleus are found in the tissue space. Needle biopsy, HE, ×400.

Fig. 31.

A 13-year-old male, HBsAg+. The wall of the central vein is thickened and homogenous and harbors mononuclear cells. Needle biopsy, HE, ×200.

Fig. 32. Chronic active hepatitis.

With early cirrhosis. A 14-year-old male, HBsAg + . Note the widened portal space and the unsharp border between the portal tract and the parenchyma. Passively formed reticulin fibers connect the portal with the portal and the portal with the central zones. Highly regenerative parenchyma is beginning to be surrounded by a passive septum. Needle biopsy, HE, ×100.

Fig. 33.

With early cirrhosis. A 14-year-old male, HBsAg+. Note the passive reticulin collapse and the young fibrotic septation dissecting the parenchyma, forming regenerative nodules. Needle biopsy, HE, ×100.

Fig. 34. Cirrhosis.

A 12-year-old female, HBsAg+. Note that the gland-like hepatocytes are surrounded by reticulin and hard collagen fibers. Inflammmatory cells are predominantly macrophages, but lymphocytes are occasionally found. Wedge biopsy, HE, ×200.

Fig. 35.

A nine-year-old male. Note the group of foam-clear hepatocytes isolated by stroma mainly composed of proliferated bile ductules. Wedge biopsy, HE, ×200.

Fig. 36.

A 14-year-old male. In one area, hepatocytes have almost disappeared and collapse of a large extent is noted where the reticulin framework shows a new formation of fibers, including hard collagen. A few islands of hepatocytes of a pseudoglandular shape are scattered. Needle biopsy, HE, ×100.

Fig. 37.

A 10-year-old male, HBsAg-. The collapse where hepatocytes have disappeared, varies in extent and stage. In one part, the reticulin framework shows passive collapse with inflammation and the other part reveals hard collagen. Needle biopsy, HE, ×200.

Fig. 38. Biopsy specimen of an asymptomatic case of an adult showing chronic active hepatitis of a spotty necrotic type.

A higher magnification, showing two acidophilic bodies and a focal necrosis replaced by inflammatory cells. HE, ×400.

Fig. 39.

The biopsy specimen shows severe portal inflammatory reaction with an unsharp border between the portal tract and the parenchyma (piecemeal necrosis) and the beginning of the formation of a connective tissue septa. HE, ×200.

Fig. 40.

The biopsy specimen shows a regenerating nodule surrounded by inflammatory septum. HE, ×100.

5 CIRCUMSCRIBED HEPATIC NECROSIS: A PATTERN OF PROGRESSION

Whan Kook Chung, M.D., Ph.D.

Chronic active or aggressive hepatitis (CAH), in which periportal inflammation (piecemeal necrosis) is associated with progression, potentially to cirrhosis, implies little concern with intra-lobular necroinflammation as a process responsible for aggravation and progression. Some published observations, however, refer to episodes of acute necrotizing bouts ("subacute hepatic necrosis") (1,2). For technical reasons, relatively few sequential biopsy studies of chronic viral hepatitis B are available; particularly, initial acute hepatitis B is barely documented, since biopsies are now rarely performed in the acute stage of hepatitis. Moreover, most published sequential studies are complicated by therapeutic interventions.

In general, chronic hepatitis B in Western countries seems to have less tendency to progression (3) than in the Orient, which might explain the particularly unfavorable response to steroid therapy there (4). The availability of Korean serial biopsy specimens, obtained over a period of more than twenty years, encouraged the description of a seemingly characteristic circumscribed necrotizing lesion within the lobular parenchyma, observed during the course of chronic hepatitis B.

Patients

For this study, 15 patients were selected on the basis of CHN detected by subsequent biopsies after the initial biopsy revealed various stages of hepatitis

(Table 5-1). They showed histologic progression during the follow-up studies (1958–1981) at a Korean Army Hospital and St. Mary's Hospital in Seoul. The ages of the 15 patients (11 men and four women) ranged from 21 to 44 years with an average of 34.8 years. Twelve of these had tests for hepatitis B virus antigen; eleven showed hepatitis B surface antigen (HBsAg) in sera and only the remaining one had anti-HBsAg. None of the patients had been exposed to hepatotoxic drugs, chemicals, alcohol abuse or steroid therapy during the year preceding the first biopsy or the period of the follow-up observation.

This study is a revision of our previous study with new additional cases and further follow-up (5).

Definition of Circumscribed Hepatic Necrosis (CHN)

In circumscribed portions of the parenchyma (Figs. 41, 42, see page 38), the hepatocytes showed conspicuous hydropic swelling and cytoplasmic clumping. They were arranged in the form of acini, i.e., usually dilated bile canaliculi were lined on cross-section by four or eight hepatocytes and, in most instances, contained small bile plugs to indicate cholestasis (Figs. 43, 44, see page 38). The hepatocytes were surrounded by layers of reticulin and sometimes even hard collagen fibers, which separated the acinar hepatocytes to varying degrees (Fig. 45, see page 38). Inflammatory cells were predominantly macrophages but, occasionally, lymphocytes were found, while segmented leukocytes were seen only in the presence of cholestasis (Figs. 46, 47, see pages 38, 39). In some areas the acinar hepatocytes had disappeared and collapse of different extent was noted where the reticulin framework showed new formation of fibers, including hard collagen. Usually these foci involved the periportal area, and only exceptionally the central (perivenous) zone, when the lobular architecture was sufficiently preserved to judge the location in the lobule (Fig. 48, see page 39). The foci often involved one-third to one-half of the lobule extending contiguously into the neighboring lobules. Of the 13 biopsies which showed CHN, seven had some degree of collapse and six showed predominant collapse. In the areas not affected by circumscribed lesions, the features of CAH were noted (Fig. 49, see page 39) although the uninvolved lobular parenchyma was sometimes hardly altered. In other instances, focal necrosis with acidophilic bodies (five specimens) and steatosis were observed. Ground glass cells were seen twice (Fig. 50, see page 39). Oncocytic hepatocytes (excess of mitochondria) were also observed near the portal tracts. In ten instances, transition to cirrhosis was seen. Mild lesions were noted in only three patients. No delta-Antigen was detected in the seven biopsy specimens which were obtained from the liver at the time of CHN.

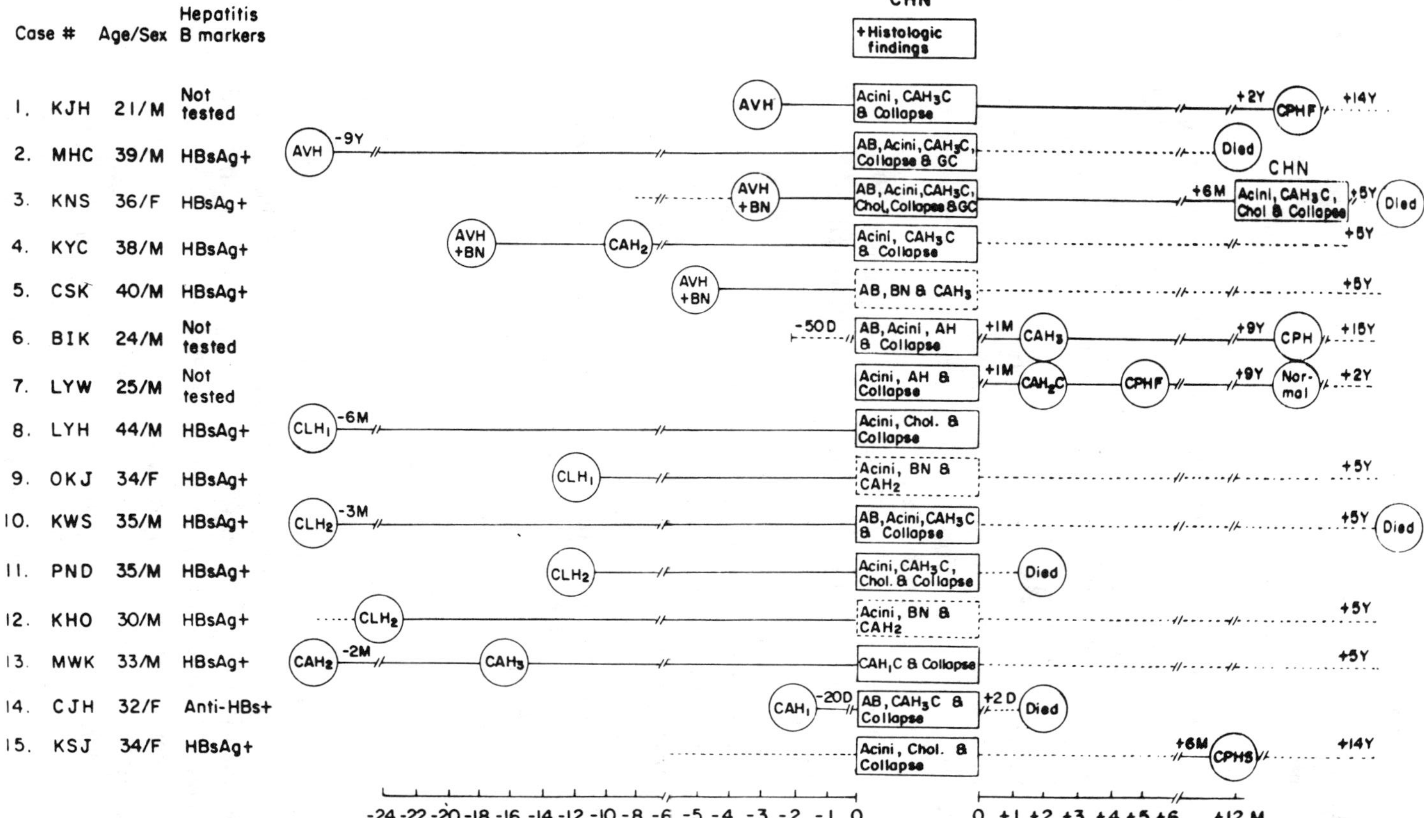

Table 5-1. Histologic Precursors and Outcomes of CHN in the Evolution of Chronic Viral Hepatitis B

AB = Acidophilic bodies; AH = Acute viral hepatitis; BN = Bridging necrosis; CAH = Chronic active hepatitis (1 = mild, 2 = moderate, 3 = severe); CAHC = CAH with Cirrhosis; CHN = Circumscribed hepatic necrosis; Chol. = Cholestasis; CLH = Chronic lobular hepatitis (1 = mild, 2 = moderate, 3 = severe); CPH = Chronic persistent hepatitis; CPHF = CPH with fibrotic septa; GC = Groundglass cells; [solid box] = CHN; [dashed box] = Not overt but mild features of CNH; ——— = Histological follow-up; ------ = Clinical follow-up

(Some cases are from Chung, W.K., Cha, S.B. and Moon, S.K. Bulletin Clinical Res. Institute 12:1–11, 1984, with permission)

Sequential Development of Histologic Lesion (Table 5-1)

CHN Lesions. Of the 15 patients, 12 exhibited CHN on one or two occasions during the follow-up serial biopsies; in one patient, two successive bouts were observed one year apart. The remaining three did not show overt features of CHN but had similar mild lesions.

Precursor Lesions of CHN. Of 12 patients who were available for biopsy before the stage of CHN, five had had acute hepatitis (AH) previously, two, three months before, one, five months before, one, 18 months before, and one, 11 years before. Five had had chronic lobular hepatitis (CLH) 12–30 months before and two, CAH 20 days and 16 months before, respectively. In two patients, two biopsies preceded the stage of CHN, both specimens showing CAH; in one, CAH was preceded by AH and, in the other, the CAH became aggravated. There were no intervening biopsies in four patients who initially had AH and in five patients who previously had CLH.

Outcomes of CHN. Five patients were available for subsequent biopsy: one showed CHN one year later; two, histologic regression to CPH with increased fibrosis one and three years later, respectively; and two, regression to CPH or normal through the stage of CAH with cirrhosis during the follow-up (10 years in both). Clinical follow-up observations ranged from two days to 16 years (mean 5.1 years) after the last biopsy showing CHN. Five of the 15 patients died, two within two months, one, one year later, and two, six years later. Ascites developed suddenly in six cases and hepatic coma in three at the time of demonstration of CHN. Ascites was transient in four patients as was hepatic coma in two. Rise in the activities of serum aminotransferase and serum bilirubin, prolonged prothrombin time and abnormal elevation of alpha-Fetoprotein level, were common at the time of CHN. HBsAg was usually present in the sera.

Typical Case Reports

Case 3—with AH at the initial biopsy. A 36-year-old housewife was admitted to St. Mary's Hospital because of dark urine and jaundice. She had been well until ten days prior to admission. She denied previous jaundice. She had mildly icteric sclerae. The liver edge was minimally tender. Serum aspartate aminotransferase (SAST), serum alanine aminotransferase (SALT) and serum bilirubin were conspicuously elevated and declined to the normal range at the end of the fourth month of hospitalization, but slowly rose again thereafter and reached a peak in the sixth month. SAST, SALT and serum bilirubin again fell to the normal range four months after the peak, but slowly rose again thereafter, and a second peak occurred one year later. The prothrombin time was prolonged during the second peak. Transient ascites appeared at both peaks. Three liver biopsies were performed: the first during the first bout; the second during the convalescence three months after the first biopsy, and the third during the second bout one year after the second biopsy. The first biopsy specimen showed AH, which progressed to CHN with cirrhosis. In the third biopsy specimen, CHN, which progressed to cirrhosis later, was still present (Fig. 51, see page 39). The first biopsy specimen was subjected to study for Delta-antigen but none was detected. This patient died due to esophageal variceal bleeding and hepatic failure six years after the onset of the disease.

Case 10—with CLH at the initial biopsy. A 35-year-old man was admitted because of easy fatigability and jaundice which had started 15 days before the admission. He had moderately icteric sclerae and a tender, palpable liver edge. SAST, SALT and bilirubin levels were elevated initially, and fluctuated for eight months and gradually fell thereafter. Jaundice recurred 20 months later. A prolonged prothrombin time persisted after the appearance of jaundice. Liver biopsy was performed two months after the initial observation and, again, two years and three months after the first biopsy or eight months after the recurrence of jaundice. CLH (Figs. 52, 53, 54, see page 39) was observed in the first biopsy specimen and CHN with cirrhosis in the second (Fig. 55, see page 40). Delta-Antigen was absent in the first specimen. HBsAg was positive in the serum at the time of the first and second biopsy but was once absent in between. The spleen size gradually increased and he died due to esophageal variceal bleeding six years after the onset of the disease.

Case 15 (Table 5-2)—with CHN at the initial biopsy. A 34-year-old woman was admitted because of jaundice and ascites. The patient, who had been well, began to have jaundice 55 days before her admission. The serum aminotransferase activity and the bilirubin levels were elevated until two months after the admission. Thereafter, however, they gradually decreased and reached normal levels. Two biopsies were done one year apart: the first performed on admission showed CHN with cirrhosis, and the second, done 12 months after the first, demonstrated CPH with a mild increase of fibrosis. In this instance, clinical and histologic restoration was maintained for 15 years.

Comments

The main purpose of this presentation is to put in focus a lesion developing in the course of chronic hepatitis B. The circumscribed lesion is characterized by degeneration of hepatocytes, which assume an acinar arrangement, and is associated with perihepatocellular inflammation progressing to conspicuous fibrosis and eventual collapse. The lesion seems to develop during the stage of CAH. It appears to be common in Korea. In agreement with other reports from Oriental countries, for example, Taiwan and Hong Kong (4), chronic hepatitis B in Korea has a far more progressive course than in Western countries (6). Such a lesion, however, has been occasionally encountered in Western mate-

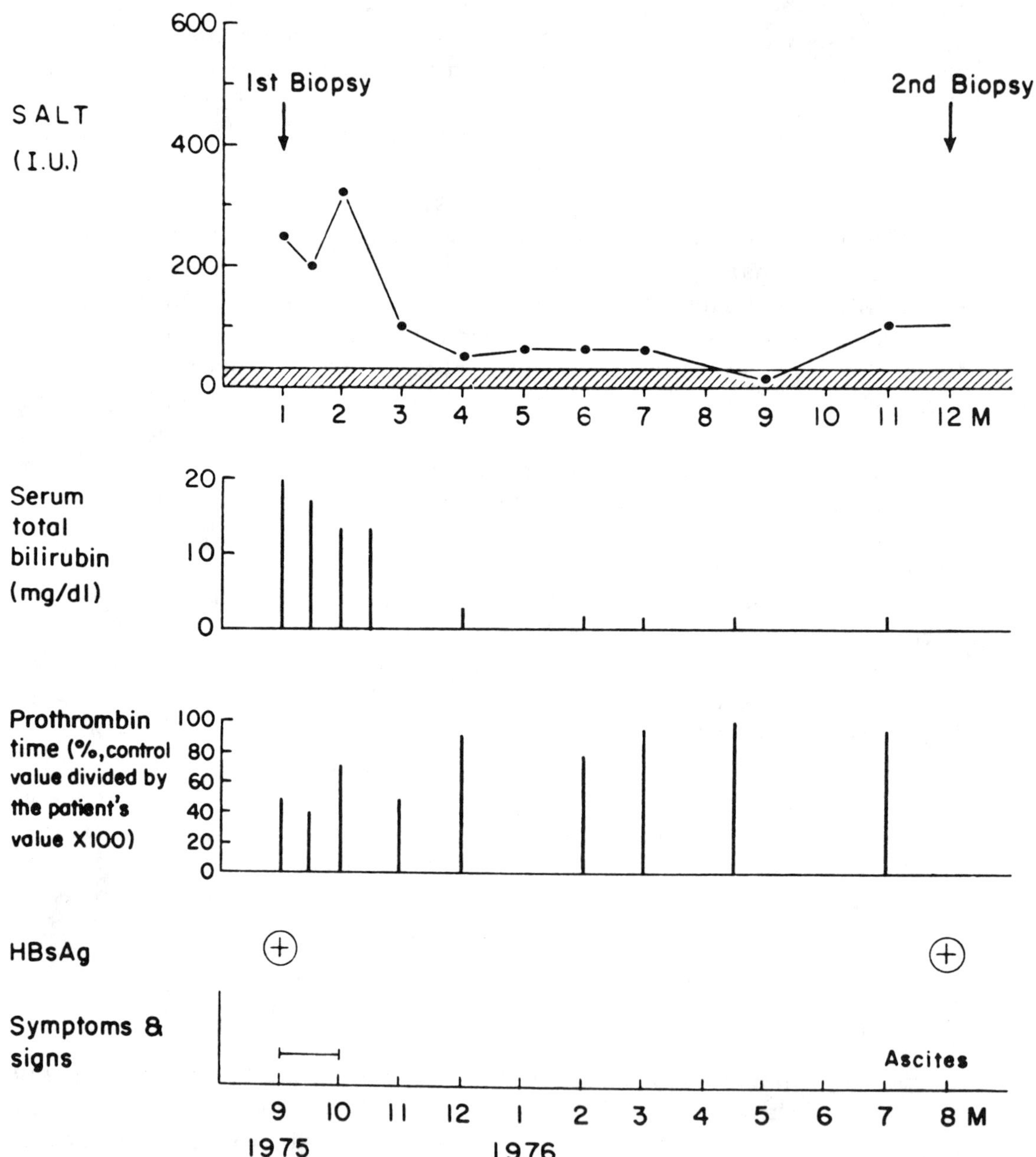

Table 5-2. Summary of Laboratory and Clinical Data of Case 15

rial. The circumscribed lesion contrasts with other portions of the parenchyma which show changes commonly associated with CAH and/or SHN.

Sequential biopsies permit the author to put CHN into the conventional framework for classification of hepatitis. In some instances, acute viral hepatitis is histologically documented as the initial lesion. This acute hepatitis frequently shows histologic features which, in the past, have indicated transition to chronicity, because of conspicuous periportal necroinflammation and portal central necrotic bridges (7). Recent evidence, however, denies these features' predictive value in hepatitis B, since they were observed at the height of acute hepatitis B in medical personnel who completely recovered with the clearing of surface antigen (8). HBsAg- containing ground glass cells are the only accepted morphologic indicator of transition to chronicity in acute hepatitis B (9). I encountered a number of cases that developed chronic lobular hepatitis before CHN. This contradicts the common Western assumption that CLH does not progress (10). This may be related to the greater tendency to progression in the Orient but also calls for caution in Western material. CHN is not only more severe than CLH but is also circumscribed, while CLH involves the entire liver more or less uniformly. Chronic persistent hepatitis was seen in the examined material only rarely and usually followed more severe lesions similar to those observed during the improvement of CAH following immunosuppressive treatment (11).

CHN was associated with transition to cirrhosis in the majority of the cases studied and may be considered a major factor in this development. In most instances, CHN coincided with significant clinical deterioration reflected in the biochemical observations, and was sometimes associated with the sudden onset of ascites and hepatic coma. These acute bouts of hepatic insufficiency associated with CHN may recur, and eventually be followed by death or recovery with prolonged survival. In my study, one instance showed clinical and histologic restoration 15 years later. The temporary disappearance of HBsAg in one case may reflect extensive destruction of hepatic parenchyma since it was reported in fulminant hepatitis (8,12). Ground glass cells, presumably reflecting deposition of large amounts of HBsAg, were encountered only in a few instances during the development of chronic hepatitis.

The pathogenesis of acute bouts of circumscribed hepatic necrosis, usually associated with evidence of hepatic failure, remains problematic. It may be the result of an exacerbation of hepatitis B, presumably associated with increased viral replication which may even reappear after a preceding period of absent viral replication. Cases were reported (13–15) that showed dramatic improvement including clearance of HBsAg, following immunosuppressive therapy, but were aggravated after the withdrawal of therapy. However, recent reports indicate that superinfection of HBV virus carrier chimpanzees with hepatitis A, non-A, non-B and Delta-agent result in severe aggravation of the histologic features (16–19). This suggests the possibility that such superinfections may account for the described bouts in the setting of hepatitis B infection. Characteristically, under these circumstances, replication of HBV is suppressed. Although Delta-antigen infection was originally described in Italy (17), recent observations suggest a far wider distribution; it seems to be rare in the Far East. In this study, seven biopsies, which were obtained at the time of acute bouts of CHN, were subjected to study for Delta-antigen but no Delta-antigen was detected.

Further investigation is needed to clarify whether replication of viral DNA is depressed or elevated in CHN, whether immune reactivity is changed, whether superinfection can be established and, finally, whether such a lesion is found only in hepatitis B infection.

Whatever the results of these studies, reported experiences focus on the importance of lesions in the lobular parenchyma in the classification and evaluation of chronic hepatitis.

Summary

Thirty-seven sequential biopsy specimens obtained from 15 Korean adult patients over periods ranging from 20 days to 11 years were studied in correlation with clinical findings. In twelve, severe circumscribed alterations of lobular parenchyma were noted and in three others minor degrees of a similar lesion. The circumscribed hepatic necrosis showed an acinar arrangement of altered hepatocytes surrounded by increased connective tissue, progressing to collapse. The lesion frequently followed histologically documented acute viral hepatitis, but it was found in the presence of chronic active hepatitis, and was also preceded by chronic lobular hepatitis, which differs from the emphasized circumscribed lesion by diffuse lobular development. The lesion, frequently associated with transition to cirrhosis, is presumed to be a factor in this process. It is usually accompanied by clinical manifestations of hepatic failure and is often followed by the death of the patient during observation, but cases of recovery are also recorded. The pathogenesis of the lesion, which is relatively rare in Western countries, requires further exploration. The observations presented suggest a major role of parenchymal changes in the evolution of chronic viral hepatitis B.

References

1. Selmair, H., Vido, I., Wildhirt, E., et al. Die chronisch-nekrotisierende Hepatitis. Dtsch Med Wochenschr 95. 1397–1401, 1970.

2. Baggenstoss, A.H., Summerskill, W.H.J. and Ammon, H.V. The morphology of

chronic hepatitis. In: Schaffner F, Sherlock S, Leevy CM, eds. The liver and its diseases. New York: International Medical Book Corporation, 199–206, 1974.

3. Hoofnagle, H.J. and Seeff, L.B. Natural history of chronic type B hepatitis. In: Popper H, Schaffner F, eds. Progress in Liver Diseases, Vol VII. New York: Grunn & Stratton, Inc. 469–480, 1982.

4. Lo, K.J., Tong, M.J., Chien, M.C., Tsai, Y.T., Liaw, Y.F., Yang, K.C., Chian, H.C. and Lee, S.D. The natural course of hepatitis B surface antigen-positive chronic active hepatitis in Taiwan. J Infec Dis 146: 205–210, 1982.

5. Chung, W.K., Cha, S.B. and Moon, S.K. Circumscribed hepatic necrosis developing in the course of chronic hepatitis B. Bulletin Clinical Res Institute 12: 1–11, 1984.

6. International Group. Morphological criteria in viral hepatitis. Review by an international group. Lancet 1: 333–337, 1971.

7. Vanstapel, M.J., van Steenbergen, W., de Wolf-Peeters, C., Desmyter, J., Fevery, J., De Groote, J. and Desmet, V.J. Prognostic significance of piecemeal necrosis in acute viral hepatitis. Liver 3: 46–57, 1983.

8. Tabor, E., Krugman, S., Weiss, E.C. and Gerety, R.J. Disappearance of hepatitis B surface antigen during an unusual case of fulminant hepatitis B. J Med Virology 8: 277–282, 1981.

9. Houthoff, H.J., Niermeijer, P., Gips, C.H., Arends, A. and Hofstee, N. Hepatic morphologic findings and viral antigens in acute hepatitis B. Virchows Arch (Pathol Anat) 389: 153–166, 1980.

10. Wilkinson, S.P., Portmann, N.B., Cochrane, A.M., Tee, D.E. and Williams, R. Clinical course of chronic lobular hepatitis. Q J Med 47: 421–429. 1978.

11. Soloway, R.D., Summerskill, W.H.J., Baggenstoss, A.H., Geall, M.G., Gitnick, G.L., Elveback, L.R. and Schoenfield, L.J. Clinical biochemical and histological remission of severe chronic active liver disease: a controlled study of treatments and early prognosis. Gastroenterology 63: 820–833, 1972.

12. Tabor, E., Gerety, R.J., Hoofnagle, J.H. and Barker, L.F. Immune response in fulminant viral hepatitis, type B. Gastroenterology 71: 635–640, 1976.

13. Davis, G.L., Hoofnagle, J.H. and Waggoner, J.G. Spontaneous reactivation of chronic type B hepatitis. Gastroenterology 84:1370, 1983.

14. Galbraith, R.M., Eddleston, A.L.W.F., Williams, R. and Zuckerman, A.J. Fulminant hepatic failure in leukemia and choriocarcinoma related to withdrawal of cytotoxic drug therapy. Lancet 2: 528–530, 1975.

15. Hoofnagle, J.H., Dusheiko, G.M., Schafer, D.F., Jones, E.A., Micetich, K.C., Young, R.C. and Costa, J. Reactivation of chronic hepatitis B virus infection by cancer chemotherapy. Ann Intern Med 96: 447–449, 1982.

16. Dienes, H.P., Purcell, R.H., Popper, H., Bonino, F. and Ponzetto, A. Simultaneous infection of chimpanzees with more than one hepatitis virus. Hepatology 1: 506, 1981.

17. Rizzetto, M., Canese, M.G., Arico, S., Crivelli, O., Trepo, C., Bonino, F. and Verme, G. Immunofluorescence detection of a new antigen-antibody system (delta/anti-delta) associated with hepatitis B virus in liver and serum of HBsAg carriers. Gut 18: 997–1003, 1977.

18. Rizzetto, M., Verme, G., Recchia, S., Bonino, F., Farci, P., Arico, S., Calzia, R., Picciotto, A., Colombo, M. and Popper, H. Chronic hepatitis in carriers of hepatitis B surface antigen, with intrahepatic expression of the delta antigen. An active and

progressive disease unresponsive to immunosuppressive treatment. Ann Intern Med 98: 437–441, 1983.

19. Verme, G., Rizzetto, M. and Bonino, F. (eds). Delta infection and viral hepatitis. New York: Alan R, Liss, 1983.

Legends

Fig. 41. Boundary of circumscribed lesion.

Circumscribed hepatic necrosis is attached directly on the noninvolved parenchyma (arrows) showing a sharp border. Needle biopsy, HE, ×400.

Fig. 42.

The lesion of CHN (left) is separated from noninvolved parenchyma by a thin fibrous capsule. CHN involves up to a central vein (CV). Needle biopsy, HE, ×100.

Fig. 43. Cholestasis.

Conspicuous hydropic swelling and cytoplasmic clumping of hepatocytes form acini. The dilated bile capillary contains a small bile plug (arrow). Needle biopsy, HE, ×400.

Fig. 44.

Bile plugs (arrows) are seen in the lumen of bile ductules. Needle biopsy, HE, ×200.

Fig. 45. Fibrogenesis.

Hard collagen separating acinar hepatocytes to varying degrees is demonstrated. Needle biopsy, HE, ×100.

Fig. 46. Inflammatory cell infiltration.

The intralobular, pericellular inflammatory cells are predominantly macrophages but occasionally lymphocytes. Needle biopsy, HE, ×400.

Fig. 47.

Interlobular and intralobular inflammatory cells are predominantly macrophages and lymphoid cells but segmented leucocytes are occasionally seen. Needle biopsy, HE, ×400.

Fig. 48. Extent of CHN.

A higher magnification of the central vein in a CHN case, showing thickened and inflammatory infiltration of the vascular wall of the central vein. Needle biopsy, HE, ×200.

Fig. 49. Unaffected areas.

Subacute hepatic necrosis (SHN) accompanied by vigorous chronic inflammatory infiltration and collapse is noted. Inflammatory exudate is scanty in part. Needle biopsy, HE, ×100.

Fig. 50.
Note many ground glass-appearing cells. Needle biopsy, HE, ×200.

Fig. 51. Biopsy specimens from a case with AH at the initial biopsy (Case 3).
The third biopsy specimen obtained one year after the second biopsy during the second bout, showed CHN with extensive collapse. Diffuse perihepatocellular fibrosis with acinar arrangement of hepatocytes is noted. Needle biopsy, HE, ×200.

Fig. 52. Biopsy specimens from a case with CLH at the initial biopsy (Case 10).
The first biopsy specimen obtained two months after the initial observation, showing inflammatory reaction of central vein (CV) and mild variation of hepatocytes and scattered single cell necrosis. Disarray of liver cell plates is mild but more than one cell thick. Needle biopsy, HE, ×200.

Fig. 53.
The same biopsy specimen illustrated in Fig. 52, showing conspicuous sinusoidal cell reaction. HE, ×200.

Fig. 54.
The same biopsy specimen illustrated in Fig. 52, showing widening inflammatory cell reaction of the portal tract. HE, ×200.

Fig. 55.
The second biopsy specimen obtained 27 months after the first, showing isolation of cell groups by a band of collapsed fibrous tissue. Needle biopsy, HE, ×200.

6 CHRONIC HEPATITIS: CLASSIFICATION AND ITS PROGNOSIS

Whan Kook Chung, M.D., Ph.D.

In Korea, chronic hepatitis (CH) is so common that it is now one of the major causes of death. Statistics for the causes of death released in 1982 by the National Bureau of Statistics, the Economic Planning Board, ROK, indicate that in Korea the death rate of CH and CH-related diseases, including cirrhosis and hepatocelluar carcinoma (HCC), is 79.3/1,000 deaths(1). CH ranks fourth among the causes of death, and Korea has one of the highest CH death rates in the world.

CH is presumed to have several etiologies but, in Korea, the hepatitis B carrier state represents a major factor in the etiology of CH (Figs. 56, 57, see page 40).

Of 32 cases of biopsy-proven chronic anicteric hepatitis, detected by a mass-screening survey performed with serum aspartate aminotransferase (SAST) in Korea in 1962 (see Chapter 3), nine showed "serum hepatitis antigen" in liver cells(2). Sera from eight of the nine patients had HBsAg, emphasizing the significance of the carrier state in the etiology of CH in Korea(3). Of 397 patients with biopsy-proven CH, in whom HBsAg, HBeAg, anti- HBs, anti-HBe and anti- HBc were measured by radioimmunoassay at St. Mary's Hospital, Seoul, during 1979–1983, 286 had HBsAg (72%), 177 HBeAg (45%), 64 anti-HBs (16%), 64 anti-HBe (16%) and 389 had anti- HBc (98%)(4). Thus, at least one marker for hepatitis B was found among 389 of the 397 CH cases (98%), suggesting active or resolved infection with hepatitis B virus (HBV) in almost all cases (4).

Non-A, non-B hepatitis can lead to CH in Korea. 79% of post-transfusion hepatitis cases are HBsAg-negative. Recently, we tested these HBsAg-negative samples for antibody to hepatitis C virus (anti-HCV) using the Abbott enzyme immunoassay method (5). Among 57 HBsAg-negative patients with post-transfusion hepatitis, 38 (66.7%) were positive for anti-HCV. Of 85 HBsAg-negative patients with sporadic chronic hepatitis, 42 (49.4%) were positive for anti-HCV(5).

These data suggest that, of the above-mentioned 397 patients with CH, some may, in addition to hepatitis B, have non-A, non-B viral infection which may cause or contribute to CH.

HISTOLOGIC TYPES

Much progress has been made in the past decade in the classification of CH syndrome due to the clarification of correlation between specific histologic features and progressive liver cell destruction(6–8).

This study was designed to evaluate the diagnostic and prognostic value of histologic criteria on the basis of biopsy findings. 342 cases (286 males and 56 females between the ages of 17 and 73 years, with an average age of 36 years) of biopsy-proven CH were followed-up by needle biopsy and/or clinico-laboratory evaluation from 1958 to 1990 at an Army Hospital and St. Mary's Hospital in Seoul. None of these patients had exposure to hepatotoxic drugs, alcohol abuse or steroid therapy.

Conventional Types

The conventional classification of CH (Table 6–1) distinguishes persistent (portal) (CPH; Types Ia and Ib) from chronic active or aggressive (periportal) hepatitis (CAH; Types IIa and IIb) (6,9). Lobular hepatitis (CLH; Type IIIa) is considered a rarer, independent type, in which the manifestations of acute hepatitis (AH) persist for more than six months, the conventionally accepted time of onset of CH. CLH is said to subside with only minor sequelae.

In establishing the distinction between CPH, in which inflammation is restricted to the portal tracts, and active or aggressive hepatitis, in which periportal inflammation (piecemeal necrosis) is often associated with progression to cirrhosis, little attention has been paid to intralobular inflammation as a process responsible for aggravation and progression. Some published observations, however, refer to acute necrotizing bouts (subacute hepatic necrosis, SHN; Type IIIb) (10,11).

Availability of serial biopsy specimens, obtained from Korean patients

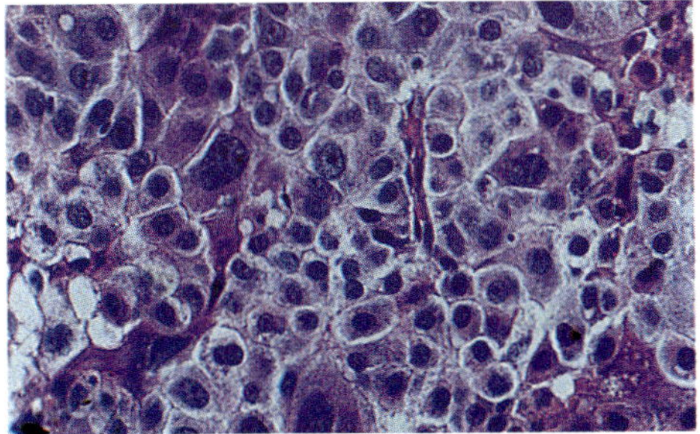

Fig. 77 See Legend page 104.

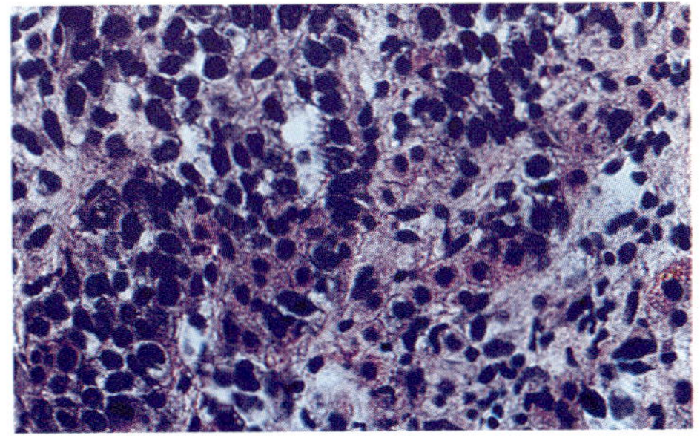

Fig. 78 See Legend page 105.

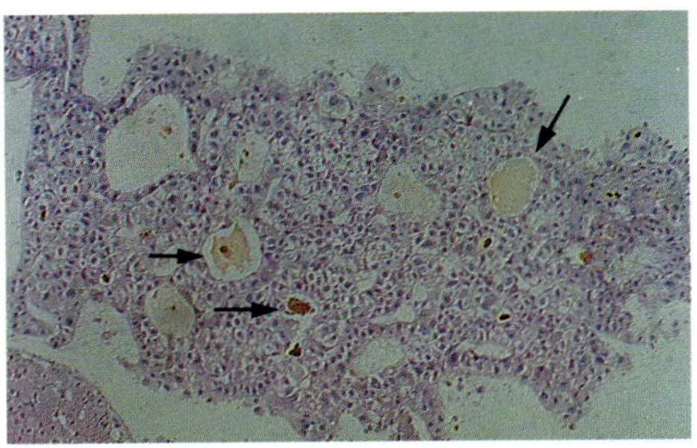

Fig. 79 See Legend page 105.

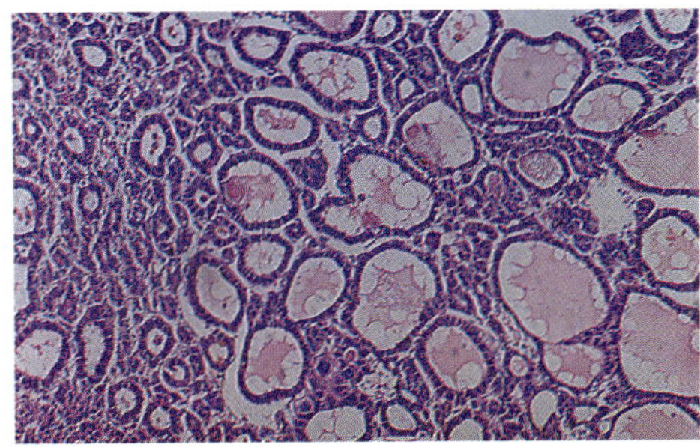

Fig. 80 See Legend page 105.

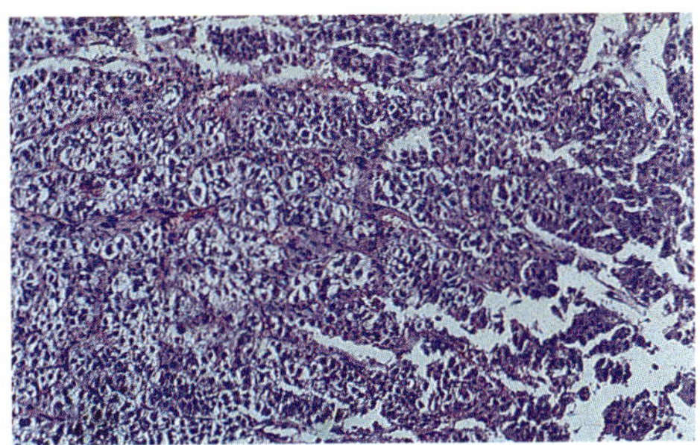

Fig. 81 See Legend page 105.

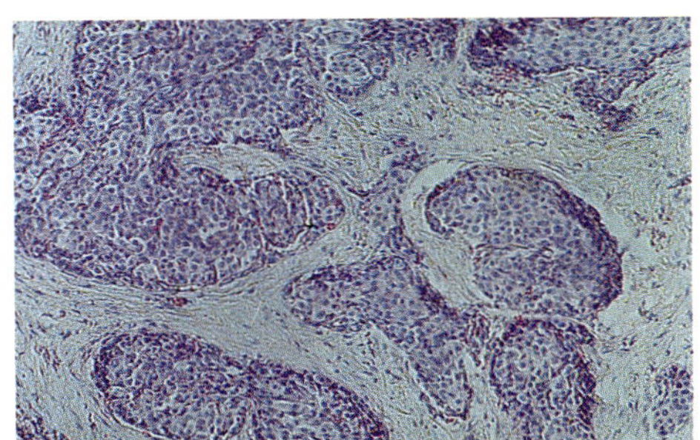

Fig. 82 See Legend page 105.

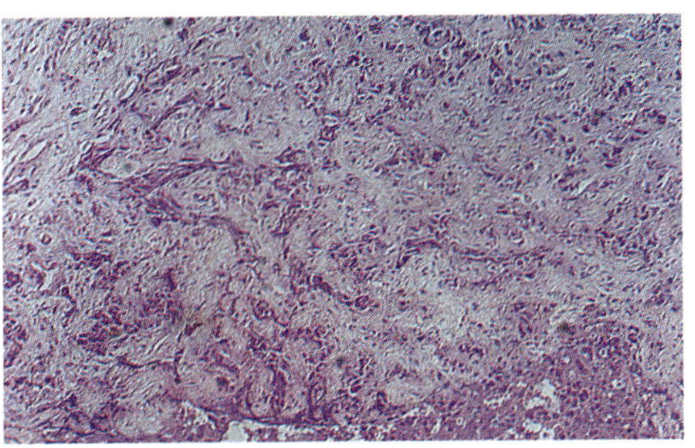

Fig. 83 See Legend page 105.

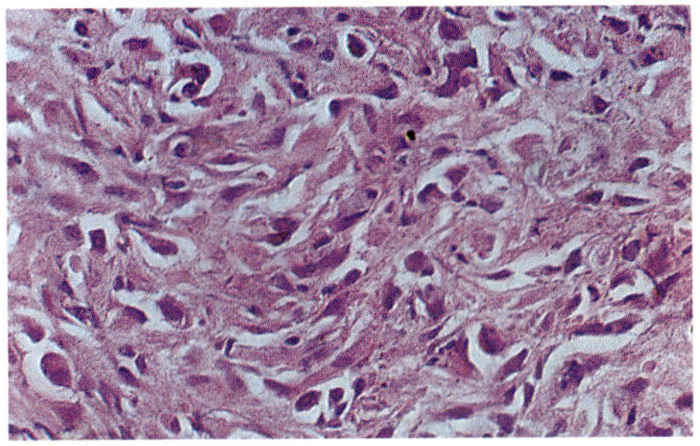

Fig. 84 See Legend page 105.

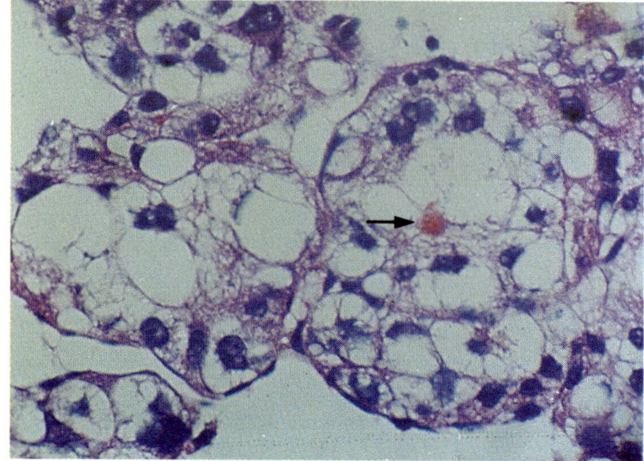

Fig. 85 See Legend page 105.

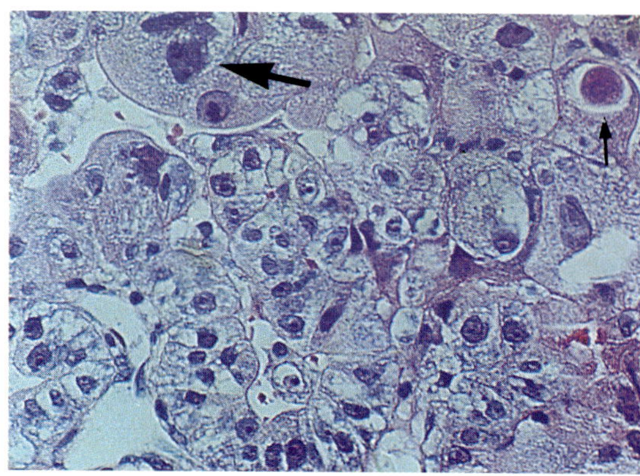

Fig. 86 See Legend page 105.

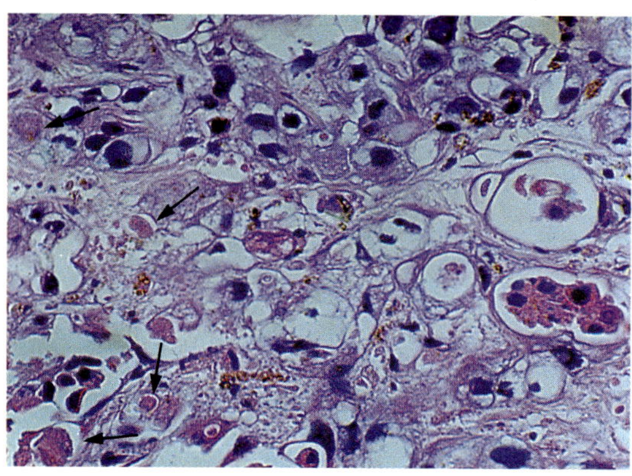

Fig. 87 See Legend page 106.

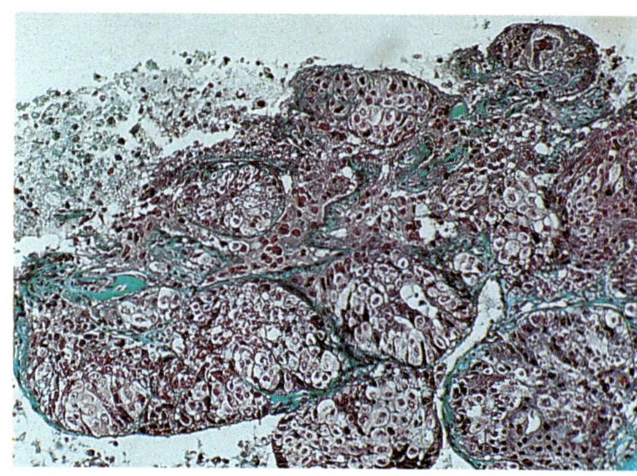

Fig. 88 See Legend page 106.

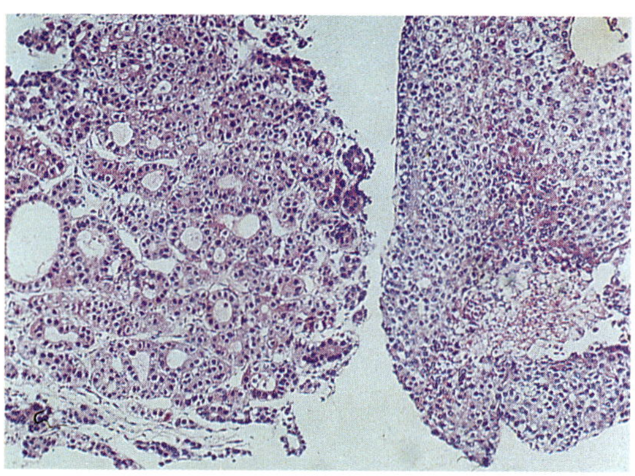

Fig. 89 See Legend page 106.

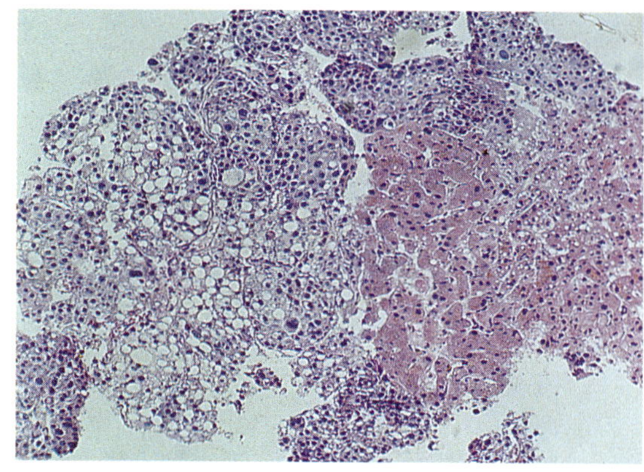

Fig. 90 See Legend page 106.

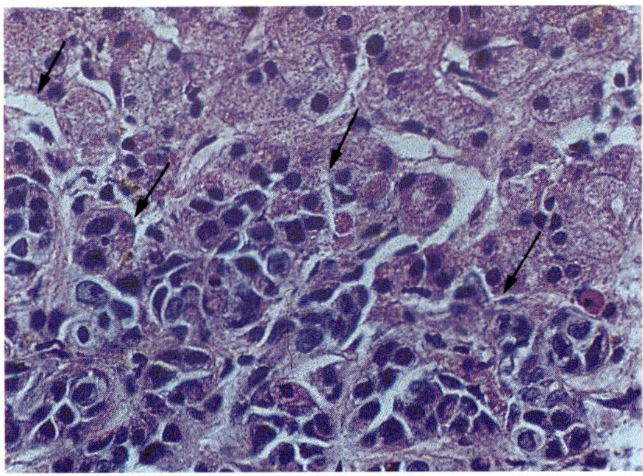

Fig. 91 See Legend page 106.

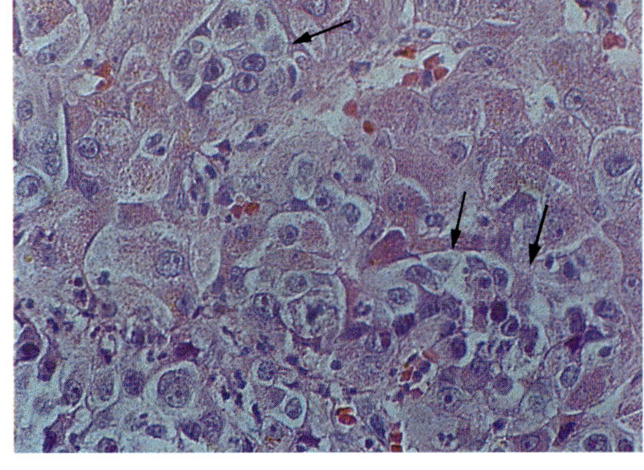

Fig. 92 See Legend page 106.

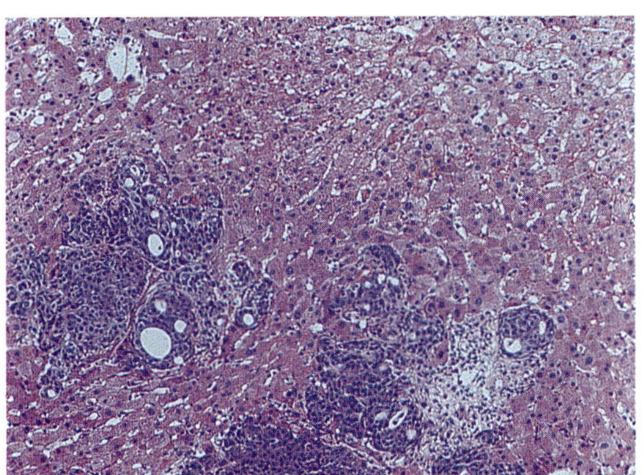

Fig. 93 See Legend page 106.

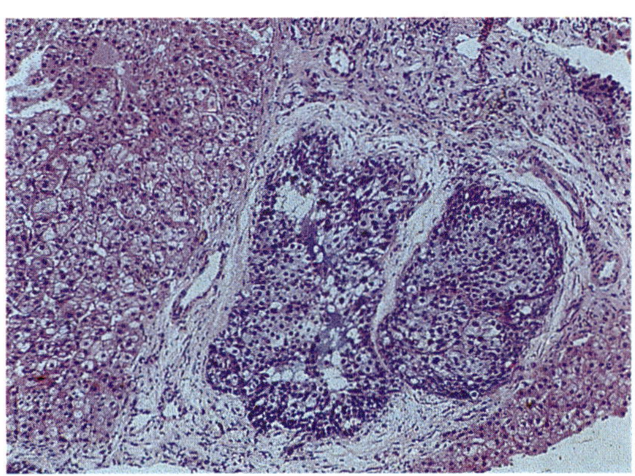

Fig. 94 See Legend page 106.

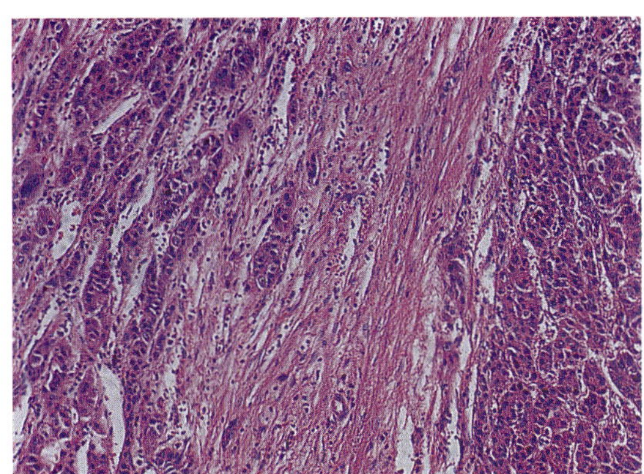

Fig. 95 See Legend page 106.

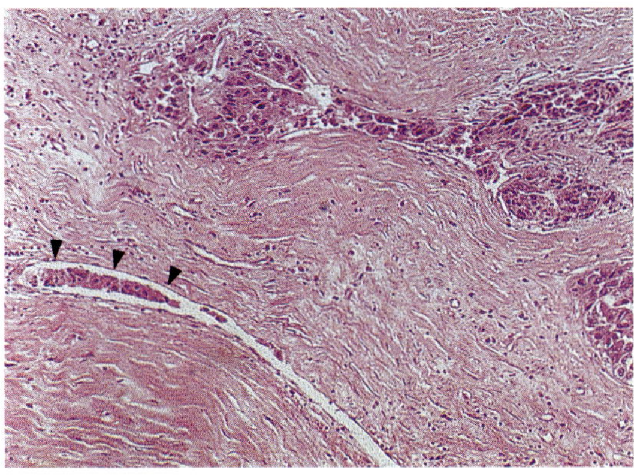

Fig. 96 See Legend page 106.

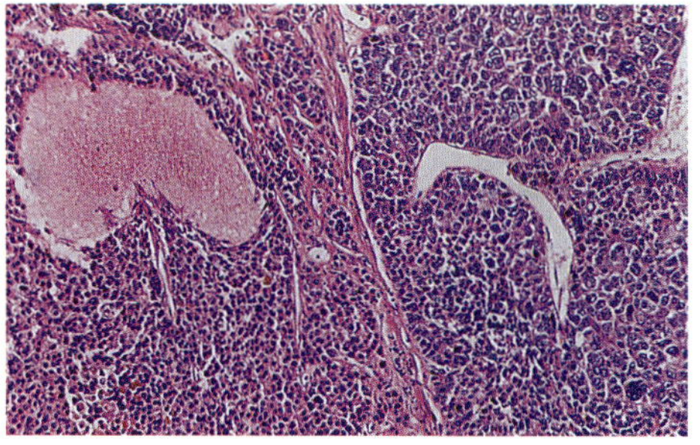

Fig. 97 See Legend page 107.

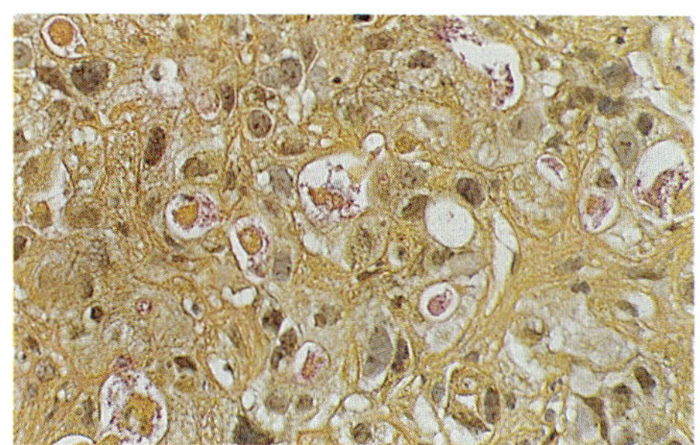

Fig. 98 See Legend page 107.

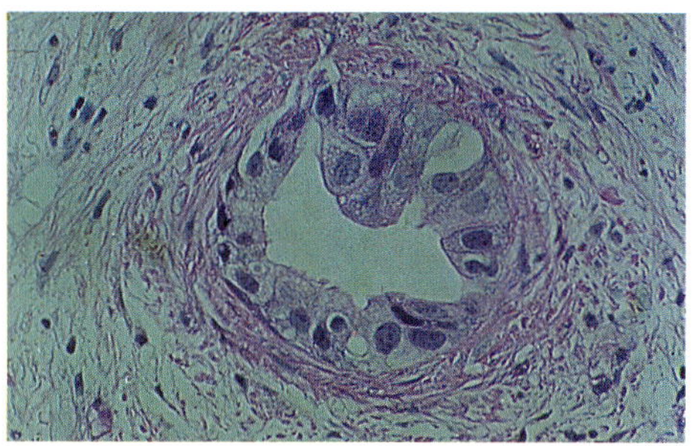

Fig. 99 See Legend page 107.

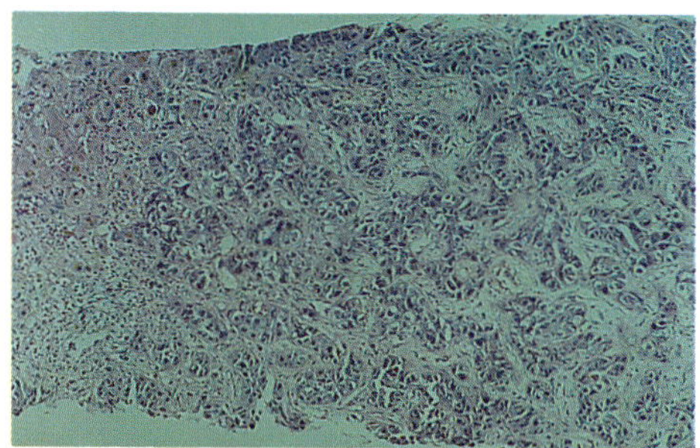

Fig. 100 See Legend page 107.

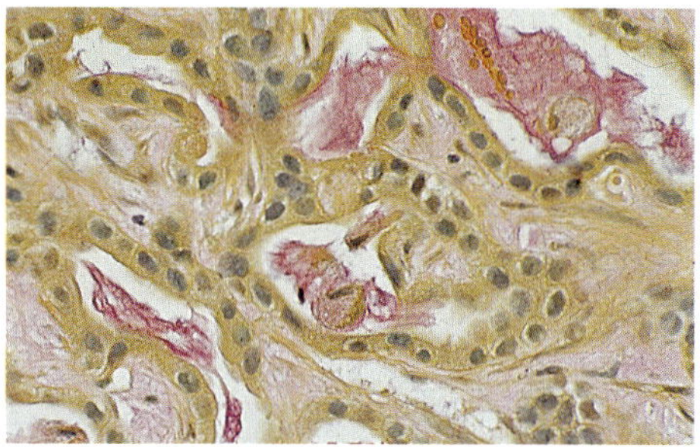

Fig. 101 See Legend page 107.

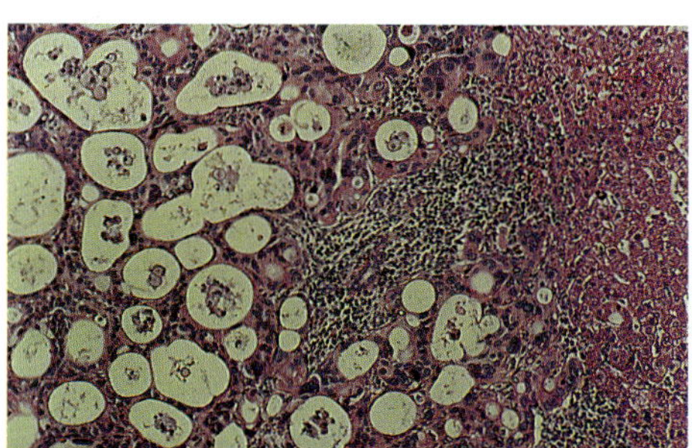

Fig. 102 See Legend page 107.

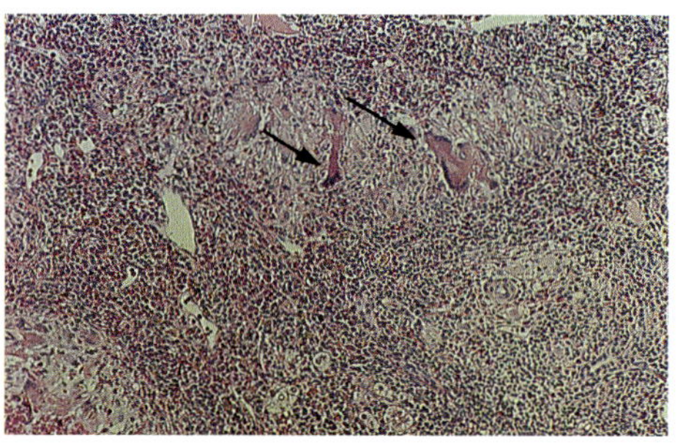

Fig. 103 See Legend page 107.

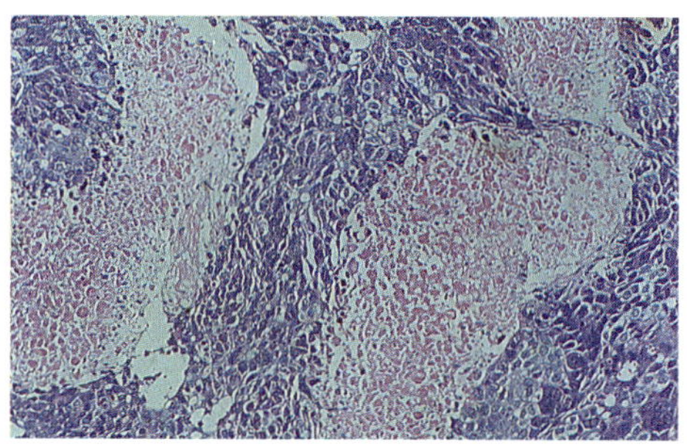

Fig. 104 See Legend page 107.

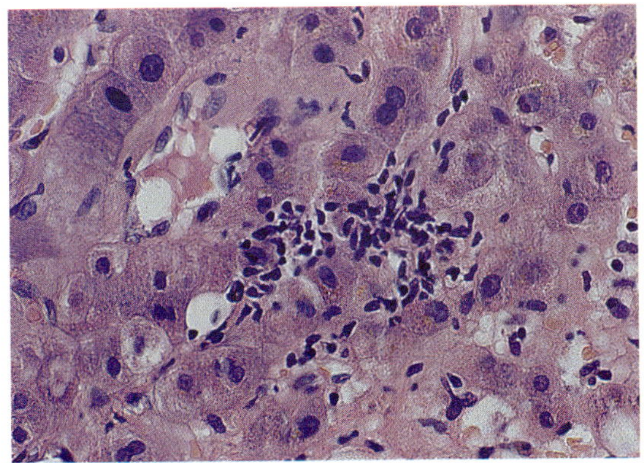

Fig. 105 See Legend page 123.

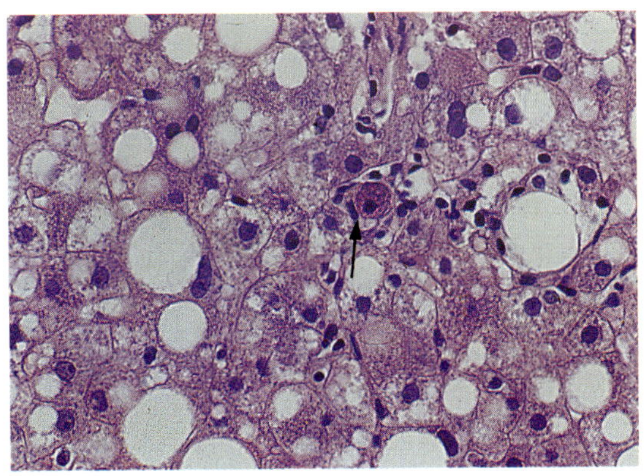

Fig. 106 See Legend page 123.

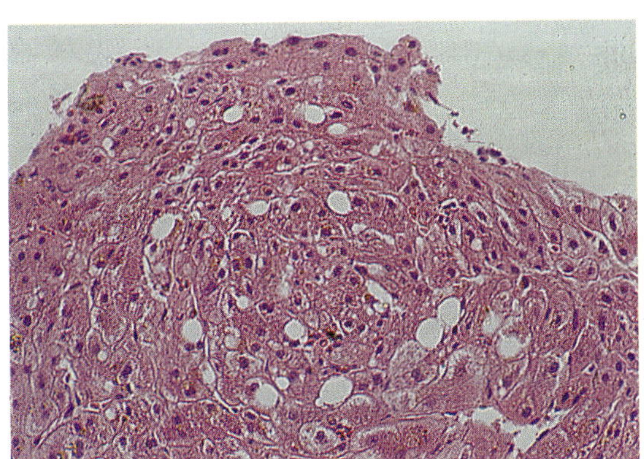

Fig. 107 See Legend page 123.

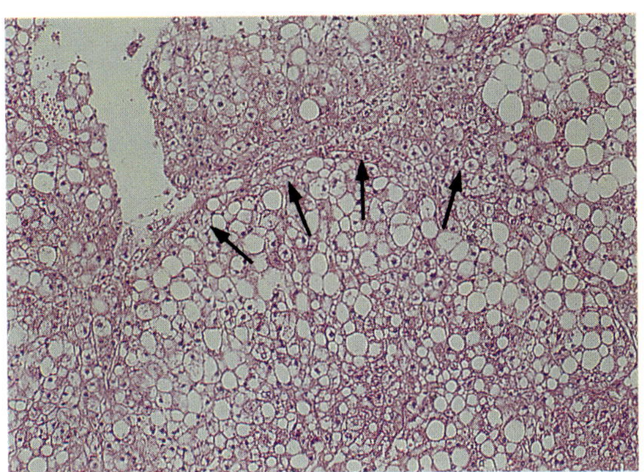

Fig. 108 See Legend page 123.

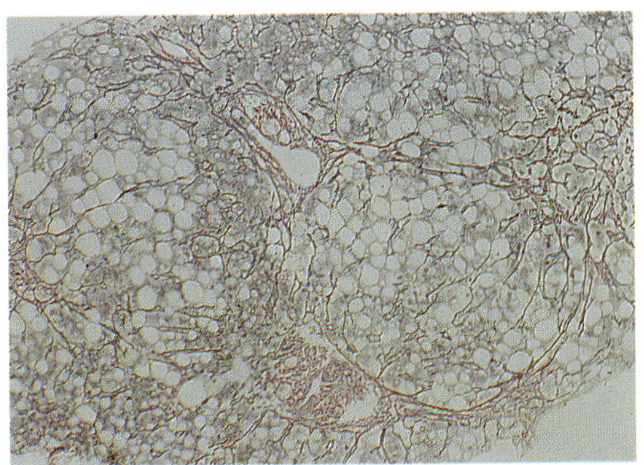

Fig. 109 See Legend page 123.

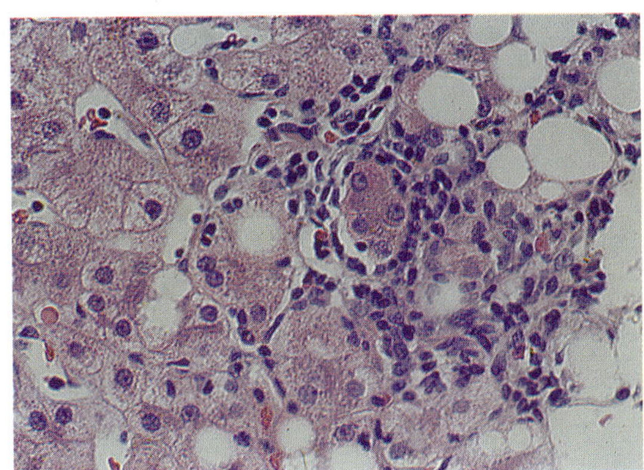

Fig. 110 See Legend page 123.

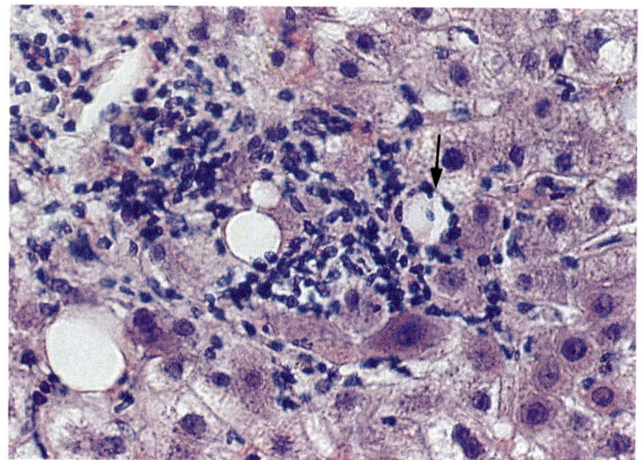

Fig. 111 See Legend page 124.

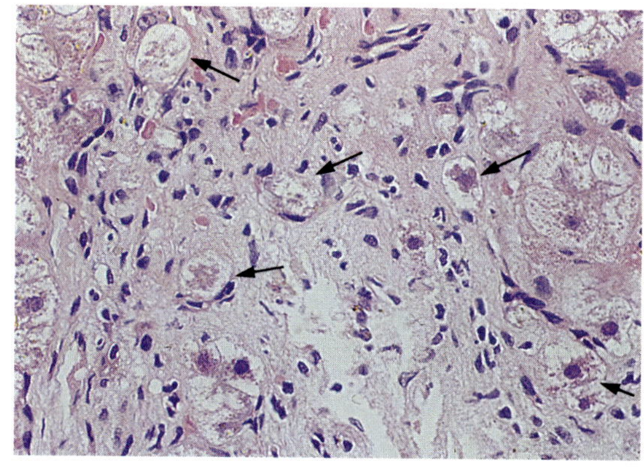

Fig. 112 See Legend page 124.

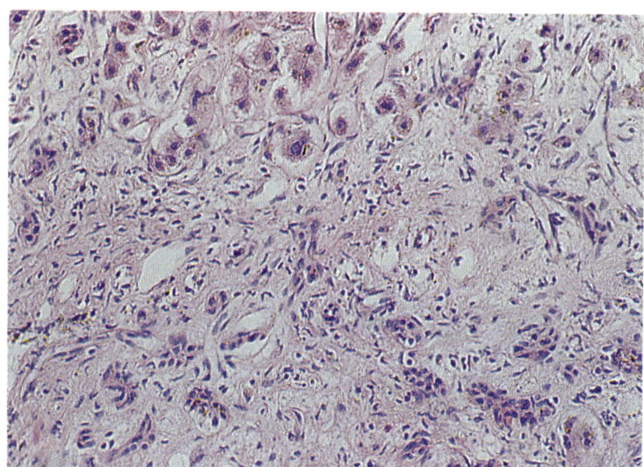

Fig. 113 See Legend page 124.

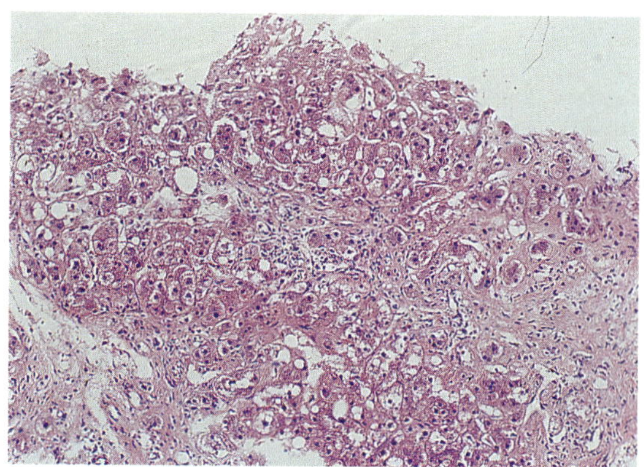

Fig. 114 See Legend page 124.

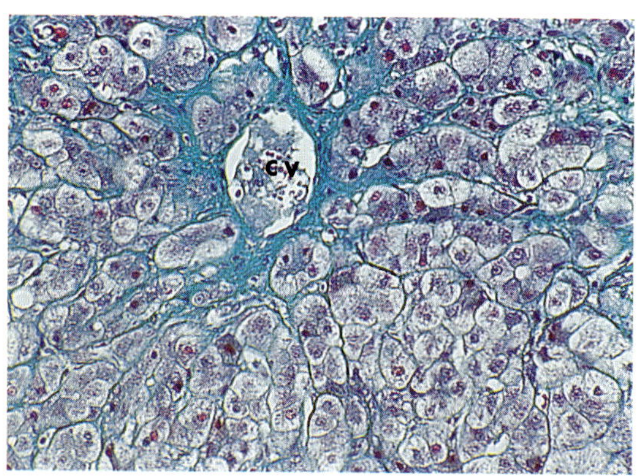

Fig. 115 See Legend page 124.

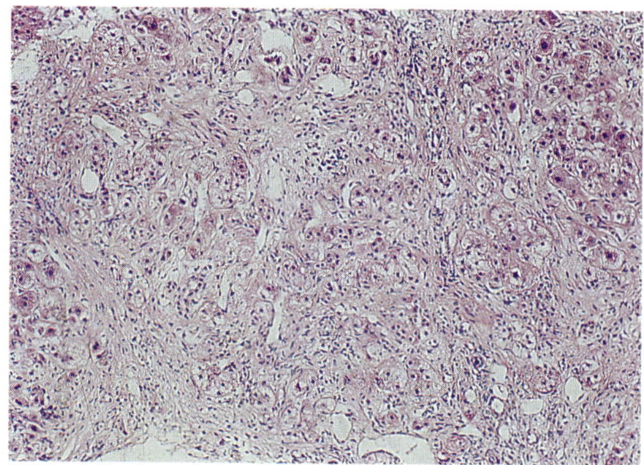

Fig. 116 See Legend page 124.

over a period of more than 20 years, permitted the description of a seemingly characteristic, circumscribed hepatic necrosis (CHN) (see Chapter 5) within the lobular parenchyma, observed during the course of CH, B, and its placement in the conventional framework of classification of CH (see Chapter 5).

Present Author's Classification of CH

The histologic features of the initial biopsy specimens permitted the author to divide them into three types with seven subtypes (Table 6–1).

I. Portal inflammation

CPH—Somewhat expanded portal tracts contain many mononuclear cells which are restricted to the surrounding parenchyma (Type Ia). In addition, increased portal fibrosis is present to varying degrees (Type Ib) (Fig. 58, see page 40).

II. Periportal inflammation

CAH—The portal tracts contain conspicuous exudate of predominantly mononuclear cells intermixed with a few segmented leukocytes. They extend into the surrounding periportal parenchyma where hepatocytes have disappeared (piecemeal necrosis) (Type IIa) (Fig. 59, see page 40) as well as into connective tissue septa radiating from the portal tract and extending into the parenchyma, frequently linking portal tracts. The septa also reach the central zone and cirrhotic changes begin (Type IIb) (Figs. 60, 61, see pages 40, 73). The ductules are proliferating. A few hepatocytes are trapped in the portal and periportal infiltration. Lobular alterations are mild.

III. Intralobular necroinflammation

CLH—The lesions are essentially identical to AH, but they are usually less severe and less uniform in different parts of the specimen.

SHN—The lesions are a parenchymal confluent necrosis so extensive as to involve the contiguous lobule (multilobular necrosis) or link the centrilobular areas to the portal tracts (bridging necrosis). These passively formed septa contain little collagen and relatively few inflammatory cells at first (12).

CHN, Type (IIIc) (Fig. 62, see page 73)—Upon random examination of many liver biopsy specimens, the author was impressed by frequent severe lobular changes in CH in Korea. Such lobular changes as CHN are characterized by degeneration of hepatocytes that assume an acinar arrangement and are associated with perihepatocellular inflammation progressing to conspicuous fibrosis and eventual collapse. They are usually associated with transition to cirrhosis (see Chapter 5).

TABLE 6–1.

Histologic Classification of Chronic Hepatitis

Types	*Histologic characteristics*	*SALT (Karmen Units)*	*Incidence of HBsAg (%)*	*Number of Cases*
Portal and periportal inflammation				
I. Persistent hepatitis (CPH)	Chronic inflammation restricted to the portal tract			
Ia. Without increased fibrosis		67.3± 40.2	43	56
Ib. With increased fibrosis	Thin incomplete fibrotic septation or increased portal fibrotic scar in addition to type Ia	49.2± 12.5	43	42
II. Chronic active hepatitis (CAH)	Periportal inflammation (piecemeal necrosis) in association with progression			
IIa. Without cirrhosis		175.6±101.3	89	17
IIb. With cirrhosis		190.8±116.9	52	124
III. Intralobular necroinflammation				
IIIa. Chronic lobular hepatitis . (CLH)	Diffuse parenchymal spotty necrosis (acute viral hepatitis picture); persist longer than 6 months	331.6±132.7	76	41
IIIb. Subacute hepatic necrosis (SHN)	Acute bridging and/or multilobular necrosis without acinar arrangement of hepatocytes	277.6±230.2	100	23
IIIc. Circumscribed hepatic necrosis (CHN)	Acinar arrangement of altered hepatocytes surrounded by increased connective tissue, progressing to collapse, and usually associated with transition to cirrhosis	133.4± 60.4	87	39

NATURAL COURSE

Our knowledge of the natural history of CH is rather limited because few sequential studies including biopsies are available. Most of the sequential studies published are about cases complicated by therapy. However, the author had an opportunity to conduct a long-term follow-up study of the aforementioned 342 patients with CH by means of liver biopsy and/or clinical and laboratory evaluation.

Long-term Follow-up Study

In the former study (4), a follow-up study was made on 260 patients with 384 liver biopsy specimens over a period of two months to 20 years (average 7.3 years). The most common terminal events were hepatic failure, cirrhosis and HCC. The survival curves (13)(14) extended from the time of the first biopsy up to 20 years; Type IIa patients had the shortest curve (12 years) (Table 6-2). The cumulative proportion of survival was highest in Types Ia, IIa, and IIIa, and lowest in Types IIb and IIIc, with a significant difference between Type IIIc and Types Ia or Ib ($P<0.001$). Of the types with low survival rates, Type IIIc had a significantly lower rate than Type IIb ($P<0.001$). While the curve dropped very rapidly in Types IIb, IIIb, and IIIc from the beginning, the curve dropped slowly in Types Ia, Ib, IIa, and IIIa. The differences between the curves of Type IIIc and Type Ia or Ib in the 1st, 5th, and 10th year were significant ($P<0.001$). The mortality rate of Type IIIc was 28% within one year, with half of the patients surviving longer than five years after the initial biopsy; however, only 40% passed the 10-year limit.

During the follow-up study of the 342 patients, 35 developed HCC, one to 22 years later. The initial histologic findings (precancer stage) of liver tissue from the 35 patients showed chronic inactive hepatitis including nonspecific reactive hepatitis and CPH in five cases, CAH with cirrhosis in 19 and SHN and/or CHN in 10. The remaining one case had CLH. Of these, 27 cases were tested for HBsAg: 21 were positive for HBsAg (see Chapter 7).

The remaining six HBsAg-negative patients might have been infected by hepatitis C virus (5).

Table 6-3 is a summary diagram of the evolution of CH. The pathway to the left is favorable (Fig. 63, see page 73), and the pathway to the right is unfavorable (Figs. 64, 65, 66, 67, 68, see page 73). Most of the cases of CH originated from anicteric hepatitis. Type IIb was the most frequent CH that was seen in hospitals and occasionally developed into HCC (15%), but the mortality was highest in Type IIIc during the follow-up. HCC developed most frequently in Type IIIc (20%) (see Chapter 7).

Type IIIc frequently followed histologically documented AH, but was also

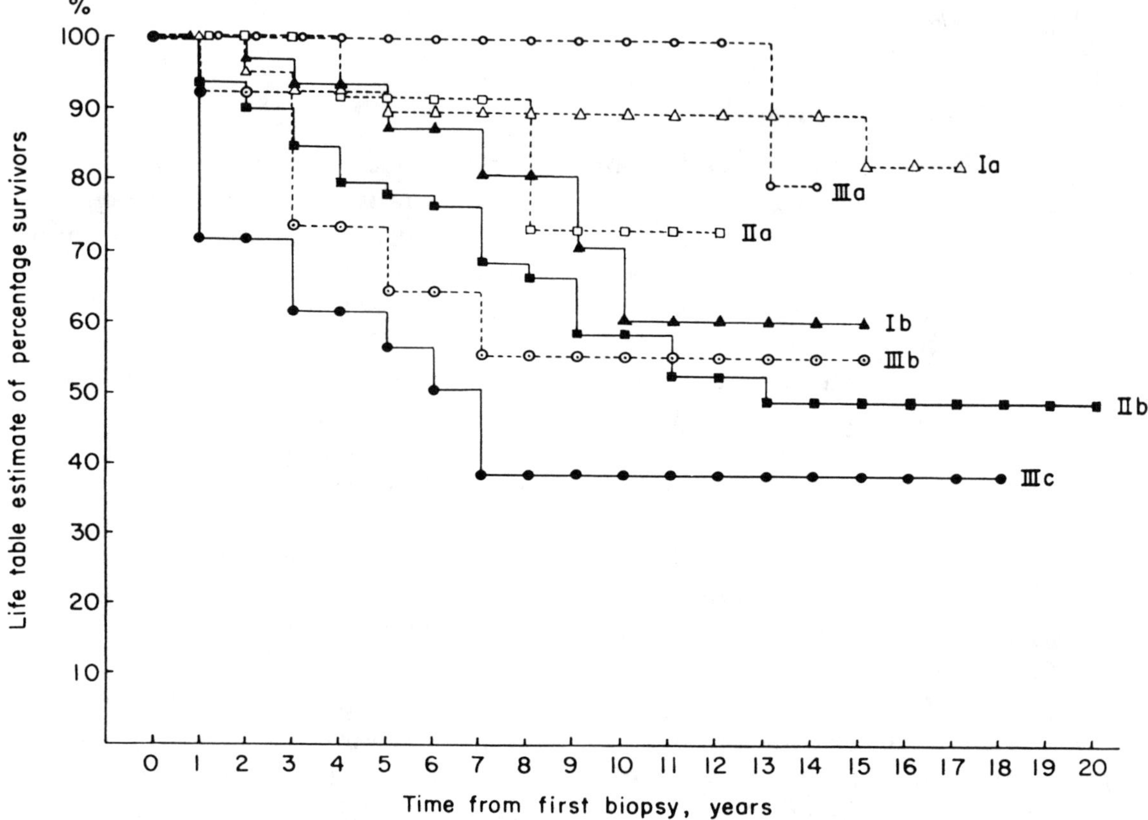

Table 6-2. Cumulative Survival Curves

The initial total 260 patients comprised 43, 38, 15, 99, 30, 14 and 21 for groups Ia, Ib, IIa, IIb, IIIa, IIIb and IIIc, respectively. Using the technique of Kaplan and Meier, life-table estimates of the cumulative proportion of survival were computed for each group separately and plotted (13). A test of Gehan, which takes into account the overall pattern of survival curves compared, was done and it confirmed a significant difference ($p<0.001$) in survival curves (14). (Reproduced from Chung, W.K., Progress in Liver Diseases, Vol VIII, Page 480, 1986, with permission)

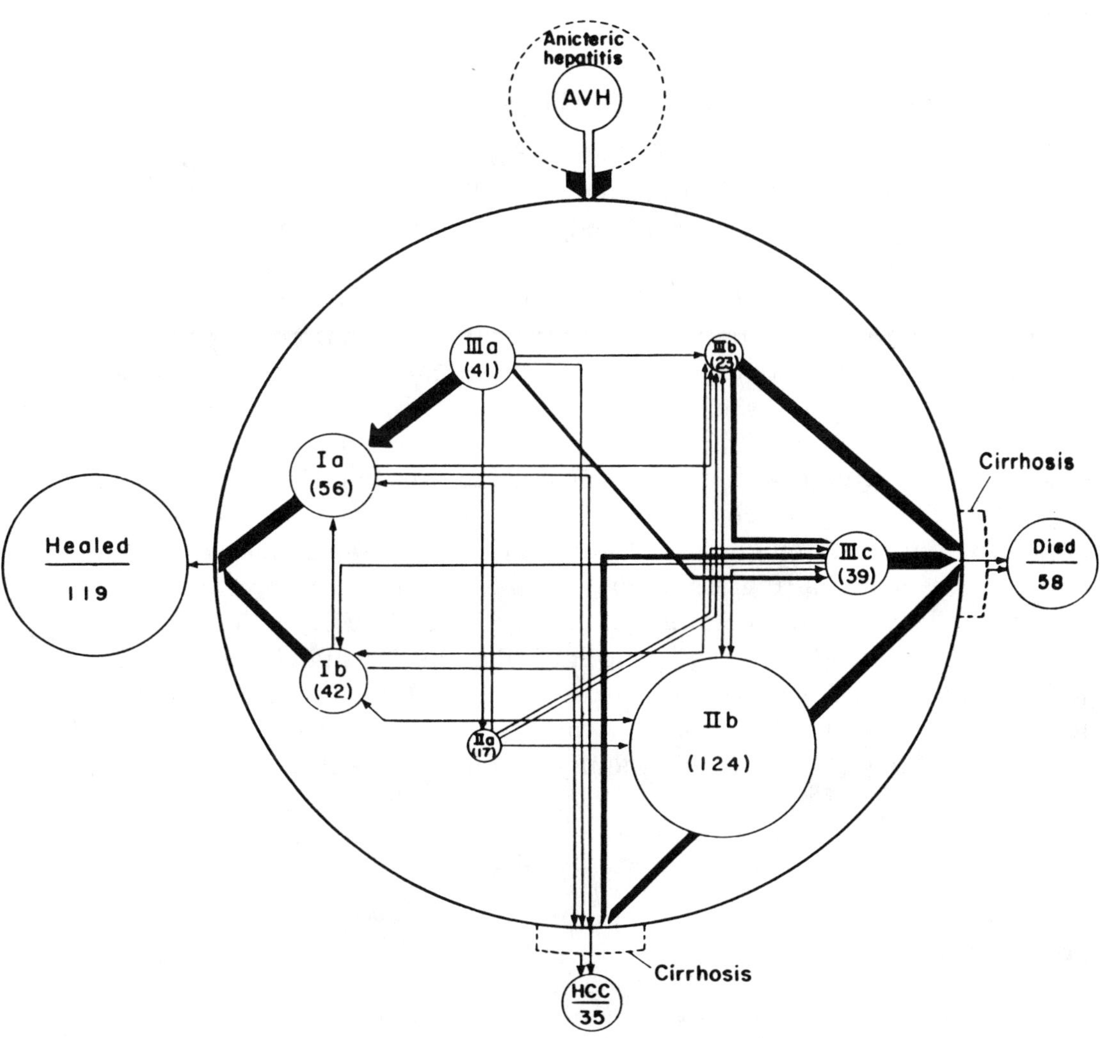

Table 6-3. Summary of Natural Evolution of Chronic Hepatitis as Evidenced by Long-term Follow-up Study

found at the time of or after CAH; it was sometimes preceded by CLH (see Chapter 5). The lesion was frequently associated with transition to cirrhosis. This leads the author to presume that such a lesion may induce cirrhosis.

Of the 342 cases with CH, 119 cases (35%) regressed and 58 cases (17%) died during the follow-up.

Problems of Histologic Classification by Biopsy

The diagnosis of CH from biopsy alone is not always correct because of inter- and intraobserver error and sampling variability.

CPH (Type Ia) has been considered a benign condition and, on rare occasions, it develops histologic features of relatively mild CAH (15). CLH (Type IIIa) is also said to subside with only minor sequelae (16). In this study, however, around 10% of both groups (Types Ia and IIIa) developed hepatic failure or progressed to cirrhosis. By contrast, complete regression was observed in cases with active or aggressive hepatitis characterized by piecemeal necrosis and intralobular fibrosis. Such histologic classification does not indicate etiology. Predicting from which histologic precursor HCC results is not always possible. HCC often developed among cases combined with cirrhosis (Type IIb), but rarely among cases without cirrhosis (Types IIa and IIIa), and among cases showing regression (Types Ia and Ib). In the precancer stage, significant hepatocytic necroinflammation (SHN of CHN) followed by collapse, and occasionally with episodic clinical bouts, is usual. Most of the cases that developed HCC were HBsAg chronic carriers. Even when histologic findings improve, the initial offenders, which are potential causes of HCC, still remain (See Chapter 7). Accordingly, any histologic classification can be faulty when etiologies are not taken into consideration. Nonetheless, liver biopsy remains the best way to identify progression or regression of CH pending clarification of etiology and pathogenesis of all forms of CH.

PROGNOSIS

Sometimes, predicting the outcome only on the basis of liver biopsy slides is difficult. Even when histologic findings indicate severe CHN, recovery is a possibility (Fig. 69, see page 74) (see Chapter 5). Conversely mild CLH can progress to cirrhosis due to repeated episodes of lobular necroinflammation (Figs. 67, 70, see pages 73, 74). However, with proper sampling and good histologic interpretation, accurate prognosis can be predicted by liver biopsy, provided that the natural history of subgroups has been well defined.

References

1. Shin, Y.J. International comparison of major causes of death. Edited by Y.J. Shin: Cause of Death Statistics. Republic of Korea, National Bureau of Statistics, Economic Planning Board, PP. 94–97, 1982.

2. Prince, A.M., Fuji, H. and Gershon, R.K. Immunohistochemical studies on the etiology of anicteric hepatitis in Korea. Am J Hygiene 79: 365–381, 1964.

3. Prince, A.M. and Gershon, R.K. The etiology of chronic active hepatitis in Korea. Yale J Biol Med 52: 159–167, 1979.

4. Chung, W.K. Chronic hepatitis in Korea. Edited by H. Popper and F. Schaffner: Progress in Liver Diseases, Vol VIII. New York, Grune & Stratton, PP. 469–483, 1986.

5. Chung, K.W., Sun, H.S., Chung, W.K., Shin, H.K., Park, C.K., Yoo, J.Y., Di Bisceglie, A.M., Waggoner, J.J. and Hoofnagle, J.H. A preliminary report on the prevalence of type C hepatitis in Korea. Korean J Intern Med 38: 750–753, 1990.

6. de Groote, J., Desmet, V.I., Gedick, P., Korb, G., Popper, H., Poulsen, H., Scheuer, P.J., Schmid, M., Thaler, H. and Uehlinger, E. A classification of chronic hepatitis. Lancet 2: 626–628, 1968.

7. Popper, H. and Schaffner, F. Nonsuppurative destructive chronic cholangitis and chronic hepatitis. Edited by H. Popper and F. Schaffner: Progress in Liver Diseases, Vol III. New York, Grune & Stratton, pp. 336–354, 1970.

8. Summerskill, W.H.J. Chronic active liver disease reexamined: Prognosis hopeful. Gastroenterology 66: 450–464, 1974.

9. Popper, H. and Schaffner, F. The vocabulary of chronic hepatitis. N Engl J Med 284: 1154–1156, 1971.

10. Selmair, H., Vido, I., Wildhirt, E., et al. Die chronisch-nekrotisierende Hepatitis. Dtsch Med Wochenschr 26: 1397–1401, 1970.

11. Bagenstoss, A.H., Summerskill, W.H.J. and Ammon, H.V. The morphology of chronic hepatitis. Edited by F. Schaffner, S. Sherlock, C.M. Leevy: The Liver and its Diseases, New York, International Medical Book, pp. 199–206, 1974.

12. Boyer, J.L. and Klatskin, G. Pattern of necrosis in acute viral hepatitis. Prognostic value of bridging (subacute hepatic necrosis). New Engl J Med 283: 1063–1071, 1970.

13. Kaplan, E. and Meier, P. Nonparametric estimation from incomplete observations. J Am Stat Assoc 53: 457–481, 1958.

14. Gehan, E. A generalized Wilcoxon test for comparing arbitrarily singly-censored samples. Biometrika 52: 203–224, 1965.

15. Chadwick, R.G., Galizzi, J, Jr., Heathcote, J., Lyssiotis, T., Cohen, B.J., Scheuer, P.J. and Sherlock, S. Chronic persistent hepatitis. Hepatitis B virus markers and histological follow-up. Gut 20: 371–377, 1979.

16. Wilkinson, S.P., Portmann, N.B., Cochrane, A.M.G., Tee, D.E. and Williams, R. Clinical course of chronic lobular hepatitis. Q J Med 47: 421–429, 1978.

Legends

Fig. 56. HBsAg and HBcAg in Hepatocytes.

HBsAg is found in the cytoplasm of hepatocytes. Needle biopsy, fluoresceinated antiserum to HBsAg, ×400.

Fig. 57.

Chronic active hepatitis. HBcAg is demonstrated in the nucleus (thin arrow) as well as in the cytoplasm (thick arrow) of hepatocytes. Needle biopsy, PAP method for HBcAg followed by hematoxylin stain, ×200.

Fig. 58. Type Ib.

Biopsy findings of a case showing Type Ib. A sharp border between portal inflammation and parenchyma is noted. Incomplete strand septal fibers radiate from the portal tract into the parenchyma. The arrangement of parenchymal cell plates is almost intact. Needle biopsy, HE, ×100.

Fig. 59. Type IIa.

A biopsy specimen from a case with the features of Type IIa. Note the severe portal reaction, pronounced piecemeal necrosis and little scarring. Needle biopsy, HE, ×200.

Fig. 60. Type IIb.

Laparoscopic findings of a case of chronic active hepatitis with cirrhosis (Type IIb). The left lobe shows an uneven, irregular surface with a papuloid-shape nodularity and several dells. Peritoneal adhesion of the edge is seen. The right lobe looks similar to the left, but rather atrophic and thin fibrotic flecks are seen on the surface. The edge is sharp and irregular.

Fig. 61.

A biopsy specimen from the case illustrated in Fig. 60. Note the diffuse and striking post-collapse septal fibrosis and irregular regenerative nodules. Chronic portal tract inflammation with piecemeal necrosis is noted. Needle biopsy, HE, ×100.

Fig. 62. Type IIIc.

A biopsy specimen from a case with circumscribed hepatic necrosis (Type IIIc). The lobular architecture is completely distorted. Isolated groups of liver cells, which often assume a rosette-like appearance, are separated by fibrotic septa. Needle biopsy, HE, ×200.

Fig. 63. A reversed case with chronic lobular hepatitis.

The first biopsy specimen showing extensive spotty parenchymal necrosis with a moderate to marked degree of chronic portal inflammation and multifocal piecemeal necrosis (Type IIIa). Parenchymal cells vary somewhat in size and staining quality. Needle biopsy, HE, ×100.

Fig. 64. A case of acute hepatitis that later developed into CHN.

A third biopsy specimen obtained 16 months after acute hepatitis, showing CHN with extensive collapse. Diffuse perihepatocellular fibrosis with an acinar arrangement of altered hepatocytes is noted. Needle biopsy, HE, ×200.

Fig. 65. A case of CPH that later developed into SHN.

A third biopsy, obtained two years after the finding of CPH. The portal exudate of predominantly mononuclear cells extends into the surrounding periportal parenchyma up to the central zone where hepatocytes disappeared and portal fibrosis radiates from the portal tract into parenchyma. Needle biopsy, HE, ×200.

Fig. 66. A case of Type IIa that later developed into Type IIIb.

A second biopsy specimen, obtained 27 months after one that showed CAH. The bulk of the liver parenchyma has undergone necrosis. A few hepatocytes are trapped in inflammatory exudate. Proliferated bile ductules are seen. Needle biopsy, HE, ×200.

Fig. 67. A case of Type IIIa that later developed into Type IIIc.

The first biopsy specimen, obtained two months after the initial observation, showing a mild variation of hepatocytes and scattered single cell necrosis. The disarray of liver cell plates is mild but more than one-cell thick. Needle biopsy, HE, ×100.

Fig. 68.

The second biopsy specimen, obtained 27 months after the first, showing an isolation of cell groups by a band of collapsed fibrous tissue. Needle biopsy, HE, ×100.

Fig. 69. Type IIIc, reversible.

Circumscribed hepatic necrosis, showing an acinar arrangement of altered hepatocytes isolated by increased pericellular inflammatory fibrosis and collapse. The patient recovered from illness and maintained a healthy condition for 20 years. Needle biopsy, HE, ×400

Fig. 70. A case of Type IIIa that later developed cirrhosis.

Chronic lobular hepatitis. Focal spotty necrosis with occasional acidophilic bodies (arrow) and Kupffer cell mobilization in the sinusoidal space are seen. A little variation of hepatocytes in size and staining quality is noted. Somewhat widened portal spaces with mononuclear cell infiltration and a mild erosion of limiting plates are seen. The patient developed cirrhosis and died four years after the initial biopsy. Needle biopsy, HE, ×100.

7 PRECURSOR LESIONS OF HEPATOCELLULAR CARCINOMA

Whan Kook Chung, M.D., Ph.D

Which hepatocytes are premalignant cells in hepatocarcinogenesis in humans is not clear. Liver cell dysplasia, as defined by Anthony et al. (1), indicates increased risk of malignant transformation. Another presumed precursor lesion of hepatocellular carcinoma (HCC) is circumscribed conspicuous hyperplasia of hepatocytes in the form of adenomatous nodules (2). Strong relationships between those precursor lesions and hepatitis B surface antigen (HBsAg) positivity are shown (1,3).

This study was designed to evaluate histologic lesions of HCC in Korea, focusing attention specifically on precancerous lesions in the liver. The author has also attempted to evaluate the role of risk factors, serologically and immuno-morphologically, particularly hepatitis B virus (HBV) infection.

Initial histologic findings of liver tissue from 35 patients at the precancer stage showed chronic inactive hepatitis in five cases and chronic active hepatitis (CAH) in 30 cases, including 19 cases of CAH with cirrhosis, one case of chronic lobular hepatitis, three cases of subacute hepatic necrosis and seven cases of circumscribed hepatic necrosis resulting from occasional episodic bouts of parenchymal necroinflammation (4).

Independent needle biopsy specimens were obtained by laparoscopy from uninvolved portions and tumors of the liver in 33 patients with HCC(cancer stage), and from nontumorous livers in 12 patients, in whom HCC developed one–13 years later (mean 6.5 years) (precancer stage). Routine microscopy revealed cirrhotic changes 21 times (64%) in the surrounding liver tissue, ground glass hepatocytes (Fig. 71, see page 74) nine times, dysplastic hepatocytes 19 times and adenomatous nodules 17 times. In total, potential precursor lesions (dysplasia and adenomatous nodules) were found in 76% of the cases in the cancer stage and in 42% in the precancer stage (Table 7-1).

Dysplastic cells in HBsAg-positive patients, as observed by micromorphometry, could be classified into two types—large dysplastic cells and small dysplastic cells. Small dysplastic cells were closer to hepatocellular carcinoma cells in size and nuclear-cytoplasmic ratio. This was more evident in patients with liver cancer (Fig. 72, see page 74) (Table 7-2) (5). CAH was found only four times while the tumor was present, and eight times before the tumor was found, suggesting common regression of CAH at the cancer stage (Table 7-1). According to the peroxidase-antiperoxidase method for HBsAg, α-1-Antitrypsin and α-fetoprotein followed by hematoxytin stain, HBsAg was seen 68%, α-1-Antitrypsin 44% and α-fetoprotein 11% in the surrounding liver tissue. HBsAg-containing hepatocytes were sometimes dysplastic or contained in adenomatous nodules (Figs. 73, 74, see page 74) (Table 7-3).

Blood specimens obtained from the 30 patients at the precancer and/or the cancer stage were tested for hepatitis B virus (HBV) immune markers by means of radioimmunoassay. Serologic tests for HBV immune markers showed that 21 out of 27 cases in the precancer stage had HBsAg and the remaining six cases had antibody to HBsAg (anti- HBs), and 90% of these HBsAg did not change until the cancer stage.

Of 18 cases followed-up for hepatitis B e antigen (HBeAg) and antibody to HBeAg (anti-HBe) status from the precancer to the cancer stage, 10 were positive for HBeAg in the precancer stage, of whom seven (70%) became negative later. Of these seven cases, six showed seroconversion to anti-HBe at the cancer stage. The remaining three cases had persistent HBeAg until the cancer stage and showed histologic characteristics of severe parenchymal necroinflammation in the precancer stage. Thus, the viral replication is relatively low in the cancer stage, but sometimes viral replication persists. It is evidenced by our former studies together with this result(6,7).

Non-A, non-B hepatitis can lead to HCC. According to this report on the distribution of antibody to hepatitis C virus (anti-HCV) in patients with HBsAg-negative HCC in Korea, of 27 patients with HBsAg-negative HCC, 13 (24.1%) were positive for anti-HCV. Some of the HCC may thus have non-A, non-B viral infection in addition to HBV infection (8). DNA-polymerase activity was significantly reduced in the cancer stage (41.2%) from the precancer stage (chronic hepatitis without HCC) (77.4%) ($P<0.005$). The serum aminotransferase activity also decreased in the cancer stage compared with the precancer stage. Alpha-fetoprotein levels usually increased in the cancer stage compared with the precancer stage, with a few exceptions.

TABLE 7–1.

Histologic Findings of Nontumorous Liver in 33 Patients with HCC and of Liver in 12 Patients in Whom HCC Developed Later

Histologic findings	*Cancer stage*		*Precancer stage*		*P value (x)*
	Positivity No. times	*%*	*Positivity No. times*	*%*	
Chronic active hepatitis	4	12	8	67	< 0.01
Parenchymal collapse	2	6	5	42	< 0.05
Cirrhosis	21	64	3	25	
(Evidenced by laparoscopy)	(22)	(67)			
Presence of dysplastic hepatocytes (D) and adenomatous nodule (A)	25	76	5	42	< 0.05
(With cirrhosis)	(20)	(61)	(1)	(8)	< 0.01
(Without cirrhosis)	(5)	(15)	(4)	(34)	
D alone	8	24	3	25	
(With cirrhosis)	(6)	(18)	(1)	(8)	
(Without cirrhosis)	(2)	(6)	(2)	(17)	
A alone	6	18	2	17	
(With cirrhosis)	(4)	(12)	(0)	(0)	
(Without cirrhosis)	(2)	(6)	(2)	(17)	
Combination of D and A	11	33	0	0	
(With cirrhosis)	(9)	(27)			
(Without cirrhosis)	(2)	(6)			
Absence of D and A	8	24	7	58	
(With cirrhosis)	(1)	(3)	(2)	(16)	
(Without cirrhosis)	(7)	(21)	(5)	(42)	
Ground glass cells	9	27	1	8	
(With D alone)	5	15	1	8	
(With A alone)	2	6	0	0	
(Combination of D and A)	2	6	0	0	

TABLE 7–2.

Micromorphotometric Findings of Size (mean) of Cells and Nuclei, and Nucleocytoplasmic Ratio (mean) in Dysplastic and Carcinoma Cells of Liver

	Nucleus (μm)	*Cytoplasm (μm)*	*Nucleocytoplasmic ratio*
NH in HBsAg (−) cases	6.5	18.5	0.35
LDC in HBsAg (+) patients without HCC	*10.2	*27.5	0.37
LDC in HBsAg (+) patients with HCC	*10.7	*29.1	0.37
SDC in HBsAg (+) patients without HCC	7.3	15.5	∞0.47
SDC in HBsAg (+) patients with HCC	7.5	14.1	∞0.53
HCCC in HBsAg (+) patients	8.0	14.4	∞0.56

Key: HCC, hepatocellular carcinoma; HCCC, HCC cells; LDC, large dysplastic hepatocytes; NH, normal hepatocytes; SDC, small dysplastic hepatocytes; *, the difference or the mean size of nucleus and cytoplasm in the normal hepatocytes and large of small dysplastic cells ($P<0.01$); ∞, the difference of the nucleocytoplasmic ratio in the normal hepatocytes and large or small dysplastic cells ($P<0.01$). (Reproduced from Choi, K.Y. and Chung, W.K., J. Catholic Medical College, 37 : 467–482, 1984, with permission)

TABLE 7–3.

HBsAg, HBcAg, α 1-Antitrypsin and α-fetoprotein Evidenced by Peroxidase-antiperoxidase Method in Nontumorous Liver Cells in Patients with Hepatocellular Carcinoma

Tests	*No. tested*	*Positivity (%)*
HBsAg	19	68
HBcAg	19	0
α 1-Antitrypsin	18	44
α-fetoprotein	19	11

Key: HBsAg, hepatitis B surface antigen; HBcAg, hepatitis B core antigen

Summary

In Korea, HCC is almost always associated with HBV infection. It usually follows chronic hepatitis B, and has characteristic cytologic precursor lesions which are closely related to HBV infection.

In the precancer stage, significant hepatocytic necroinflammation in chronic hepatitis, occasionally with episodic bouts accompanied by conspicuous acinar transformation of hepatocytes resulting in collapse, is usual, while the histologic pattern is sometimes inactive. However, inflammatory liver disease activity referable to viral hepatitis and viral replication is relatively low in the cancer stage, but sometimes viral replication persists.

References

1. Anthony, P.P., Vogel, C.L. and Barker, A.F. Liver cell dysplasia: A premalignant condition. J Clin Path 26: 217–223, 1973.

2. Peters, R.L. Pathology of hepatocellular carcinoma, In; Okuda, K. and Peters, R.L. eds. Hepatocellular Carcinoma. New York: John Wiley & Sons, pp. 107–168, 1976.

3. Chen, M.L., Gerber, M.A., Thung, S.N., Thornton, J.C. and Chung, W.K. Morphometric study of hepatocytes containing hepatitis B surface antigen. Am J Path 114: 217–221, 1984.

4. Jeong, J.W. and Chung, W.K. Relation of hepatitis B virus infection to hepatocellular carcinoma in Korea; histologic and serologic evaluation. J Catholic U Med Coll 41: 291–303, 1988.

5. Choi, K.Y. and Chung, W.K. A histologic study on precursor lesions of hepatocellular carcinoma. J Catholic University Medical College 37: 467–477, 1984.

6. Chung, W.K., Sun, H.S., Park, D.H., Minuck, G.Y. and Hoofnagle, J.H. Primary hepatocellular carcinoma and hepatitis B virus infection in Korea. J Med Virology 11: 99–104, 1983.

7. Sjoegren, M.H., Lemon, S.M., Chung, W.K., Sun, H.S. and Hoofnagle, J.H. IgM

antibody to hepatitis B core antigen in Korean patients with hepatocellular carcinoma. Hepatology 4: 615–618, 1984.

8. Chung, K. W., Sun, H. S., Chung, W.K., Shin, H.K., Park, C.K., Yoo, J.Y., Di Bisceglie, A.M., Waggoner, J.J. and Hoofnagle, J.H. A preliminary report on the prevalence of type C hepatitis in Korea. Korean J Intern Med 38: 750–753, 1990.

(The outline of this paper was presented at the IIIrd Biennial Scientific Meeting of the Asian-Pacific Association for the Study of the Liver, Hong Kong, 1982).

Legends

Fig. 71. Ground glass cells and slightly dysplastic cells. Needle biopsy, HE, ×400.

Fig. 72. Nontumorous area of HCC. Small dysplastic cells are arranged in an irregular and multiple cell-thick plate pattern. Needle biopsy, HE, ×100.

Fig. 73. HBsAg in cytoplasm of dysplastic cells. Needle biopsy, peroxidase-antiperoxidase (PAP) method for HBsAg followed by hematoxylin stain, ×400.

Fig. 74. HBsAg in cytoplasm of many hepatocytes in a nodule and only in scattered hepatocytes outside the nodule. Needle biopsy, PAP method for HBsAg followed by hematoxylin stain, ×100.

8 HEPATOCELLULAR AND CHOLANGIOCELLULAR CARCINOMA: HISTOLOGIC TYPES AND GROWTH PATTERNS

Whan Kook Chung, M.D., Ph.D.

I. HEPATOCELLULAR CARCINOMA (HCC)

HCC has become a major cause of death in Korea. Statistics for the causes of death released in 1988 by the National Bureau of Statistics, Economic Planning Board, ROK, indicate that, in Korea, the death rate of HCC is 33/1,000 deaths. HCC ranks second among the causes of death from malignant tumors in males and Korea has one of the highest HCC death rates in the world.

HCC death rate in Korea has gradually increased with the passing years. In the 1960's, among Koreans who died from a malignancy, 9% were from HCC and, in comparison, in the 1980's the rate has increased to 16%.

The relationship between persistent hepatitis B virus (HBV) infection and HCC, which usually develops decades after onset of the infection, has been well documented by both epidemiologic and clinical observations.

Korea went through the great tragedy of the Korean War some 40 years ago. As a result, tens of thousands of people were wounded and numerous people contracted diseases through contaminated blood and blood products. At that time, due to the extremely difficult socio-economic conditions of this country, type B hepatitis became prevalent, almost to the extent of being endemic. Since then, the economic condition and the living standard of the people have remarkably improved. However, the disease, once it gained its prevalency, has not shown any sign of decline. As a result, chronic hepatitis and HCC related to type B hepatitis have now, four decades after the Korean War, become common and major diseases in this country (1). This has caused me to have great concern for the study of HCC and to perform liver biopsies on many cases of HCC.

In order to perform liver biopsies, the instruments and methods I used from the late 1950's until the early 1970's were the Vim-Silverman type needle and the Menghini type needle for blind biopsy only through the intercostal approach. After that, from the late 1970's, in addition to blind biopsy, liver biopsy under laparoscopic observation has also been employed. Also, the author has occasionally had surgical wedge biopsy specimens made available.

Though ultrasonography or computerized tomography guided needle biopsy has recently become possible, there often are sampling errors when blind needle biopsy is performed on space-occupying hepatic lesions like HCC. Also, there are anatomical limitations in biopsies carried out while being observed through laparoscopy. In addition, HCC tissue is often hypervascular, the hepatic vein is often obstructed by the tumor thrombus, congestion is severe in HCC bearing nontumorous liver and complications like massive bleeding can occur. There is also the danger of transplanting the tumor tissue into other tissues. Notwithstanding, the very best method for confirming HCC is the histologic analysis and interpretation of tissue obtained by biopsy.

HCC may show a variety of appearances but there is little evidence that these morphological features have clinical, biological or epidemiologic significance. Several histologic patterns and cytologic features are, however, worthy of note.

A. Histological Classification

A classification of HCC was originally proposed in the latter part of the 19th century by Hanot and Gilbert (2) but was supplemented by a detailed and classic work of Edmondson and Steiner (3). The best developed and worldwide accepted morphological characterization of HCC is the WHO classification which appeared in 1978 (4). In Japan, Nakajima and Kojiro have recently proposed a classification of HCC, using the WHO classification as a basis (5). The author has attempted to employ a slightly modified version of the WHO classification.

1. Edmondson-Steiner Classification

Grade I Carcinoma. The most differentiated HCC (Fig. 75, see page 74).

The tumor cells reveal a resemblance to normal hepatic cells and are arranged usually in a thin trabecular pattern.

Grade II Carcinoma. Moderately differentiated HCC (Fig. 76, see page 74). While the tumor cells reveal a resemblance to normal hepatic cells, the nuclei are large and more hyperchromatic than usual. The cytoplasm, however, is still abundant and acidophilic. Tumor cells are arranged usually in the acinar pattern with bile, but associated frequently with trabecular structure.

Grade III Carcinoma. Poorly differentiated HCC (Fig. 77, see page 75). Larger and more hyperchromatic nuclei than in Grade II are seen. The nucleus occupies a relatively large proportion of the cell. Bile and acinar formation are noted less frequently. Giant tumorous cells are frequent in this type.

Grade IV Carcinoma. The most poorly differentiated HCC (Fig. 78, see page 75). The nucleus is markedly hyperchromatic and occupies the greater part of the cell. The cytoplasm is often scanty and contains fewer granules. The growth in the liver is more medullary and trabeculae are few. Many of the cell masses appear to lie loosely and freely without cohesion. Bile is extremely rare in this type.

2. Author's Classification

Trabecular (sinusoidal) type

The tumor cells grow in a liver-like fashion, i.e., in a trabecular or plate-like fashion; these vary in thickness.

a. Microtrabecular (finger-like) pattern. This type of HCC is the most familiar and the most common. The well-differentiated neoplastic trabecula is made up of linear columns of hepatocytes of a thickness of one or more cells. The trabeculae are separated from blood by sinusoids lined by flat and inconspicuous endothelial cells. Kupffer cells are not usual components. Other than endothelial cells, there is little accompanying stroma in the microtrabecular carcinoma and the orderly trabecula often gives the impression of a mesh formed in clear space.

b. Macrotrabecular pattern. Occasionally, a macrotrabecular pattern of HCC develops, multiple cells thick and each trabecula is widened to a plump peninsular structure.

Pseudoglandular (acinar) type

A variety of gland-like structures may be seen. When the canaliculus is retained, the tumor cells arranged radially about it have an acinar appearance on cross-section (Figs. 76, 77, see pages 74, 75). Canaliculi, with or without bile, are often recognizable (Fig. 79, see page 75). Many variations are produced when the canaliculus is greatly dilated. Occasionally, a follicular, thyroid-like appearance is produced (Fig. 80, see page 75). A peliosis-like pattern is rarely also present.

Compact (solid) type

The sinusoid may be made inconspicuous by compression, and the tumor made to appear solid. Usually, the tumor cells have a cobble-stone appearance.

Scirrhous type

Trabecular HCC is typically characterized by lack of stroma.

Rarely, however, peritrabecular, sinusoidal thin fibrosis (capillarization) can be seen (Fig. 81, see page 75). The areas with abundant fibrous stroma separating nodules of tumor cells, which may be the result of tumor infarction and subsequent scar formation, show a cirrhotomimetic pattern (Fig. 82, see page 75). HCC, in which the pattern is acinar, pseudoglandular or adenoid, often has a varied amount of stroma. Occasionally, the stromal response may be dense enough to be called sclerosing hepatic carcinoma (Fig. 83, see page 75). The cords, because of the surrounding collagen, resemble the duct structure (Fig. 83, see page 75).

Sarcomatous type

In cases with a sarcomatous appearance, it is difficult to conclude whether the sarcomatous appearance is caused by sarcomatous change of part of the tumor tissue or by the coexistence of HCC and sarcoma. In a case from my series, the tumor, consisting mainly of spindle-shaped sarcomatous cell and a transitional form of the tumor cell between a trabecular arrangement and a sarcomatous arrangement, was observed (Fig. 84, see page 75).

Clear cell type

The tumor tissue may also contain clear cell areas and the tissue is rarely wholly or predominantly composed of such cells. In some instances, this is due to excess of fat, but storage of glycogen is the commonest cause (Fig. 85, see page 76).

Free-cell type

This type is similar to Edmondson-Steiner Grade IV carcinoma. Many of the tumor cells are free without cohesion (Fig. 78, see page 75).

Pleomorphic type

Cytological variant. There are marked nuclear variability, multi-nucleation and cellular enlargement. Bizarre pleomorphic tumor cells may constitute a part or most of the tumor tissue and the trabecular pattern may be lost over large areas (Figs. 86, 87, 88, see page 76).

Areal variant. HCC often varies in cell type and the degree of differentiation from one area to another as evidenced by a tiny needle biopsy specimen (Figs. 83, 89, 90, see pages 75, 76).

B. Distribution of Sex, Age and Histologic Types of HCC

For the purpose of documenting the structural characteristics of HCC, histological analysis was performed on 275 cases of biopsy-proven HCC.

Of 262 HCC patients, 216 (83%) were men and 46 women, ranging in age from 19 to 74 (mean 49.5) years.

Serologic evidence of the ongoing HBV infection was found in 74% of the HCC patients. Abnormal elevation of serum alpha-fetoprotein level (over 50 ng/ml) was seen in 69 of 98 patients (70%).

The analysis of a variety of histologic features in HCC cases is shown in Table 8-1.

TABLE 8–1.

Histologic Analysis of Hepatocellular Carcinoma

Histologic finding	*No. cases observed*	*Positivity*	
		No. cases	*Rate*
Trabecular pattern	273	213	78.1%
Pseudoglandular pattern	223	50	22.4%
Scirrhous type	223	55	24.7%
Sarcomatous type	223	2	0.9%
Clear cell type	223	51	22.9%
Pleomorphic type (Cytologic variant)	223	17	7.6%

In the incidence of histologic types according to the grading system of Edmondson and Steiner, Grade II type showed the highest frequency with 50%, and next came Grade IV with 21.2%, Grade III with 16% and Grade I was lowest with 13%.

On the other hand, the scirrhous pattern (24.7%), the pseudoglandular pattern (22.4%) and the clear cell type (22.9%) were the most prominent besides the trabecular pattern. Steatosis and cytologic pleomorphism were intermediate in frequency. Acidophilic inclusions, sarcomatous changes and oncocytes were rare.

C. Growth Patterns of HCC

Under this title, the growth pattern of HCC rather than the growth pattern of the tumor itself, is more concerned with how the spreading pattern of tumor cells towards surrounding nontumor tissue develops. Namely, it refers to the invasion pattern of tumor cells on the surrounding nontumor tissue.

The growth pattern can be divided into two basic categories—expansive and infiltrative. The representative example belonging to the former category is the replacing growth pattern (Fig. 91, see page 77), and that belonging to the latter category is sinusoidal (Figs. 92, 93, see page 77) or vascular invasion pattern (Fig. 94, see page 77). HCC has a marked tendency for spread via intrahepatic veins, both hepatic and portal. Thrombosis of these vessels by tumor or blood clot is a characteristic finding at autopsy. However, it is very difficult to find in a needle biopsy specimen.

In addition, an attempt was separately made to classify the extracapsular growing pattern (Figs. 95, 96, see page 77) and heterogeneous growing pattern (Fig. 97, see page 78).

II. INTRAHEPATIC BILE-DUCT CARCINOMA

Clinically, intrahepatic bile-duct carcinoma falls into two major categories. Some arise from small peripheral ducts and may resemble HCC, and others occur in or near the porta hepatis with the presentation being chronic obstructive jaundice. In this study, selection of cases with intrahepatic bile-duct carcinoma are limited to peripheral type. Histologically, two types of carcinoma are of intrahepatic bile-duct origin, namely cholangiolar (cholangiocellular) carcinoma and cholangiocarcinoma.

a. Cholangiolar carcinoma: The concept of this relatively rare carcinoma was introduced by Steiner (6) and Steiner and Higginson (7) to describe tumors that arise from the canal of Hering or cholangiole. Such tumors were found in four out of 17 cases with intrahepatic bile-duct carcinoma in this study. They retain the configuration usually associated with cholangioles, forming double-layered cuboidal epithelial cell cords that have a tiny lumen with mucus and a basement membrane (Fig. 98, see page 78). Occasionally, tumor cells grow in a vein also with destruction of the vascular wall and perivascular tissue, causing fibrotic loosening (Fig. 99, see page 78).

b. Cholangiocarcinoma: Of 292 patients with intrahepatic carcinoma in this study, 275 (94.1%) were HCC and 17 (5.9%) bile-duct carcinoma. The histologic pattern is most commonly tubular and occasionally papillary with varied degrees of differentiation (Fig. 100, see page 78). The glandular (tubular) structure with mucus is usually obvious, characterized by the presence of abundant fibrous stroma (Fig. 101, see page 78).

Cholangiocarcinoma is much less common than HCC. However, the incidence in Korea is presumed to be a little bit higher than that in Western countries. Such increase seems to be related to infestation with liver fluke (Figs. 102, 103, see page 78).

Spread: Although blood-borne spread is rare compared with HCC, sinusoidal or vascular invasion can be seen in intrahepatic bile duct carcinoma (Figs. 99, 100, see page 78).

III. COMBINED (MIXED) TYPE

Some carcinomas having predominantly ductal features in some areas and may have HCC in other areas. These have been called combined (mixed) hepatocellular cholangiocarcinomas and have been thought to arise from cells that have a potential to form either hepatocytes or duct cells. According to the evidence, however, HCC, in which some areas of the tissue show scirrhous change and tumor cells form ductal features (Fig. 83, see page 75), is often misinterpreted as a combined type. On the other hand, cholangiocellular carcinoma, in which multiple layers formed as the result of active ductal cell proliferation and are mistaken for HCC tissues, is often misdiagnosed as a mixed type. Genuine combined tumors are supposed to show unequivocal evidence of both types of carcinoma, i.e., sinusoidal pattern of growth and/or bile production plus a glandular pattern and/or mucus secretion. These are the most frequent causes of confusion.

IV. REACTIONS AND ALTERATIONS OF TUMOR

A lymph nodule-like pattern which seems to be an unusual tumor reaction can be observed. Cytoplasmic eosinophilic inclusion bodies may be present (Figs. 86, 87, see page 76). Oncocytes, which exhibit granular, deeply eosinophilic cytoplasm containing numerous densely packed mitochondria as demonstrated by electron microscopy, can rarely be seen. The sarcoid-like granulomatous reaction within malignant tumors has long been recognized (8). However, it is believed to be rare in HCC or cholangiocarcinoma (9). The author has observed only one case of cholangiocarcinoma with sarcoid-like granulomatous reaction in a patient with Clonorchis sinensis infestation (Figs. 102, 103, see page 78). While it is presumed to be a tumor reaction, a reaction due to parasites may not be ruled out.

When the soft tumor mass blocks the blood flow, canalization and vascularization can occur in the tumor tissue in parallel with the blood stream.

The tumor cells tolerate reduction of sinusoidal circulation up to a certain point. If further reduced, as after gastrointestinal hemorrhage or after severe infection or after out-flow block of blood from a tumor nodule, centronodular ischemic necrosis develops (Fig. 104, see page 78).

References

1. Chung, W.K., Sun, H.S., Park, D.H., Minuk, G.Y. and Hoofnagle, J.H. Primary hepatocellular carcinoma and hepatitis B virus infection in Korea. J Med Virology 11: 99–104, 1983.

2. Hanot, V.C. and Gilbert, A. Etudes sur les Maladies du Foie, 1888. Quoted by Rolleston HD; Disease of the Liver, Gall Bladder and Bile Ducts, 2nd ed. MacMillan, New York, PP. 474, 1912.

3. Edmondson, H.A. and Steiner, P.E. Primary carcinoma of the liver. A study of 100 cases among 48,900 necropsies. Cancer 7: 462–502,1954.

4. Gibson, J.B. Histological typing of tumors of the liver, biliary tract and pancreas. International Histological Classification of Tumors 20, World Health Organization. Geneva, 1978.

5. Nakajima, T. and Kojiro, M. Hepatocellular Carcinoma; an atlas of its pathology. Springer-Verlag, Tokyo, Berlin, Heidelberg, New York, London, Paris. 1987.

6. Steiner, P.E. Carcinoma of liver in the United States. Acta Univ Int Contra Cancer 13: 628–645. 1957.

7. Steiner P.E. and Higginson, J. Cholangiolocellular carcinoma of the liver. Cancer 12(2): 53–759, 1969.

8. Gregorie, H.B., Othersen, H.B. and Moor, M. The significance of sarcoid-like reaction in association with malignant neoplasm. Am J Surg 104:577–586, 1962.

9. Nevilde, E., Piyasena, K.H.G. and James, D.G. Granulomas of the liver. Postgrad Med J 51: 361–365, 1975.

Legends

Histologic Classification

Fig. 75. Edmondson-Steiner Classification.

Grade I. A 50-year-old male, HBsAg+, alpha-fetoprotein 0.5 ng/ml. Well-differentiated HCC. Highly differentiated tumor cells with a thin trabecular pattern. Needle biopsy, HE, ×400.

Fig. 76.

Grade II. A 56-year-old female, HBsAg+, alpha-fetoprotein 450 ng/ml. Moderately differentiated HCC. The nuclei are larger and more hyperchromatic than the cells in Fig. 75. The cytoplasm, however, is abundant and acidophilic. The acinar structure is associated with the trabecular pattern. In the center of the acinus, a bile plug is seen (arrow). Needle biopsy, HE, ×400.

Fig. 77.

Grade III. A 60-year-old male, HBsAg-. Poorly differentiated pleomorphic HCC. The nuclei are usually larger and more hyperchromatic than in Grade II. The nuclei occupy a relatively large proportion of the cell. Giant tumor cells are numerous. The tumor cells reveal a marked pleomorphism in size, staining quality and growth pattern showing a trabecular as well as acinar form. Needle biopsy, HE, ×400.

Fig. 78.
Grade IV. A 43-year-old male, HBsAg+, alpha-fetoprotein 832.4 ng/ml. The most poorly differentiated HCC. The nuclei are intensely hyperchromatic and occupy a large part of the cell. The cytoplasm varies in amount; it is often scanty but sometimes with plenty of granules. While some of the cells are arranged in a trabecular pattern, many of the cell masses seem to lie loosely and without cohesion. Needle biopsy, HE, ×400.

Author's Classification

Fig. 79. Pseudoglandular (acinar) Type.
A 65-year-old male, HBsAg-, alpha-fetoprotein 232 ng/ml. Moderately differentiated HCC, showing a typical pseudoglandular pattern with bile production (arrows). Needle biopsy, HE, ×100.

Fig. 80.
A 63-year-old male, HBsAg+, alpha-fetoprotein 43 ng/ml. Well differentiated HCC, showing a pseudoglandular pattern characterized by follicular, thyroid-like appearance. Wedge biopsy, HE, ×100.

Fig. 81. Scirrhous (sclerosing) Type.
A 51-year-old male, HBsAg+, alpha-fetoprotein 1.171 ng/ml. Moderately differentiated HCC, showing peritrabecular (sinusoidal) thin fibrosis. Needle biopsy, HE, ×100.

Fig. 82.
A 47-year-old male. Poorly differentiated scirrhous HCC, showing a cirrhotomimetic pattern. Needle biopsy, HE, ×100.

Fig. 83.
A 19-year-old female, HBsAg-, anti–HCV+. Fully developed scirrhous pattern with glandular structures of HCC. Needle biopsy, HE, × 100.

Fig. 84. Sarcomatous Type.
A 42-year-old male, HBsAg+. Note the sarcomatous appearance with spindle-shaped tumor cells. Needle biopsy, HE, ×400.

Fig. 85. Clear cell Type.
A 42-year-old male, HBsAg-. HCC is mainly made up of clear cells containing fat vacuoles. Bile is seen in the bile capillary (arrow). Needle biopsy, HE, ×400.

Fig. 86. Pleomorphic Type, Cytological variants.
A 56-year-old male. Note bizarre, multinucleated giant cells (thick arrow), cytoplasmic globular hyaline inclusion (thin arrow) and great variations of tumor cells in size, shape and staining quality. Needle biopsy, HE, ×400.

Fig. 87.

A 60-year-old male, HBsAg-, alpha-fetoprotein 39 ng/ml. Tumor cells contain various intracytoplasmic globular hyalines (arrows). Focal necrosis of tumor cells is seen. Needle biopsy, HE, ×400.

Fig. 88.

A 38-year-old male, HBsAg+, alpha-fetoprotein 981.1 ng/ml. Pleomorphic tumor cells in all nodules are surrounded by fibrotic tissue. Needle biopsy, trichrome, ×100.

Fig. 89. Area variants

A 54-year-old male, HBsAg-. Both solid-trabecular and pseudoglandular patterns are seen in the slide. Needle biopsy, HE, ×100.

Fig. 90.

A 37-year-old male, HBsAg+. Note fat metamorphosis both in the group of tumor cells and in the nontumor cells. Needle biopsy, HE, ×100.

Growth Patterns

Fig. 91. Replacing growth.

A 50-year-old male, HBsAg-. Cancer cells grow and replace the hepatocytes on the tumor-nontumor boundary (arrows). Sinusoidal spaces are seen between the cancerous tissue and the noncancerous tissue. Needle biopsy, HE, ×400.

Fig. 92. Sinusoidal growth.

A 42-year-old male. Free cell type cancer cells are growing in the sinusoids (arrows) and compressing the adjacent normal liver cell plates. Needle biopsy, HE, ×400.

Fig. 93.

A 50-year-old male, HBsAg-, alpha-fetoprotein 0 ng/ml. Multifocal sinusoidal tumor nests. They grow in the sinusoid and finally take the replacing growth pattern. Needle biopsy, HE, ×100.

Fig. 94. Vascular invasion.

A 42-year-old male, HBsAg-, alpha-fetoprotein 0 ng/ml. Organization of the tumor thrombus in the portal vein. Needle biopsy, HE, ×100.

Fig. 95. Growth through capsule.

A 25-year-old female, HBsAg+. The tumor cells beyond the capsule are separated by fibrotic tissue. It is suggested that the fibrotic capsule and intercellular fibers result mainly from the passively condensed reticulin fibers after parenchymal (tumor cell) necrosis. Wedge biopsy, HE, ×100.

Fig. 96.

Same case as that illustrated in Fig. 95. Tumor cells penetrating into a crack and a vascular space (arrow heads) of a thick fibrous capsule. HE, ×100.

Fig. 97. Heterogeneous growth.
A 25-year-old female. Poorly differentiated (Edmondson-Steiner grade IV carcinoma) HCC is divided into two parts (left and right) by a thin fibrotic septum. Tumor cells at the right are larger and more pleomorphic than those at the left. Wedge biopsy, HE, ×100.

Cholangiocarcinoma

Fig. 98. Cholangiolocarcinoma.
A 47-year-old male, HBsAg-, alpha-fetoprotein 2.3 ng/ml. Cholangiolocarcinoma showing tumor cells retain the configuration associated with cholangioles forming a double-layered cuboidal epithelial cell arrangement that has a tiny lumen. There are mucin staining materials in the canals of ductular structure. Needle biopsy, Mayer's stain, ×400.

Fig. 99.
The same case illustrated in Fig. 98. There are growing tumor cells in a vein and destruction of the vascular wall and perivascular tissue, causing fibrotic loosing. HE, ×400.

Fig. 100. Cholangiocarcinoma.
A 59-year-old male, HBsAg-. Cholangiocarcinoma with glandular structures composed of tall columnar cells and desmoplasia. Note the sinusoidal infiltration of tumor cells. Needle biopsy, HE, ×100.

Fig. 101. Cholangiocarcinoma.
A 50-year-old male, HBsAg-. Cholangiocarcinoma showing poorly differentiated tumor cells with marked fibrous stroma. Note the mucin producing in glandular structures of tumor tissue. Needle biopsy, Mayer's stain, ×400.

Fig. 102. Cholangiocarcinoma.
A 65-year-old female, HBsAg-, alpha-fetoprotein 0 ng/ml. Cholangiocarcinoma showing mucin producing adenocarcinoma with some mitosis and moderately dense fibrous stroma. Macrophages are seen in the mucus. Wedge biopsy, HE, ×100.

Fig. 103.
The same case illustrated in Fig. 102. Note the granulomatous reaction with central necrosis, multi-nucleated giant cells (arrows), and massive infiltration of eosinophiles. While it is presumed to be a tumor reaction, a reaction of Clonorchis sinensis, in spite of negative test, is suggested. HE, ×100.

Tumor Reaction

Fig. 104.
A 53-year-old female, HBsAg+, alpha-fetoprotein 0 ng/ml. Poorly differentiated HCC, showing marked necrosis in the center of the trabecula. Needle biopsy, HE, ×400.

9 ALCOHOLIC LIVER DISEASES

Whan Kook Chung, M.D., Ph.D.

As long ago as 500 B.C., it was thought that there might be a connection between excess alcohol intake and jaundice. An association between liver lesion and alcoholism has been recognized for centuries.

About 400 years ago, a Korean herb doctor by the name of Ho Chun used the term "Chudan" (alcoholic jaundice) in his book entitled, *Tonguibogam*. "Chudan" signifies jaundice caused by excessive drinking of alcoholic liquors. This disease is usually found among people who habitually drink too much alcohol and ingest too little food. In other words, the occurrence of alcoholic liver is dependent on the amount of alcohol ingested, the duration of the drinking habit and a poor diet.

In 1836, Addison reported that alcoholism might lead to fatty liver (1). The relationship between chronic alcoholism and cirrhosis has been recognized for over a hundred years and is supported by autopsy evidence.

Clinicians and pathologists have long debated the role of ethanol in the pathogenesis of cirrhosis. All things considered, the development of alcoholic liver damage is dependent on the duration and dose of alcohol intake.

The deleterious effect of alcohol may be accounted for by the toxicity of acetaldehyde which accumulates in the liver cells or by proteins and water retention. Increasing evidence that alcohol itself is hepatotoxic has diminished interest in diet as an etiologic factor. Nevertheless, improvement in liver function does not always follow alcohol abstinence if dietary protein remains low.

The occurrence of alcoholic liver has individual differences (2) as well as geographic variations (3,4). Although some attribute the individual difference to hereditary potential, others presume it to be more related to the pattern of drinking.

In Western countries, the incidence of cirrhosis can be directly related to the quantity of alcohol consumed, and alcoholic abuse constitutes a major cause of cirrhosis (5). In Korea, most cirrhosis had been blamed on viral infection. However, alcoholic hepatitis or cirrhosis are on the increase. Many reasons may be cited. With improvement of the socio-economic conditions, people have easy access to alcohol and many have formed a habit of drinking a strong alcoholic drink, "Soju". Most people who have drunk more than a bottle of "Soju" (360 ml) every day for 10 years contract alcoholic hepatitis or cirrhosis. Those who have done the same for five years have the probability of getting alcoholic hepatitis or cirrhosis. "Soju" contains 25% of ethanol, thus one bottle of "Soju" is equivalent to 90 ml of ethanol.

Since alcoholic liver disease is on the increase in Korea, the author has encountered an increasing number of cases and, accordingly, has seen more and more liver biopsies related to this disease. Liver biopsy is very important in detecting alcoholic liver diseases. It confirms the presence of liver disease and identifies alcohol abuse as the likely cause.

Liver biopsy is important for prognostic judgment. Fatty change alone is not nearly as serious as perivenular sclerosis, which is probably a precursor of cirrhosis. It is by biopsy that cirrhosis can be confirmed.

Alcoholic liver disease has classically been divided into three types on the basis of light microscopy: alcoholic fatty liver, alcoholic hepatitis and cirrhosis. In individual patients, these morphological abnormalities may coexist to varying degrees, resulting in a broad, continuous spectrum of disease.

The author treated many cases of alcoholic liver diseases, conducting liver biopsies on 65 cases. None of these 65 cases had hepatitis B surface antigen. On the basis of the biopsy findings, those cases were classified into three types—fatty liver, alcoholic hepatitis and cirrhosis, with an attempted analysis of these histologic patterns (Table 9–1).

Fatty liver

Fatty change (steatosis) was the most common hepatic abnormality seen in alcoholics in whom liver biopsy was done (Table 9-1).

In Korea before the 1970's, most of the patients admitted to hospitals because of alcoholism, even with delirium tremens, sometimes revealed simple steatosis. At that time, alcoholic hepatitis and cirrhosis were rare in Korea.

TABLE 9–1.

Histologic Manifestation in 17 Simple Fatty Liver, 36 Alcoholic Hepatitis and 12 Cirrhosis due to Alcohol Abuse

Histologic findings	*Simple fatty liver (with minute focal fibrosis, without central hyaline necrosis)* *N*	*Alcoholic hepatitis* *N*	*Cirrhosis* *N*
Fatty change			
Parenchymal			
Focal	6	24	5
Zonal	3	6	2
Diffuse	10	3	4
Mesenchymal (In fibrotic tissue)	0	1	1
Lipogranuloma	9	6	2
Cholestasis	0	4	2
Hemosiderosis	1	12	1
Mallory bodies	0	8	0
Acidophilic bodies	1	3	1
Focal necrosis	7	15	2
Confluent necrosis	0	2	1
Central reactions (Perivenular hyaline necrosis and/or sclerosis)	0	25	9
Portal reactions (Inflammation and/or fibrosis)	13	32	11
Diffuse septal fibrosis	0	19	10
Focal fibrosis	7	25	5
Polymorphonuclear leucocyte infiltration		33	9
Multiple regenerative nodules	0	0	12

In this study, the author found uncomplicated fatty change in 17 biopsies from 65 alcoholics. The fatty change ranged from vacuolation of a few liver cells, often centrilobular or mid-zonal, to severe involvement of all parts of the lobules. The liver cells usually contained a single droplet of fat which displaced the nucleus to one side of the cell.

In livers with fatty change, focal necrosis, liver cell lysis (Fig. 105, see page 79), acidophilic bodies (Fig. 106, see page 79) and lipogranuloma were occasionally seen.

Fatty liver occurred alone or in association with alcoholic hepatitis or cirrhosis. In some patients with otherwise uncomplicated fatty liver, there was portal reaction with or without fibrosis or a mild degree of fibrous septum formation related to portal tracts. Very regenerative parenchyma and hyperplastic nodules (Figs. 107, 108, 109, see page 79) were seen. The nodule was not surrounded by fibrotic tissue but by collapsed reticulin fibers which resulted from the surrounding parenchymal tissue being compressed by the nodule.

Lipogranulomas were structures comprising one or more extracellular lipid droplets surrounded by lymphocytes, histiocytes and often eosinophiles (Figs. 110, 111, see pages 79, 80). Lipogranulomas occurred focally, singly or in small groups, and were found in all parts of the lobules where liver cells contained fat. The number of lipogranulomas ranged from one or a few per biopsy to several per lobule. Lipogranulomas, when they were numerous, were usually evenly distributed throughout the biopsy specimen, although sometimes focal accumulations were seen.

In this study, lipogranulomas were found in 17 biopsy specimens from 65 alcoholics with fatty change.

Alcoholic hepatitis

The histologic diagnosis of acute alcoholic hepatitis is made classically on the basis of a triad of fatty change, degeneration and necrosis of hepatocytes with or without Mallory bodies, and an inflammatory infiltrate of polymorphonuclear leucocytes, primarily within the lobule. In addition, almost all patients with alcoholic hepatitis have an increased amount of intralobular connective tissue.

None of the changes per se are pathognomonic of alcohol injury, but the constellation of the findings is generally accepted as diagnostic.

Mallory bodies, stained with hematoxylin and eosin, showed eosinophilic and intracellular aggregates of dense proteinaceous material (Fig. 112, see page 80). Cells with Mallory bodies were swollen and had indistinct cell boundaries. The affected cells were surrounded or even infiltrated by a mixture of mononuclear cells and neutrophils. This represents focal degeneration of many cytoplasmic constitutents (2) and especially microtubles.

First described in 1911, Mallory bodies came to be closely identified with alcoholic liver injury (6), but later they were found in a variety of conditions: Wilson's disease, primary biliary cirrhosis, Indian childhood cirrhosis, intestinal bypass surgery, obesity and chronic cholestasis.

Christoffersen and Nielsen found, in a consecutive series, the incidence of Mallory bodies in chronic alcoholics with moderate to severe steatosis to be approximately 12% (7).

Baggenstoss and Stauffer (8) and Popper and Szanto (9) in a non-consecutive autopsy series of alcoholics with cirrhosis demonstrated Mallory bodies in 72 and 93%, respectively. In another series, Christoffersen and Poulsen demonstrated Mallory bodies in 45 out of 120 consecutive biopsies with cirrhosis and fatty change (10).

Thus, in Western countries, the incidence of Mallory bodies in alcoholics with cirrhosis appears to be about 40–50% in consecutive series.

In Korea, however, the author found in this study Mallory bodies only in

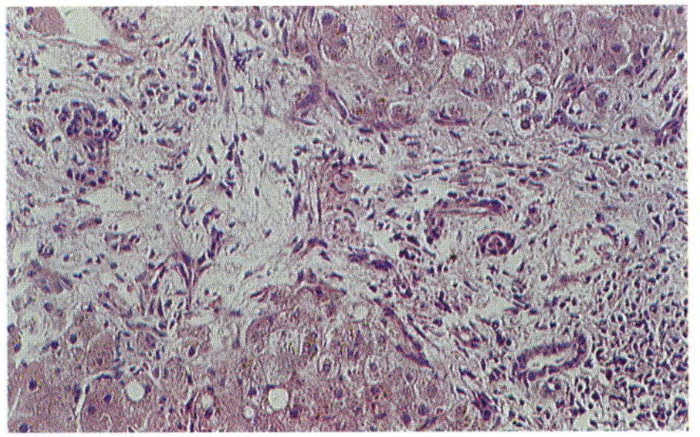

Fig. 117 See Legend page 124.

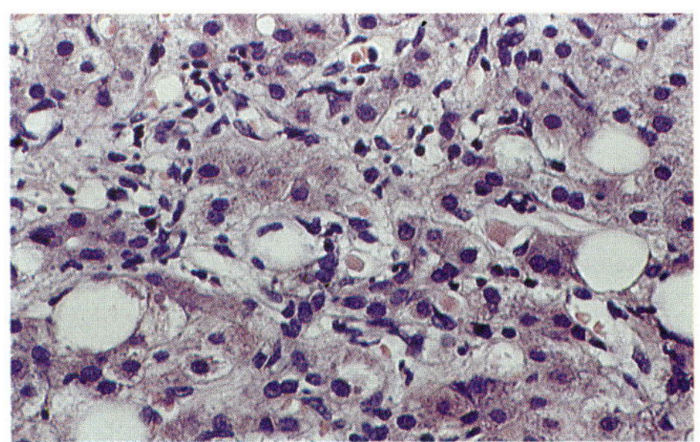

Fig. 118 See Legend page 124.

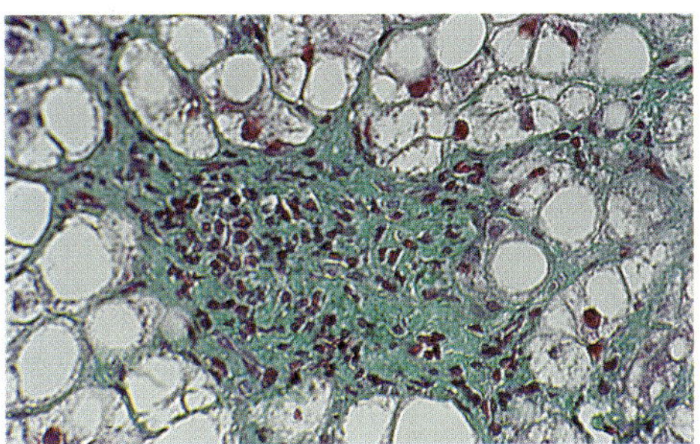

Fig. 119 See Legend page 124.

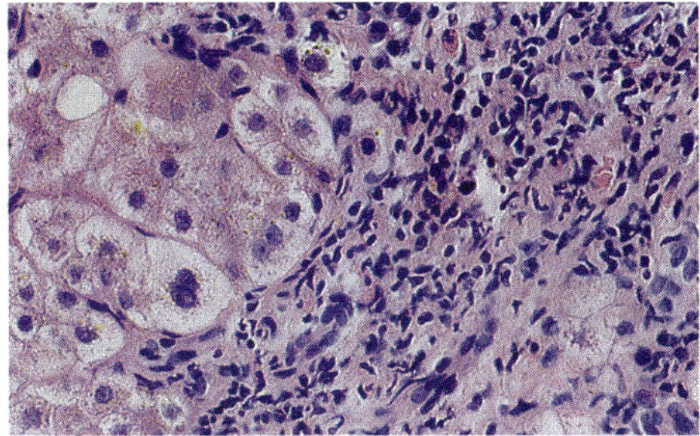

Fig. 120 See Legend page 124.

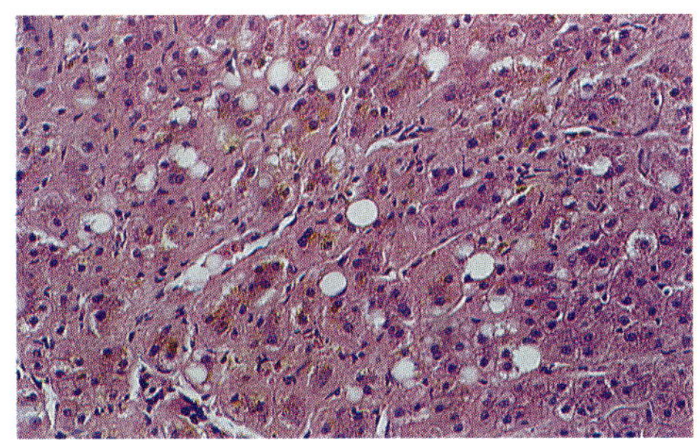

Fig. 121 See Legend page 124.

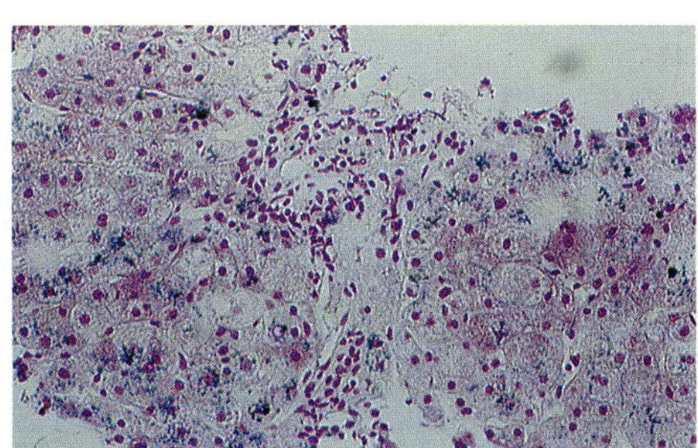

Fig. 122 See Legend page 125.

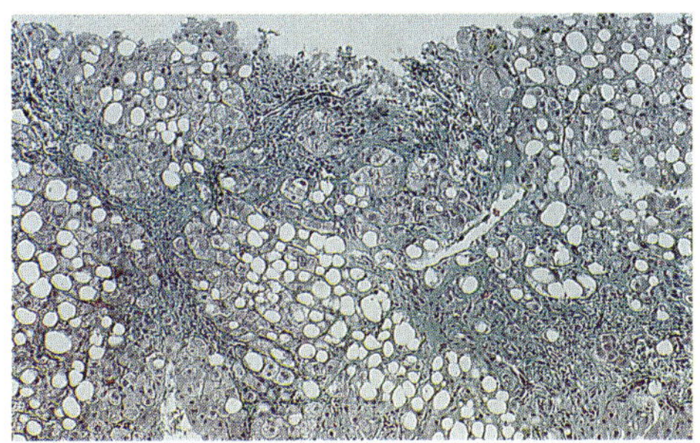

Fig. 123 See Legend page 125.

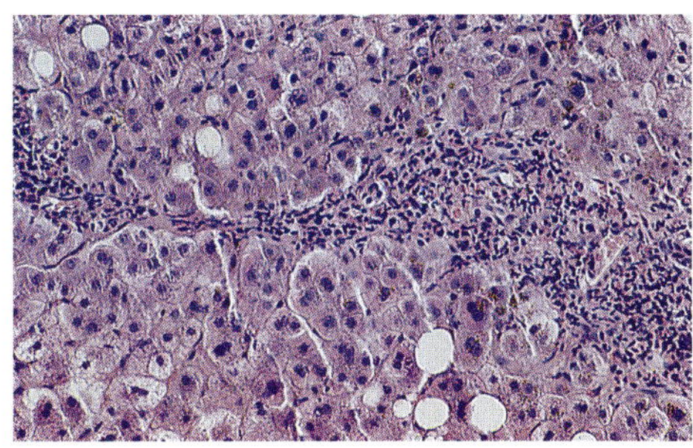

Fig. 124 See Legend page 125.

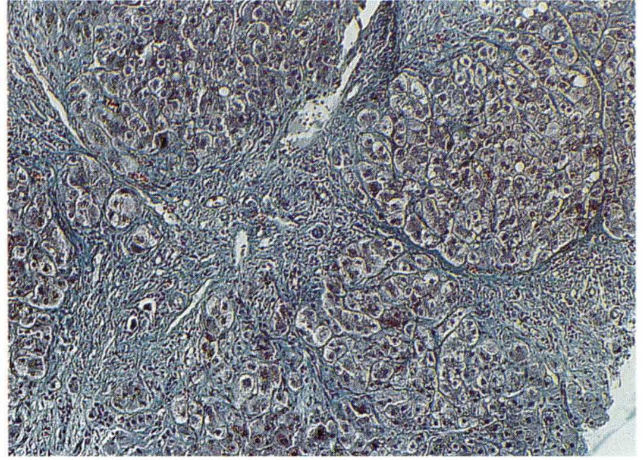

Fig. 125 See Legend page 125.

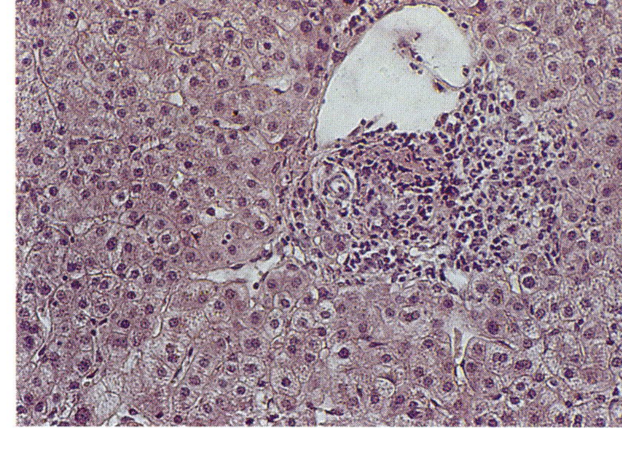

Fig. 126 See Legend page 136.

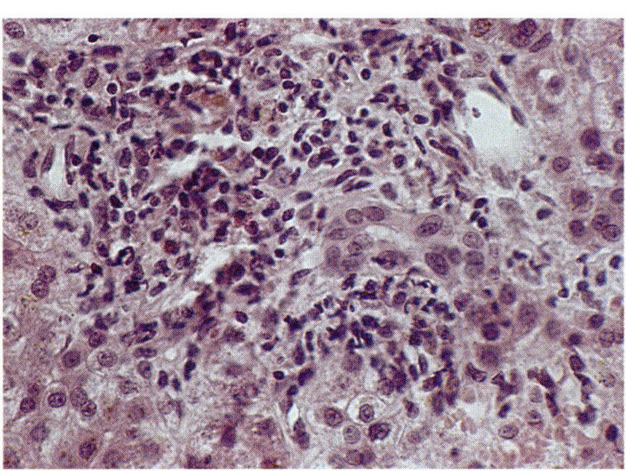

Fig. 127 See Legend page 136.

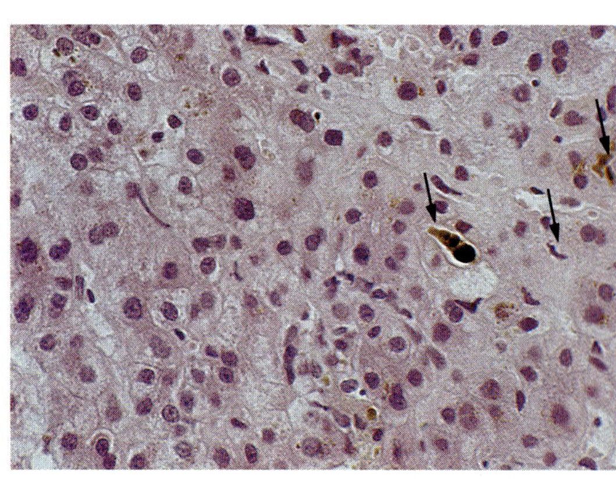

Fig. 128 See Legend page 136.

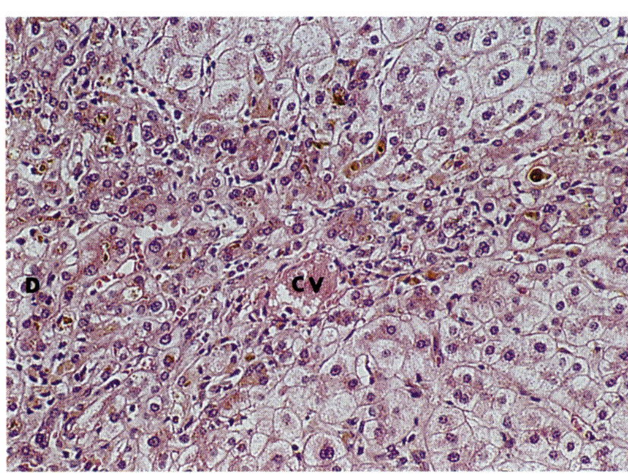

Fig. 129 See Legend page 137.

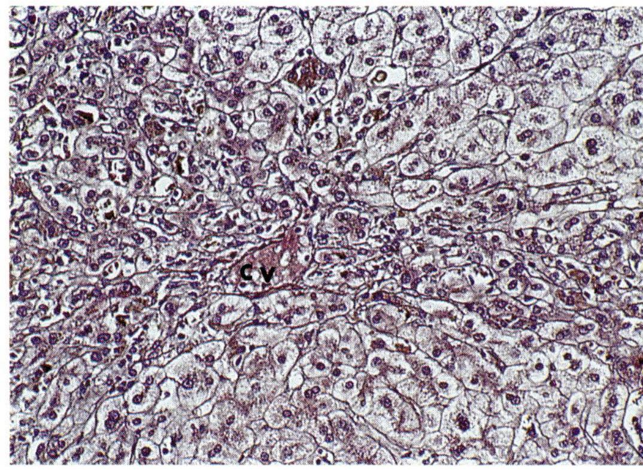

Fig. 130 See Legend page 137.

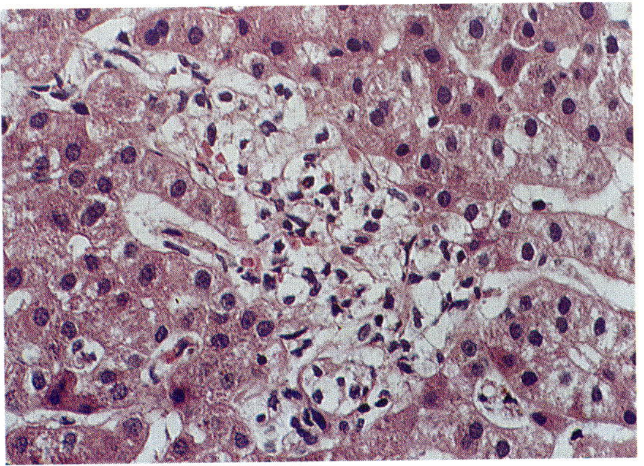

Fig. 131 See Legend page 137.

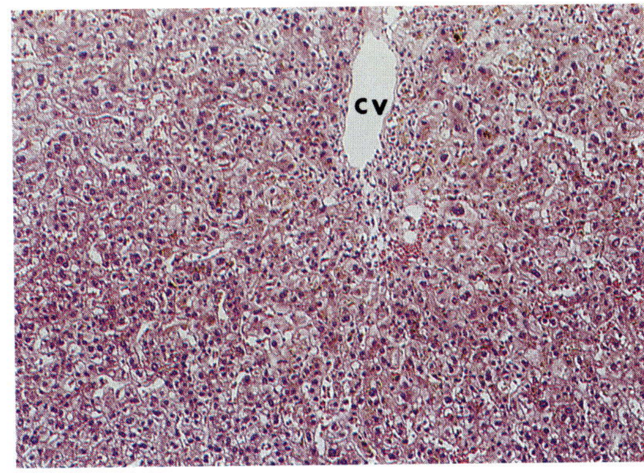

Fig. 132 See Legend page 137.

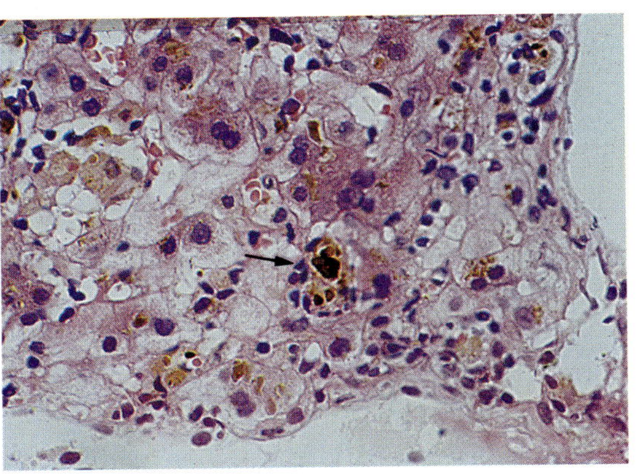

Fig. 133 See Legend page 137.

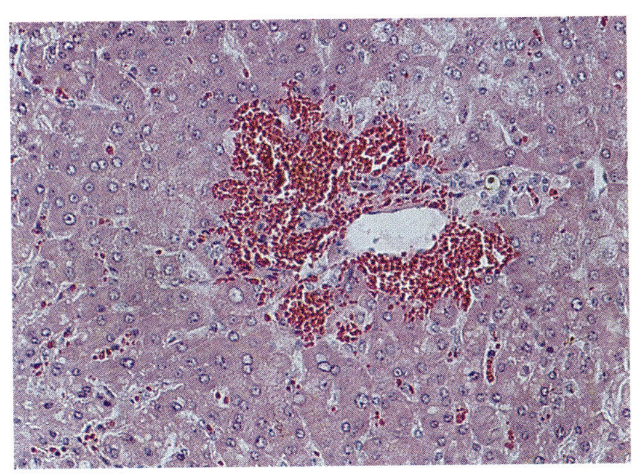

Fig. 134 See Legend page 137.

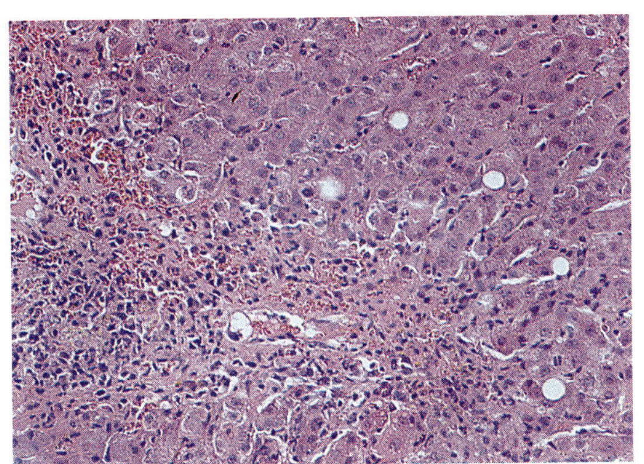

Fig. 135 See Legend page 137.

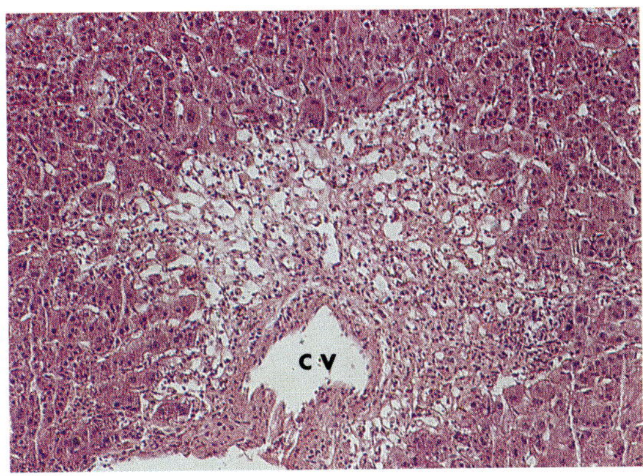

Fig. 136 See Legend page 137.

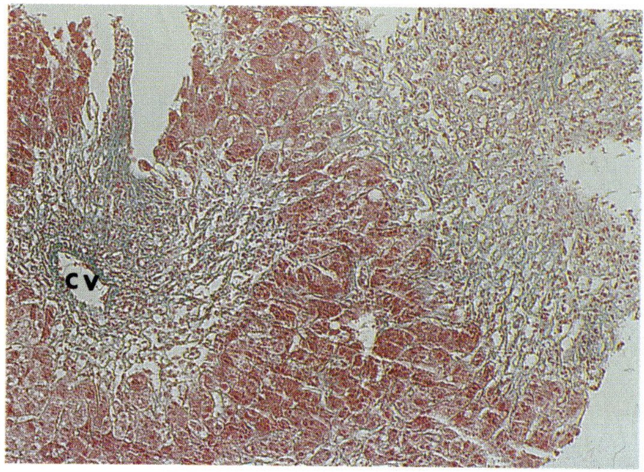

Fig. 137 See Legend page 137.

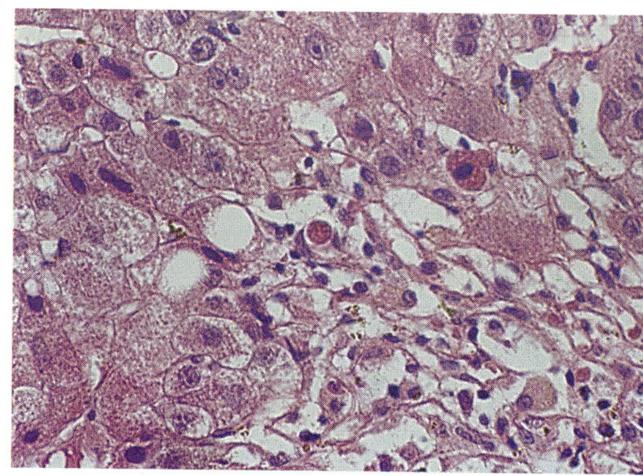

Fig. 138 See Legend page 137.

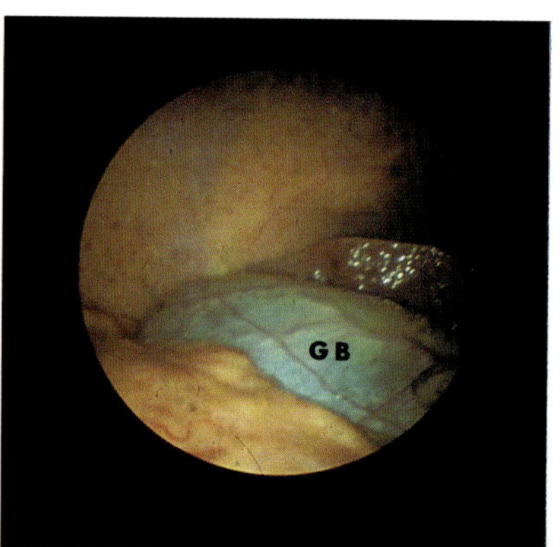

Fig. 139 See Legend page 138.

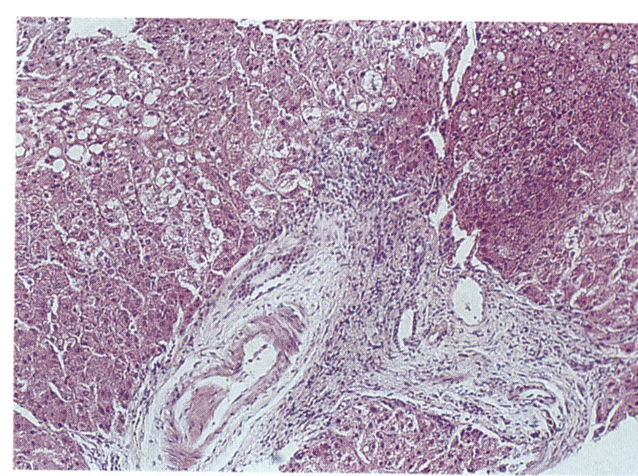

Fig. 140 See Legend page 138.

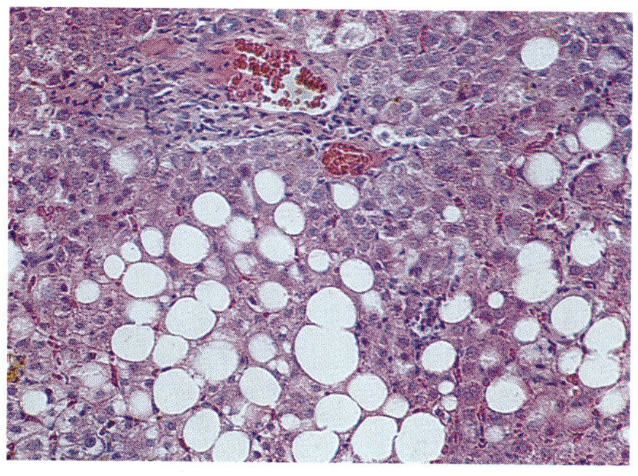

Fig. 141 See Legend page 138.

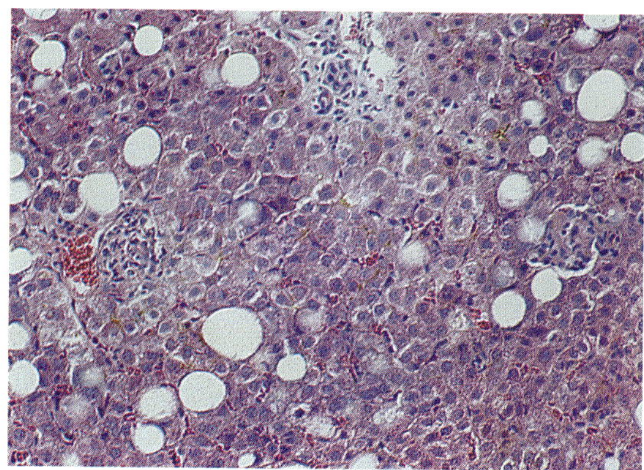

Fig. 142 See Legend page 138.

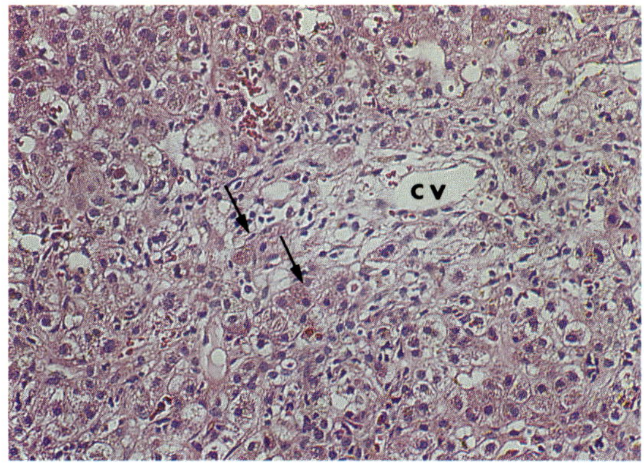

Fig. 143 See Legend page 150.

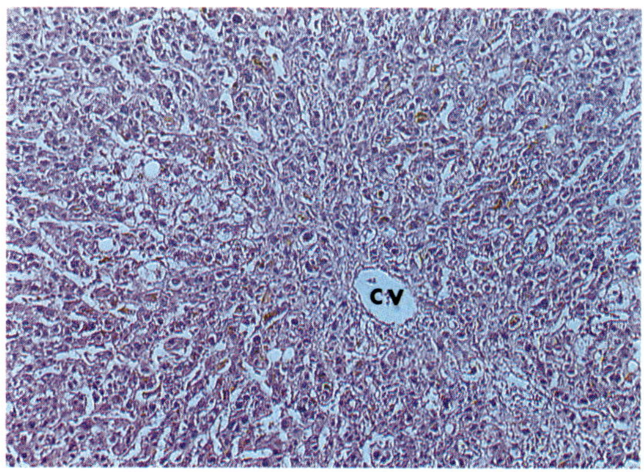

Fig. 144 See Legend page 150.

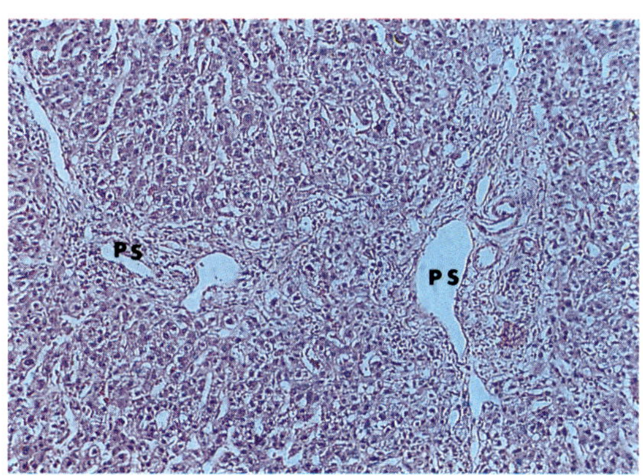

Fig. 145 See Legend page 150.

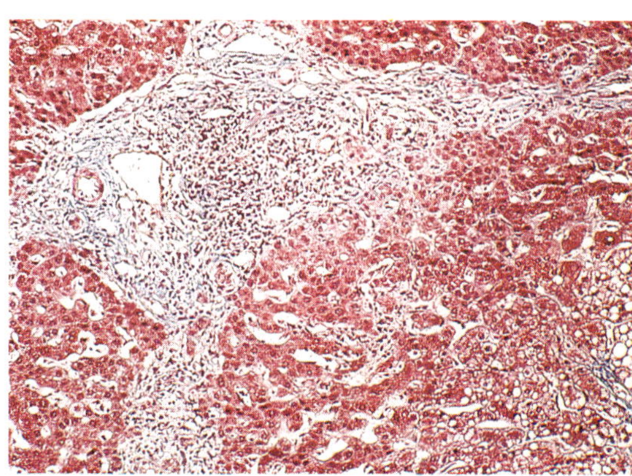

Fig. 146 See Legend page 150.

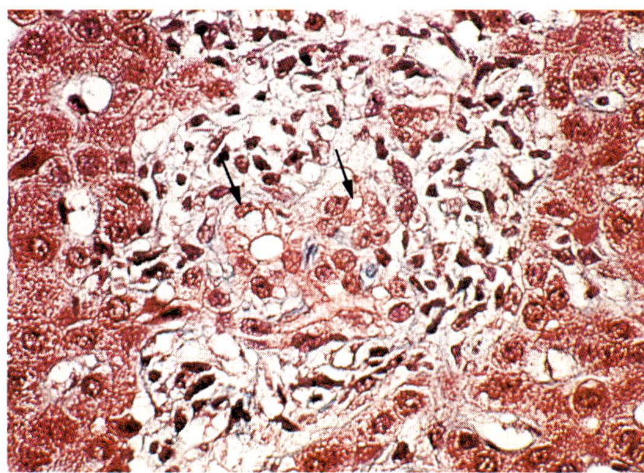

Fig. 147 See Legend page 150.

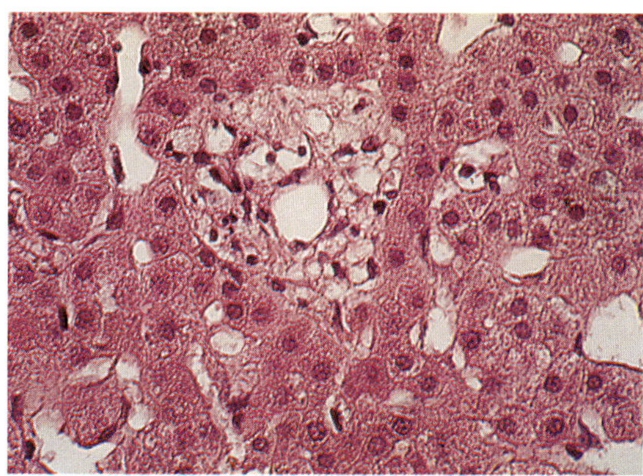

Fig. 148 See Legend page 150.

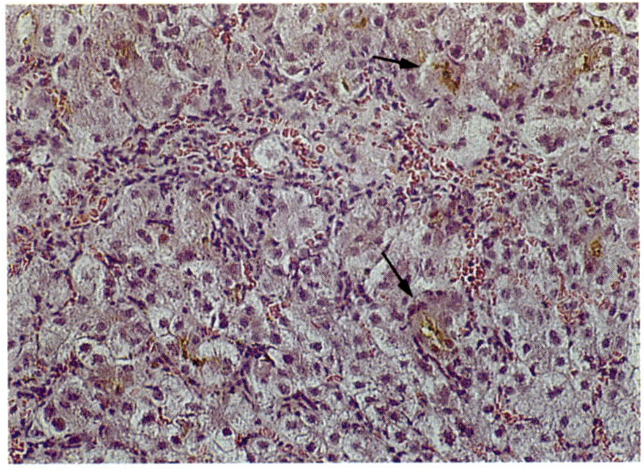

Fig. 149 See Legend page 150.

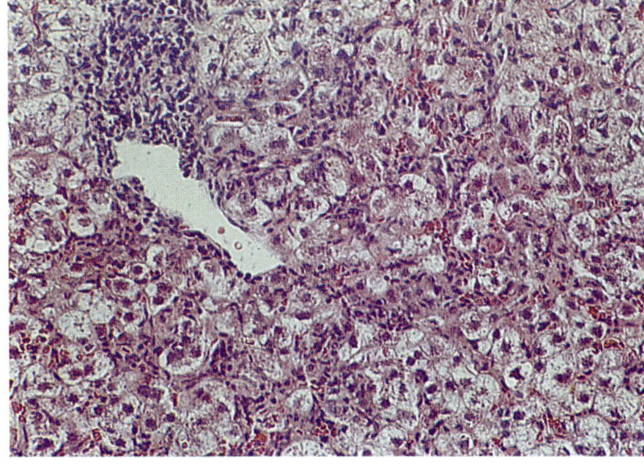

Fig. 150 See Legend page 150.

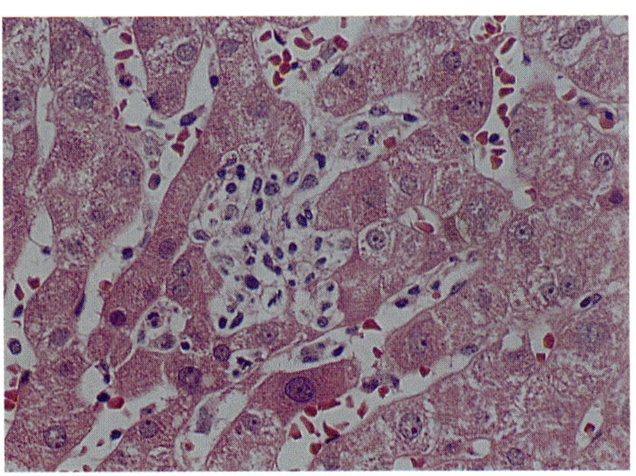

Fig. 151 See Legend page 166.

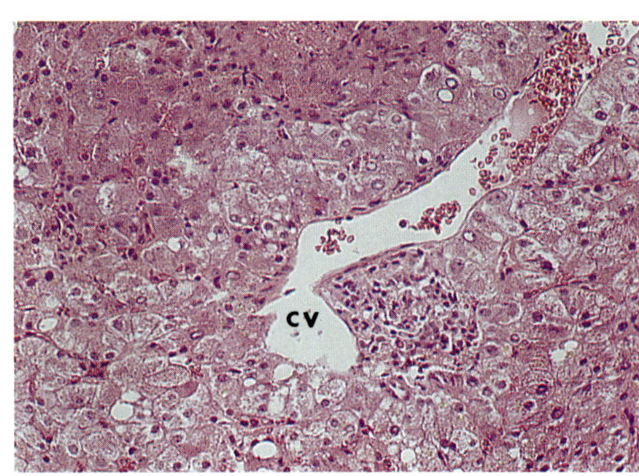

Fig. 152 See Legend page 166.

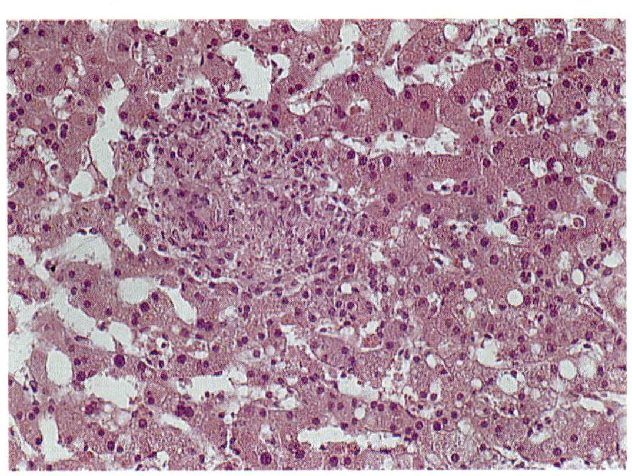

Fig. 153 See Legend page 166.

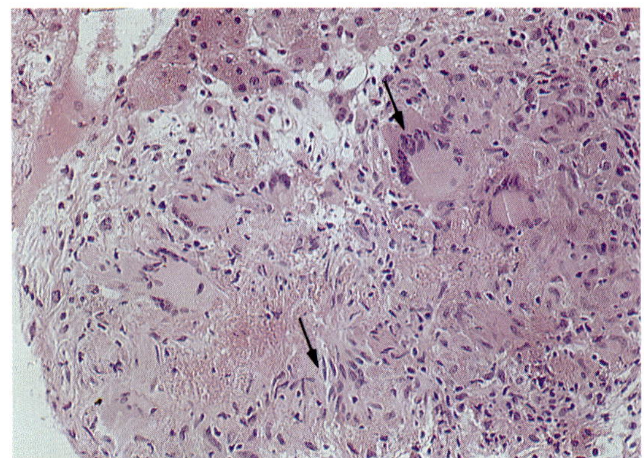

Fig. 154 See Legend page 166.

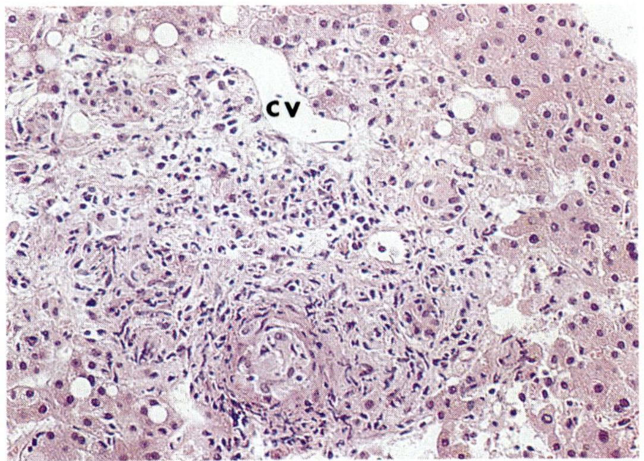

Fig. 155 See Legend page 166.

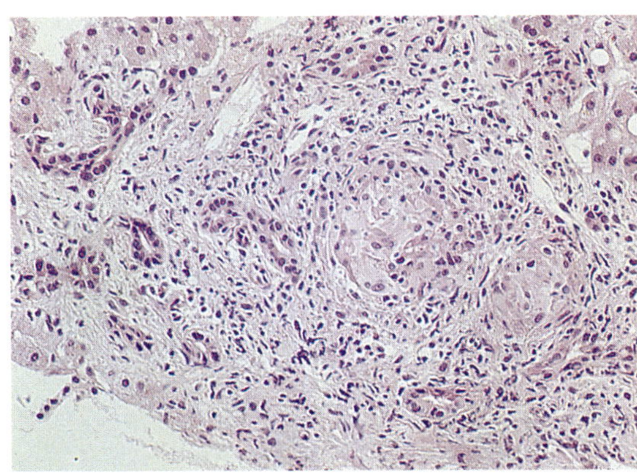

Fig. 156 See Legend page 166.

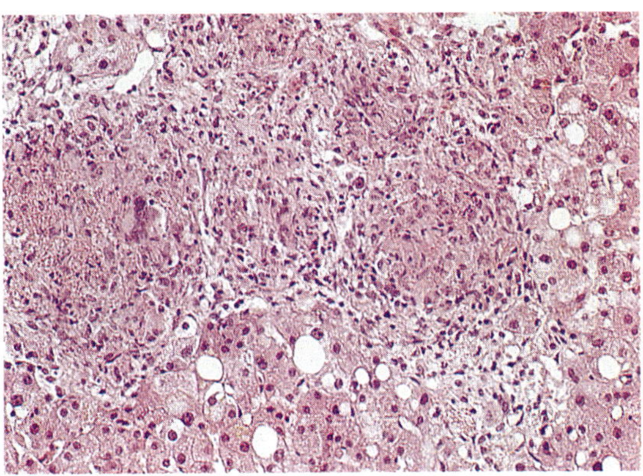

Fig. 157 See Legend page 166.

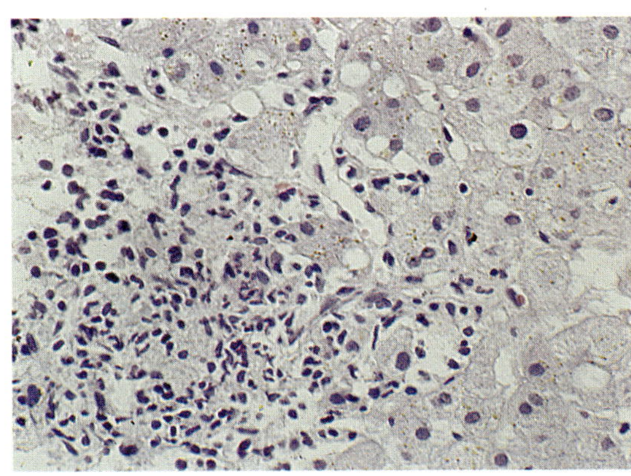

Fig. 158 See Legend page 174.

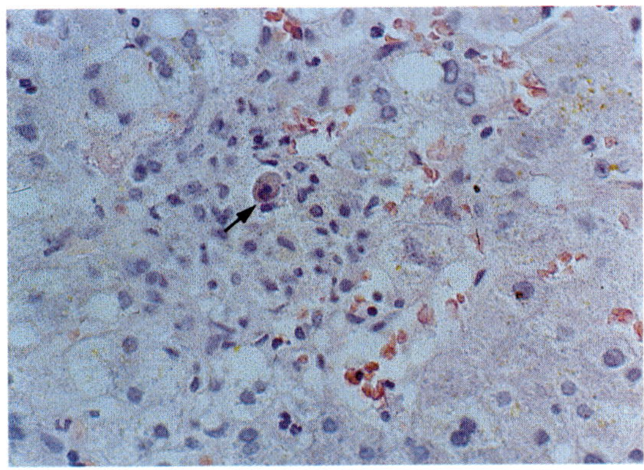

Fig. 159 See Legend page 174.

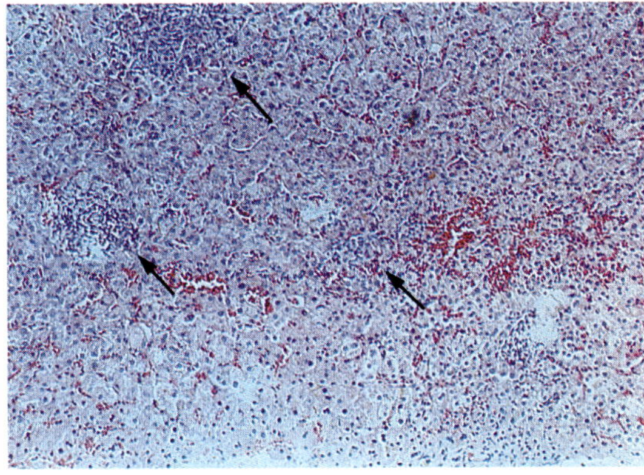

Fig. 160 See Legend page 175.

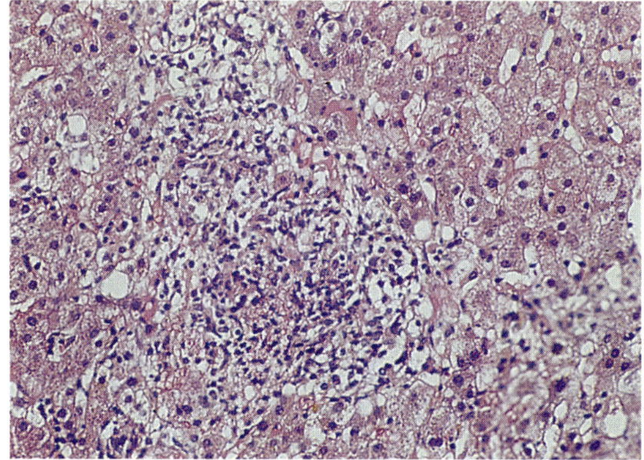

Fig. 161 See Legend page 175.

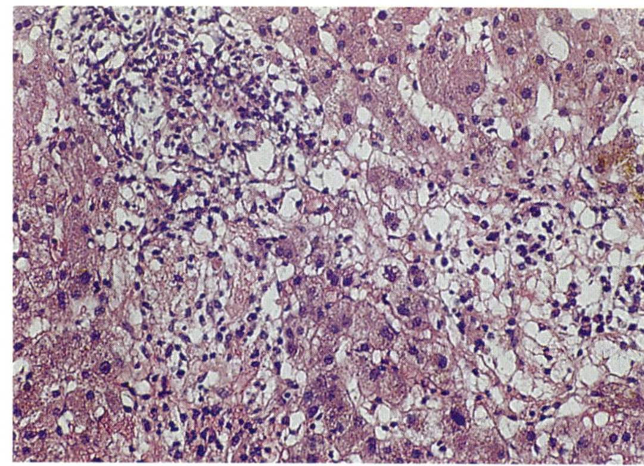

Fig. 162 See Legend page 175.

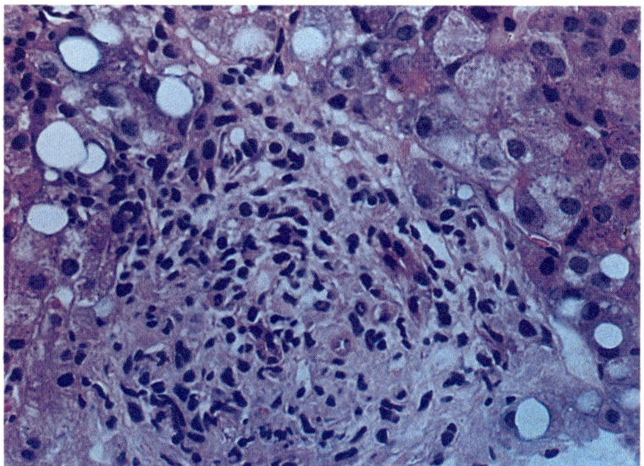

Fig. 163 See Legend page 175.

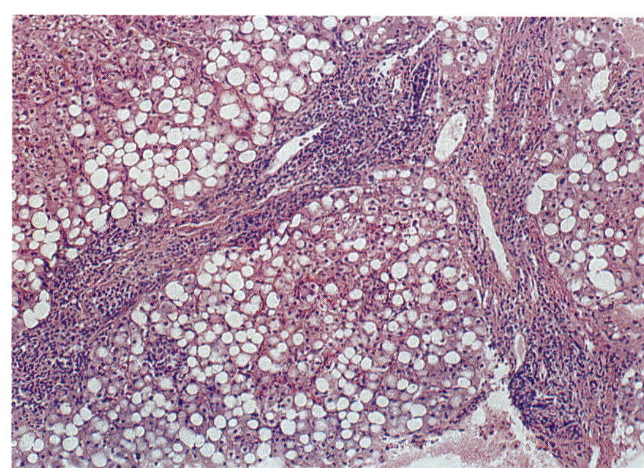

Fig. 164 See Legend page 175.

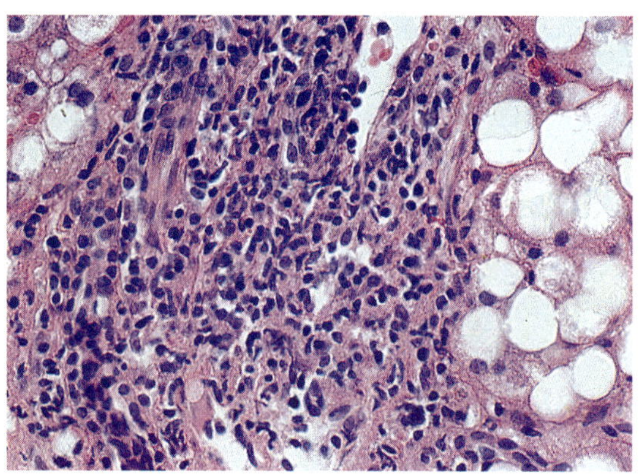

Fig. 165 See Legend page 175.

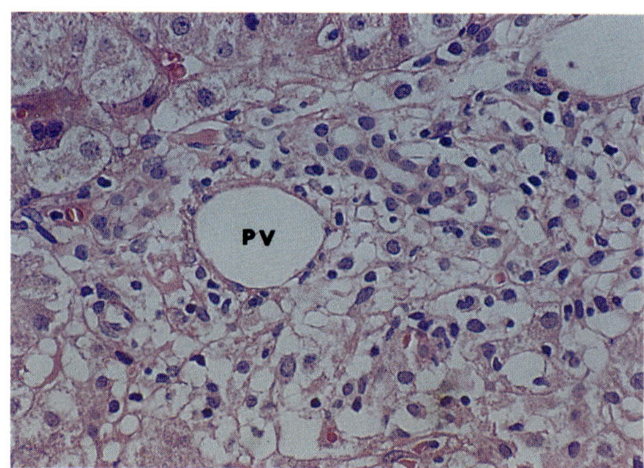

Fig. 166 See Legend page 175.

eight of 36 cases of alcoholic hepatitis, while no Mallory bodies were observed in cases with simple steatosis or cirrhosis.

It is perhaps best to regard alcoholic hepatitis as an acute process that generally heals, usually with some residual scarring. The scarring takes place in the wall of the central veins, in the space of Disse, and periportally. Repeated episodes of acute injury have been seen to eventuate in significant amounts of cumulative fibrosis, which distort the lobular architecture sufficiently to mimic cirrhosis.

"Sclerosing hyaline necrosis" is a form of alcoholic hepatitis in which the central veins become incorporated into centrilobular scar tissue. Edmondson coined the term "sclerosing hyaline necrosis" to describe a form of noncirrhotic alcoholic liver injury in which the central veins are preferentially involved by fibrosis necrosis with Mallory bodies and inflammation (11) (Fig. 112, see page 80).

In this study, the presence of considerable amounts of collagenous connective tissue could obscure the true central location of the lesion. At a superficial glance, one might suppose the area to be the portal (Fig. 113, see page 80). The central vein was recognizable in the early stage of hyaline necrosis, while the central fibrosis was not enough to obliterate the central vein. Central vein occlusion and actual obliteration may be caused by scarring of the central vein (Fig. 114, see page 80) and progressive intralobular fibrosis (Fig. 115, see page 80). In this study, at first the fibrosis was like a lattice network, and later the connective tissue condensed and became a confluent mass that was thought to produce obliteration of sinusoids, central veins and sublobular veins (Fig. 116, see page 80). Thus, central hyaline necrosis or sclerosis may produce postsinusoidal hypertension and ascites before cirrhosis develops(12).

Fibrous septa were able to connect the central and the central or the central and the portal zones (Fig. 117, see page 113) as well as to encircle hepatocytes singly or in groups. The process ultimately mimicked micronodular cirrhosis, since lobules were merged into sublobular-sized aggregates of hepatocytes in association with an impressive amount of fibrosis.

Neutrophilic leukocytes within the liver lobule should always suggest alcoholic hepatitis. In this study, polymorphonuclear leucocytes frequently surrounded liver cells (Figs. 105, 118, see pages 79, 113) (Table 9-1). The portal zone occasionally showed stellate fibrosis (Fig. 119, see page 113). Most of the portal tracts were infiltrated by a mixture of round cells and segmented neutrophilic cells (Fig. 120, see page 113).

Cholestasis was usually minimal in alcoholic hepatitis. However, it was sometimes so pronounced that bile casts were scattered in bile capillaries (Fig. 121, see page 113). Acidophilic bodies were seen in tissue space occasionally. Hemosiderosis in periportal parenchymal cells was frequent (Fig. 122, see page 113), and this may be helpful diagnostically.

Cirrhosis

Cirrhosis is the end-stage lesion of chronic alcoholic liver disease. By definition, cirrhosis is a diffuse process of fibrosis and nodular parenchymal regeneration. In its early stage, diffuse fibrosis and nodular regeneration involve every lobule. The author's materials of alcoholic cirrhosis revealed that the nodules were usually of a lobular size or smaller (Fig. 123, see page 113). Some nodules were rich in fat. Fat cysts had been formed by a mass of fatty liver cells within the fibrotic tissue.

Nodules were sometimes separated by slender septa. In most of the cases with cirrhosis, lobular architecture was unrecognizable as a result of the cirrhotic process, and efferent veins were difficult to identify. Variable acute and chronic inflammatory infiltration was present in the septa (Fig. 124, see page 113). The features of acute alcoholic hepatitis frequently coexisted with cirrhosis.

The septa became broader in the later stage and the nodules increased in size, leading to macronodular cirrhosis (Fig. 125, see page 114).

Summary

Liver needle biopsy confirms the presence of liver disease and identifies alcohol abuse as the likely cause.

Liver biopsy is important for prognostic judgment. Fatty liver change alone is not nearly so serious as perivenular sclerosing hyaline necrosis which is probably a precursor of cirrhosis. It is by biopsy that cirrhosis can be confirmed. Thus, liver biopsy is a must in a patient who is suspected of alcoholic liver disease.

The alcoholic liver injuries observed in Korea show all the histologic findings of those in Western countries. In Korea, however, the incidence of alcoholic patients is still lower than in Western countries and the hepatic lesions are also milder.

References

1. Addison, T. Observations of fatty degeneration of the liver. Guy's Hospital Reports 1: 476–485, 1835.

2. Porta, E.A., Bergman, B.J. and Stein, A.A. Acute alcoholic hepatitis. Am J Pathol 46: 657–689, 1965.

3. Bailey, R.J., Krasner, N., Eddleston, A.L.W.F., Williams, R., Tee, D.E.H., Doniach, D., Kennedy, L.A. and Batchelor, J.R. Histocompatibility antigens, autoantibodies and immunoglobulins in alcoholic liver disease. Br Med J ii: 727–729, 1976.

4. Melendez, M., Vargas-Tank L., Fuentes, C., Armas-Merine, R., Castillo, D., Wolff, C., Wegmann, M.E. and Soto, J. Distribution of HLA histocompatibility antigens, ABO blood groups and Rh antigens in alcoholic liver disease. Gut 20: 288–290, 1979.

5. Sherlock, S. Alcohol and the liver. Disease of the Liver and Biliary System, 6th Edition, Blackwell, Oxford, London. PP: 334–345, 1981.

6. Mallory, F.B. Cirrhosis of the liver. Five different types of lesions from which it may arise. Bull Johns Hopkins Hosp 22: 69–75, 1911.

7. Christoffersen, P. and Nielsen, K. Histological changes in human liver biopsies from chronic alcoholics. Acta Path Microbiol Scand, Section A, 80: 557–565, 1972.

8. Baggenstoss, A.H. and Stauffer, M.H. Posthepatitic and alcoholic cirrhosis. Clinicopathologic study of 43 cases of each. Gastroenterology 22: 157–180, 1952.

9. Popper, H. and Szanto, P.B. Fatty liver with hepatic failure in alcoholics. J M Sinai Hosp 21: 1121–1131, 1957.

10. Christoffersen, P. and Poulsen, H. Correlation of histologic features in two groups of liver biopsies with cirrhosis and fatty change, the first with and the second without Mallory bodies. Acta Path Microbiol Scand, Section A, 79: 27–31, 1971.

11. Edmondson, H.A., Peters, R.L., Reynolds, T.B. and Kuzma, O.T. Sclerosing hyaline necrosis of the liver in the chronic alcoholic. A recognizable clinical syndrome. Ann Intern Med 59: 646–673, 1963.

12. Popper, H. and Schaffner, F. Structural studies in alcohol and drug induced liver injury. In Alcoholic Cirrhosis and other Toxic Hepatopathias, ed. Engel, A. and Lucsson, T. Stockholm: Nordiska Bokhandelns Forlag PP: 15–46, 1970.

Legends

Fig. 105. Focal necrosis.

Alcohol hepatitis. Focal liver cell necrosis replaced by lymphocytes, histiocytes and segmented leucocytes. Needle biopsy, HE, ×400.

Fig. 106.

Simple fatty liver. The acidophilic body (arrow) is detached from the hepatic cell plate in the sinusoidal space and is encircled by inflammatory cells. Needle biopsy, HE, ×400.

Fig. 107. Hyperplastic parenchymal nodules.

Fatty liver. A higher magnification of hyperplastic nodule with fatty droplets. There is no fatty change in the surrounding liver. Needle biopsy, HE, ×400.

Fig. 108.

Fatty liver. A large hyperplastic nodule compresses (arrows) the surrounding tissue. Needle biopsy, HE, ×100.

Fig. 109.

Fatty liver. Condensed reticulin fibers resulted from the compression of adjacent parenchymal tissue by hyperplastic nodules. Needle biopsy, reticulin, ×100.

Fig. 110. Lipogranuloma.

Alcoholic hepatitis. Several fatty droplets and hepatocytes are surrounded by lymphocytes, histiocytes and a few eosinophiles. Needle biopsy, HE, ×400.

Fig. 111.

Alcoholic hepatitis. An extracellular lipid droplet is surrounded by inflammatory cells (arrow). Needle biopsy, HE, ×400.

Fig. 112. Alcoholic hepatitis.

Mallory bodies showing irregular eosinophilic hyaline masses (arrows) in swollen hepatic cells are scattered in an area of central hyaline necrosis. Needle biopsy, HE, ×400.

Fig. 113. Sclerosing hyaline necrosis of the central zone.

Alcoholic hepatitis. A widened central zone with hyaline necrosis and fibrosis is noted. Inflammatory cells are rare. The border between the area of hyaline necrosis and the lobular parenchyma is unsharp. The central vein is obscured by scar tissue. Bile ductule-like parenchyma is observed. It resulted from isolation and compression of liver cell plates by hyaline necrosis and fibrosis. Because of these findings, one might suppose the area to be the portal tract. Needle biopsy, HE, ×200.

Fig. 114. Alcoholic hepatitis.

Central hyaline sclerosis is seen in the right part of the photograph. Intralobular progression of fibrosis originating from the central area is noted. Needle biopsy, HE, ×100.

Fig. 115.

Alcoholic hepatitis. Fibrotic thickening of the central vein and progressive fibrosis radiating from the central vein (CV) into the parenchyma are noted. Needle biopsy, trichrome, ×200.

Fig. 116.

Alcoholic hepatitis. In addition to necrosis and inflammation, there is extensive interstitial fibrosis that involves contiguous lobule. Needle biopsy, HE, ×100.

Fig. 117. Bridging.

Alcoholic hepatitis. Central hyaline necrosis extends to the portal area and thus connects the central zone with the portal tract. Needle biopsy, HE, ×200.

Fig. 118. Alcoholic hepatitis.

Spotty necroses with conspicuous neutrophiles are noted. There are fatty vacuoles in hepatocytes. Needle biopsy, HE, ×400.

Fig. 119. Portal reaction.

Fatty liver. Stellate portal fibrosis is seen. Needle biopsy, trichrome, ×400.

Fig. 120.

Alcoholic hepatitis. There is marked portal infiltration with conspicuous segmented leucocytes. Needle biopsy, HE, ×400.

Fig. 121. Cholestasis.

Alcoholic hepatitis. Bile imbibed liver cells are distributed in the central area. Needle biopsy, HE, ×200.

Fig. 122. Hemosiderosis.

Alcoholic hepatitis. Iron staining shows iron in hepatocytes around the portal tract. Needle biopsy, Prussian blue, ×200.

Fig. 123. Alcoholic cirrhosis.

Nodules are of a lobular size or smaller and rich in fat. They are separated by slender septa. Needle biopsy, trichrome, ×100.

Fig. 124.

Acute and chronic inflammatory infiltration is present in the septa. There are fatty droplets. Needle biopsy, HE, ×200.

Fig. 125.

The septa are broader and the nodules are larger than those in Fig. 123. Needle biopsy, trichrome, ×100.

10 HEPATIC INJURY DUE TO DRUGS AND TOXINS

Whan Kook Chung, M.D., Ph.D.

The endemic prevalence of viral hepatitis in Korea makes it difficult to distinguish diagnostically between viral hepatitis and a drug reaction bearing a resemblance to viral hepatitis. Moreover, concurrent use of herbal medication by the patient often adds to the difficulty of tracing the exact cause of hepatic injury.

The purpose of this chapter is to document some cases with hepatic injury due to arsenical drugs, which were once frequent offenders, and some other cases with hepatic injury attributable to non-arsenical drugs, which are now believed to be obvious offenders of hepatic injury.

Arsenic Drug-Induced Cholestasis

1. Postarsphenamine cholestasis

The practice of using arsphenamine for the treatment of syphilis in the past is now only a matter of historical interest. This pattern of drug-induced intrahepatic cholestasis, an immunoallergic mechanism, was first postulated by Hanger and Gutman on the basis of arsphenamine-induced jaundice (1).

During the Korean War, arsphenamine was easily obtained through the Army supply route, and the prevalence of syphilis, relapsing fever, etc., resulted in the abuse of arsphenamine. As a result, the author frequently encountered patients who had developed jaundice after arsphenamine injections, in some of whom liver needle biopsy was conducted.

The clinical and pathologic features of the cases in which intrahepatic cholestasis developed were distinctive. The clinical, biochemical and histologic characteristics of this syndrome are illustrated on the basis of the three cases that follow.

Report of cases

Case 1. A 24-year-old soldier was found to have latent syphilis. He had two injections of arsphenamine at an interval of one week. On the day after the second injection, he began to have nausea, vomiting, itching and fever. Jaundice appeared one week after the second injection. On May 19, 1960, the day of admission, he had generalized pruritus. His stools were clay-colored. The liver was palpated and tender 2 cm below the right costal margin. There was severe icterus in the skin and sclerae but the other data of examination were within normal limits. Table 10-1 shows follow-up biochemical studies.

The patient's serum bilirubin level continued to increase and reached 27.9 mg/100ml on June 16 but, thereafter, began to decrease, showing 2.6 mg/100ml on September 6 (five months after the onset of the disease). However, the serum alanine aminotransferase (SALT) and the serum aspartate aminotransferase (SAST) remained 2–3 times above normal. The total cholesterol level persisted over 400 mg/100ml until August 10, four months after the onset of the disease. The serum alkaline phosphatase activity also showed an abnormal elevation until September 5. A liver needle biopsy was performed on May 19, 1960, 35 days after the onset of jaundice. The biopsy specimen showed fair preservation of the lobular architecture. No necrosis of liver cells was seen. In some areas, the liver cells and their nuclei were larger than the normal ones. There was a slight increase in fibrous tissue about the central vein and in the portal areas (Figs. 126, 127, see page 114). Conspicuous infiltration of lymphocytes with some polymorphonuclears was noted within the wall and around the central vein. The portal areas were extensively infiltrated by lymphoid cells and a moderate number of polymorphonuclears (Figs. 126, 127, see page 114). Many polymorphonuclears and some eosinophiles were observed within the walls and around the bile ductules (Figs. 126, 127, see page 114). The most striking feature of the section was the presence of patchy areas in which the bile canaliculi were markedly distended with bile thrombi (Fig. 128, see page 114). Many Kupffer cells had taken up bile pigment (Fig. 128, see page 114). Some of the liver cells in the central zone contained bile pigment.

Case 2. A 23-year-old Korean male soldier was treated at an Army hospital for syphilis. On April 2, 1960, he was given 0.1 gm of arsphenamine intravenously with no reaction. Thereafter, he received the same dose of intravenous arsphenamine injection twice a week until May 2. On the morning following his last injection, he complained of anorexia, drowsiness and weakness. He noted dark urine and itching in the skin, but was not aware of acholic stool. On May 19, the day of admission, jaundice was marked. An erythematous rash was present on the forearm. The liver was tender and enlarged to 2 cm under the right costal margin.

Blood chemical examination (Table 10-1) revealed increased bilirubin levels for at least six weeks (reaching 27.6 mg/100ml), and the serum alkaline phosphatase value was as high as 37.6 KA units, with a consistently mild elevation of amino transferase activity. The serum cholesterol level rose to over 400 mg/100ml, and persisted at least for a period of three months after the onset of jaundice.

A liver needle biopsy was done on May 28, 26 days after the onset of jaundice. The lobular architecture of the liver was normal. Considerable parenchymal cell necrosis and reticulin collapse were noted in the central zone (Figs. 129, 130, see page 114). The liver cells in this area were more intensely eosinophilic. There was a slight increase of fibrous tissue in the wall of the central vein. Some of the liver cells and Kupffer cells contained bile pigment.

Case 3. A Korean male soldier, aged 24, was treated at an Army hospital for syphilis. On March 3, 1962, the patient was given 0.1 gm of arsphenamine with no immediate reaction, but several hours later transient weakness and profuse perspiration occurred. On March 6, he received a second intravenous injection of the same dose of arsphenamine. Ten days after the second injection, jaundice was noted by his friend. When admitted to the hospital on April 17, one month after the onset of jaundice, he was deeply jaundiced and complained chiefly of itching. The liver edge was tender and palpable two finger breadths below the right costal margin. The patient's stools were clay-colored.

Blood studies (Table 10-1) revealed that the serum bilirubin value was as high as 12.5 mg/100ml on admission. The serum alkaline phosphatase increased definitely. The serum cholesterol value was 1440 mg/100ml. The SALT and SAST levels were slightly elevated. A liver biopsy was performed two days after the admission. The biopsy showed a normal architecture. Liver cells were normal but some of the cells and their nuclei showed mild variations in size. There was less cellular infiltration in the portal area and the central zone than in Case 1, but abnormal accumulations of round cells and polymorphonuclears and eosinophiles were noted. Some focal parenchymal necrosis with or without an acidophilic body were seen. There was intralobular accumulation of foamy histiocytes (Fig. 131, see page 115).

The clinical, biochemical and histologic characteristics of cases with postarsphenamine jaundice were as follows: 1) Cholestasis developed early in

TABLE 10–1.

Summary of Data in Three Males with Syphilis who Developed Postarsphenamine Cholestasis

Cases No.	Arsphenamin administration and Jaundice	Date	Total bilirubin (mg/100ml)	ALT (Sigma u.)	AST (Sigma u.)	Alkaline phosphase (B.U.)	Cholesterol (mg/100ml)
1	Jaundice developed 4 days after second injection of arsphenamine	Apr./14/1960 (onset of jaundice)					
		May/19/1960		160	100	6.4	472
		June/16/1960	27.9	80	80	10.4	400
		July/22/1960	18.1	320	90	28.0	535
		Aug./10/1960	11.4	58	29	12.3	465
		Sep./ 5/1960	2.6	95	110	21.2	
2	Jaundice developed just after 8th injection of arsphenamine. 8 injections were carried out during a period from April 2 to May 2, 1960	May/ 2/1960 (onset of jaundice)					
		May/ 2/1960		80	70	6.1	425
		June/16/1960	27.6	70	140	18.8	615
		July/22/1960	18.9	155	155	9.7	590
		Aug./10/1960	16.8	69	50	9.6	570
		Sept./ 5/1960	13.4	105	100	9.2	
3	Jaundice developed 10 days after second injection of arsphenamine	Mar./15/1962 (onset of jaundice)					
		Apr./11/1962	12.5	170	148	15.6	1440

the course of treatment with arsenicals. 2) Symptoms were precipitated by a second or multiple injections after a latent period. 3) The reaction was induced by relatively small doses of arsenic. 4) There were associated cutaneous rashes and eosinophilia. 5) Marked elevations of serum bilirubin, alkaline phosphatase and cholesterol were observed, while the SALT and SAST elevations were mild. 6) Parenchymal degeneration and necrosis were mild despite intense jaundice. 7) Inflammatory changes were observed about bile ductules and bile casts within the lumen of the bile canaliculi.

The reactions have many of the characteristics of drug hypersensitivity. Considering that parenchymal lesions are mild but not striking and that inflammatory changes about the bile ductules are apparent in these cases, probably selective involvement of cholangioles is the cause of cholestasis.

2. Postcarbarsone cholestasis

During the Korean War, intestinal amebiasis was endemic among Korean soldiers. Of the numerous arsenical compounds used for the treatment of the disease at that time, carbarsone (p-carbamidobenzine-arsonic acid) was usually conceded to be the most innocuous.

Accordingly, carbarsone was a popular drug for the treatment of intestinal amebiasis at that time. Large quantities of this preparation, alone or in combination with other agents, were used during the 1950's with surprisingly few toxic effects reported. Most doctors cautioned that it should not be used in cases with evidence of liver disease, but otherwise contraindications seemed to be absent. The reactions, during or after the use of the drugs, usually occurred in the form of skin disorders, gastrointestinal upset, neuritis or kidney damage (2). The hepatocellular and the cholestatic types of liver injury were rare; however, cases with a predominantly hepatocellular (2,3) and a cholestatic (3,4,5) pattern of injury within one month after the starting of carbarsone therapy were reported.

The purpose of this description is to document a case of cholestatic hepatitis with exfoliative dermatitis due to oral administration of carbarsone within the therapeutic range.

Case report

A 20-year-old man was diagnosed clinically to have amebic colitis. Therapy was started on January 30, 1962 with 250 mg of carbarsone three times a day. After receiving the drug for eight days, on Feb. 6, he developed headache, fatigue, dizziness and itching. The symptoms persisted and, on April 5, he was admitted to a hospital. On admission his sclerae appeared icteric, and his liver was not palpated but it was tender. Bluish brown skin eruptions were scattered all over the surface of his body. Examination revealed nothing else to be noted.

On April 11, the serum bilirubin level was 12.1 mg/100ml. The SALT and the SAST levels were 95 and 42 units, respectively. Alkaline phosphatase was 37.2 KA units and the total serum cholesterol level was 465 mg/100ml. A liver biopsy was also performed. The biopsy specimen of the liver showed a normal architecture with a slight but definite increase in fibrous tissue and inflammatory cell infiltration about the central vein (Fig. 132, see page 115). Except for sporadic cells ballooned with homogeneous eosinophilic cytoplasm and occasional feathery degeneration in the central area (Fig. 133, see page 115), the liver cells appeared to be normal. Bile plugs were present in many bile capillaries (Fig. 133, see page 115). In the portal area, there were scattered lymphocytes and occasional polymorphonuclears. This was not the histologic picture of viral hepatitis.

The clinical, biochemical and histologic patterns of this case were very similar to those of cases with postarsphenamine cholestasis.

Miscellaneous Agents

1. Halothane

Two types of halothane-induced hepatic injury can be found. One occurs in a relatively large group with mild to moderate elevations of liver enzymes, mainly serum aminotransferases, and the other in rare patients with hepatic necrosis which may result in a high fatality rate. The frequency of the latter type has been estimated at 1:6,000-1:20,000 (6). The author has encountered a case with reversible fulminant hepatitis after the initial exposure to halothane.

In a 20-year-old HBsAg-negative male patient with tuberculous peritonitis, a laparatomy was done under halothane anesthesia. Just before the surgery, liver test results were within the normal limits. Eight days after the surgery, the patient developed jaundice, showing elevation of SAST levels associated with fever and gradual development of hepatic coma.

The patient recovered from hepatic encephalopathy and the jaundice became mild. A liver biopsy was performed 23 days after halothane administration. The biopsy specimen showed severe cholestatic hepatitis.

2. Methyldopa

Stricker et al. (7) estimated the occurrence of methyldopa-induced symptomatic liver disease to be less than 0.1%, but most extensive studies give an overall incidence of approximately 5% or lower (8). The perturbation of the immune system has been found to be implicated in the pathogenesis of some methyldopa complications, particularly immune Coombs'-positive hemolytic anemia and chronic active hepatitis (9).

A 50-year-old male patient developed chronic active hepatitis during a prolonged methyldopa therapy for hypertension.

The diagnosis was confirmed by liver needle biopsy. At the time of the biopsy, the serum bilirubin was 1.8 mg/100ml, the SAST and the SALT were 300 and 290 units, respectively. HBsAg was negative. The biopsy findings were consistent with chronic active hepatitis.

3. Sulfamethoxazole (Bactrim®)

Sulfonamides may cause hyperbilirubinemia without hepatic injury by hemolysis in vulnerable persons (10).

A 41-year-old female was admitted to St. Mary's Hospital because of jaundice and purpura-like skin eruption after an injection of sulfamethoxazole for the treatment of upper respiratory infection. The total bilirubin was 3.7 mg/100ml (indirect bilirubin 3.3 mg/100ml), the hemoglobin 10 gm/100ml and the blood urea nitrogen 80 mg/100ml. Clinical diagnosis indicated a fatal hemolytic uremic syndrome. A needle necropsy was performed which showed intralobular focal hemorrhage (Fig. 134, see page 115).

4. Gold compounds

Hepatic dysfunction due to gold therapy is a rare complication and has been described only in a few cases. Liver biopsy shows mainly a cholestatic pattern (11). However, fatal hepatic necrosis has occasionally been attributed to the use of gold compounds (11).

A 32-year-old female patient developed fatal hepatic necrosis after gold sodium thiomalate (myochrysine) injection for the treatment of rheumatoid arthritis. She had been injected with myochrysine for 10 months until just before the appearance of jaundice.

A liver biopsy was carried out 25 days after the onset of jaundice. At the time of biopsy, the serum bilirubin was 9.8 mg (direct 5.7 mg and indirect 4.1 mg)/100ml, the SAST 190 units, the SALT 240 units, the prothrombin time 18% and the hemoglobin was 8.8 gm/100ml. The HBsAg was negative. The biopsy findings revealed a moderate degree of chronic active hepatitis (Fig. 135, see page 115).

The patient expired 20 days after the biopsy and a needle necropsy was performed. The necropsy specimen showed circumscribed hepatic necrosis (see Chapter 5) and predominant collapse. In the areas not affected by the circumscribed lesion, the features of chronic active hepatitis were noted.

5. Chloroquine

Chloroquine is not a hepatotoxin. When used in high doses (0.5–1 gm/day) for the treatment of porphyria cutanea tarda, it may precipitate acute reaction with elevation of serum aminotransferases (12,13) and even centrilobular necrosis (12).

A 26-year-old man took 20 tablets (250 mg/tablet) of chloroquine with the intention of committing suicide. Jaundice appeared one week later.

A liver biopsy was performed five weeks after the onset of jaundice. The biopsy specimen showed numerous multinucleated giant cells, an acidophilic body, bile pigments in Kupffer cells and traces of central necrosis and chronic portal inflammation.

6. Herbal medicine (a tonic)

Six weeks before being examined, a woman had taken herb tonic for 15 days while recuperating from a long-standing weakness.

Tension in the right shoulder, hand edema and skin rash developed 15 days after the medication. Fever began and was sustained but intermittently spiked. At the time of admission, blood culture was done but no organisms were grown. Multiple Widal tests for salmonellae were negative. On physical examination, the lungs were clear, and the heart sound was normal. There were no hepatosplenomegaly, no systemic lymphadenopathy and no dermatologic lesions.

The hemoglobin was 9.9 gm/100ml but the leukocyte count was normal. A bone marrow study showed normal findings except mild eosinophilia. The serum total protein was 6.0 gm/100ml with 3.2 gm/100ml of albumin. The total serum bilirubin showed 4.2 mg/100ml (direct, 2.3 mg/100ml). The SAST was 693 units, the SALT 340 units and the alkaline phosphatase 32 KA units. The prothrombin time was 81% of the normal. HBsAg was negative.

A liver needle biopsy was performed as part of fever study. The biopsy slide was referred for consultation to the Armed Forces Institute of Pathology in Washington, D.C. The histologic findings were reported as follows: the biopsy shows extensive necrosis and dropout of centrilobular liver cells with a milder degree of injury and regenerative changes in the remaining parenchyma (Figs. 136, 137, see pages 115, 116). The inflammatory response is relatively mild considering the extent of injury, with hypertrophied pigmented macrophages in the areas of necrosis (Fig. 138, see page 116), and several lymphocytes throughout the specimen. Portal inflammation is relatively mild and fibrosis does not appear to be significant (Figs. 136, 137, see pages 115, 116). The histologic changes are due to a severe recent hepatocellular injury, and the sharply zonal nature of the necrosis suggests that it may have been toxic in origin.

7. Lead

Although lead poisoning does not produce clinically significant changes in the liver, the nuclei of hepatocytes often contain eosinophilic, acid-fast inclusions that may be diagnostic (14). The author, along with colleagues, saw a case with chronic hepatic injury after a long-standing exposure to lead (15).

A 57-year-old male patient took herbal medicine over a period of two years for the treatment of chronic urticaria. Chemical analysis showed that the herb medicine contained 2% of lead. Because of severe abdominal colicky pain and abdominal distension, the patient was hospitalized at St. Mary's Hospital. Until then, the patient had been suffering occasionally from fatigue, dizziness, abdominal pain and abdominal distension.

No abnormality was found on physical examination except anemia and abdominal distension. Liver test results remained in the normal range. The lead concentration of blood was 135.8 ug/100ml. The urine contained 825 ug/L of lead, 166.4 ug/L of coproporphyrin and 10.1 mg/L of δ-aminolevulinic acid. The hemoglobin showed 7.8 gm/100ml and the reticulocyte count was 7.2%. The erythrocytes showed pink cytoplasm that was stippled with many fine and coarse blue granules. Radiological study of barium enema showed megacolon. Therefore, the patient had lead intoxication with hemolytic anemia.

A liver biopsy was done under peritoneoscopic observation. The liver surface was finely nodular (Fig. 139, see page 116) and the biopsy specimen demonstrated a moderate degree of steatosis and chronic portal inflammation and fibrosis (Fig. 140, see page 116). No inclusion bodies were found in the nuclei.

8. Agricultural pesticide

A 28-year-old male patient was admitted to St. Mary's Hospital because of increasing indigestion and nausea for three days prior to the admission. He had been exposed to the spray of agricultural pesticide (main compound presumed to be a malathion).

Physical examination revealed icteric sclerae and a tender and palpable liver 2 cm below the right costal margin. The hemoglobin was 13.0 gm/100ml. The white-cell count was 3,500 with 48% neutrophils, 47% lymphocytes, 2% monocytes and 3% eosinophils. The platelet count was 164,000. The serum protein was 8.8 gm (albumin 3.7gm and globulin 5.1 gm)/100ml, the bilirubin 10.4 mg (direct 4.7 mg and indirect 5.7mg)/100ml, the total cholesterol 325 mg/100ml, the SALT 248 units, the SAST 470 units and the alkaline phosphatase 5.2 KA units. A liver biopsy was performed two days after the admission. The biopsy specimen showed cholestatic hepatitis with diffuse steatosis and portal sclerosis (Figs. 141, 142, see page 116).

Summary

1) Mild parenchymal degeneration and necrosis were noted in postarsphenamine cholestasis despite intense jaundice and hepatic bile stasis.

2) Although conspicuous phlebitis and perivenular necroinflammation of the central vein were found, the principal lesion was inflammation around the bile ductules in postarsphenamine cholestasis. Selective involvement of cholangioles seemed to be the cause of cholestasis and the central vein reaction was a secondary response of cholestasis.

3) The clinical, biochemical and liver biopsy findings of postcarbarsone cholestasis were very similar to those of postarsphenamine cholestasis.

4) The patterns of reaction, due to arsphenamine injection or administration of carbarsone by mouth within the therapeutic range, showed many of the characteristics of drug hypersensitivity.

5) Hepatic injury resulting from the miscellaneous agents is unusual. While such agents can be the cause of the injury, the reason may be found elsewhere. This documentation has been made in the hope that further light may be shed on this matter in the future.

References

1. Hanger, F.M. and Gutman, A.B. Postarsphenamine jaundice. JAMA 115: 263–271, 1940.

2. Epstein, E. Toxicity of carbarsone; acute fatty degeneration of the liver, exfoliative dermatitis and death following its administration. JAMA 106: 769–772, 1936.

3. Nelson, R.S. Hepatitis due to carbarsone. JAMA 160: 764–767, 1956.

4. Radke, R.A., Washington, E. and Baroody, W.G. Carbarsone toxicity: a review of the literature and report of 45 cases. Ann Intern Med 47: 419–427, 1957.

5. Schwartz, H.J. and Donnenfeld, H. Arsenic toxicity with "high" doses of carbarsone. JAMA 191: 678, 1965.

6. Inman, N.H.N. and Mashin, N.W. Jaundice after repeated exposure to halothane: a further analysis of reports to the Committee on Safety of Medicine. Br Med J 2: 1455–1456, 1978.

7. Stricker, B.H.CH. and Spoelstra, P. Methyldopa in Drug-Induced Hepatic Injury. Elsevier, Amsterdam-New York-Oxford, Vol. 1, Page 97, 1985.

8. Rodman, J.S. Deutsch, D.J. and Gutman, S.I. Methyldopa hepatitis: a report of six cases and review of the literature. Am J Med 60: 941–948, 1976.

9. Shalev. O., Mosseri, M., Aricl, I. and Stalnikowicz. Methyldopa-induced immunohemolytic anemia and chronic active hepatitis. Arch Intern Med 143: 592–593, 1983.

10. Stricker, B.H.CH. and Spoelstra, P. Sulfonamides in Drug-Induced Hepatic Injury. Elsevier, Amsterdam-New York-Oxford, Vol., 1, Page 177, 1985.

11. Howrie, D.L. and Gartner, Ir. C. Gold-induced hepatotoxicity: case report and review of the literature. J Rheumatology 9: 727–729, 1982.

12. Taljaard, J.J.F., Shanley, B.C., Stewart-Wynne, E.G., Deppe, W.M. and Joubert, S.M. Studies on low dose chloroquine therapy and the action of chloroquine in symptomatic porphyria. Br J Dermatology 87: 261–269, 1972.

13. Sweeney, G.D., Saunders, S.J., Dowelle, E.B. and Eales, L. Effects of chloroquine on patients with cutaneous porphyria of the "symptomatic" type. Br J Med 1: 1281–1285, 1965.

14. Wachstein, M. Lead poisoning diagnosed by the presence of nuclear acid-fast inclusion bodies in kidney and liver. Arch Path 48: 442, 1949.

15. Kim, G.S., Lee, O.J., Kwon, Y.Y., Sun, H.S., Chung, W.K. and Lee, J.M. A case of an acquired megacolon and toxic hepatitis in a patient with chronic lead poisoning. Korean J Int Med 21: 1061–1066, 1978.

Legends

Fig. 126. A needle liver biopsy was performed six weeks after the last injection of arsphenamine.

The portal area is extensively infiltrated by lymphoid cells and a moderate number of polymorphonuclears. Needle biopsy, HE, ×200.

Fig. 127.

Many polymorphonuclears and some eosinophiles are observed within the wall and around the bile ductules. Needle biopsy, HE, ×400.

Fig. 128.

Many bile plugs (arrows) appear in the markedly dilated bile canaliculi. Bile pigments in Kupffer cells are noted. Needle biopsy, HE, ×400.

Fig. 129. A needle liver biopsy specimen obtained from a patient with jaundice following multiple injection of arsphenamine.

Considerable parenchymal cell necrosis is noted in the central zone (CV). The liver cells in this area are stained more intensely in eosin. Bile pigments are in the liver cells and Kupffer cells. Needle biopsy, HE, ×200.

Fig. 130.

Reticulin collapse in the central area (CV) is demonstrated. Needle biopsy, reticulin, ×200.

Fig. 131. A liver biopsy specimen obtained from a patient with jaundice that occurred two weeks after the second injection of arsphenamine.

There are intralobular accumulation of foamy histiocytes. Needle biopsy, HE, ×400.

Fig. 132. A liver biopsy specimen obtained from a patient with jaundice that followed carbarsone administration.

There is a slight but definite increase in fibrous tissue and inflammatory cell infiltration about the central vein (CV). Needle biopsy, HE, ×100.

Fig. 133.

Hepatic cells are ballooned with homogeneous eosinophilic cytoplasm, and some feathery degeneration in the central area. A bile plug (arrow), which is surrounded by inflammatory cells, is located in a dilated bile capillary. Needle biopsy, HE, ×400.

Fig. 134. A liver biopsy specimen obtained from a patient with jaundice and purpura-like skin eruption that occurred after an injection of sulfamethoxazole.

Marked focal hemorrhage is noted in the central area. Needle biopsy, HE, ×200.

Fig. 135. A liver biopsy specimen obtained from a patient with fatal fulminant hepatitis after prolonged gold therapy for rheumatoid arthritis.

A zone of extensive necrosis and collapse and a more vigorous inflammatory reaction that extends beyond the confines of the lobule. Needle biopsy, HE, ×200.

Fig. 136. A liver needle biopsy specimen obtained from a patient with jaundice that developed after administration of herb medicine.

Extensive necrosis and drop-out of centrilobular (CV) liver cells with a milder degree of injury and regenerative changes in the remaining periportal parenchyma. Needle biopsy, HE, ×100.

Fig. 137.

A mildly collapsed reticulin framework in the area of centrizonal (CV) necrosis. No significant fibrosis is seen in the centrizonal necrosis. Needle biopsy, trichrome, ×100.

Fig. 138.

Hypertrophied pigmented macrophages and acidophilic bodies in the area of necrosis. Needle biopsy, HE, ×400.

Fig. 139. A patient with lead poisoning.
Peritoneoscopy discloses a finely nodular surface with a sharp liver edge above the gall bladder (GB).

Fig. 140.
Approximation of the portal tract and the central vein without an intervening area of parenchymal cells is noted. This is presumed to be due to parenchymal confluent necrosis. Needle biopsy, HE, ×100.

Fig. 141. A liver needle biopsy specimen obtained from a patient with cholestasis following exposure to agricultural pesticides.
A little altered lobular architecture and diffuse steatosis are noted. The hepatic cell plates are many cell-thick. Needle biopsy, HE, ×200.

Fig. 142.
Intralobular lipogranulomas are seen. Needle biopsy, HE, ×400.

11

MORPHOLOGIC AND BIOCHEMICAL STUDIES OF BENIGN RECURRENT INTRAHEPATIC CHOLESTASIS: COMPARATIVE STUDIES OF RECURRENT AND PERSISTENT TYPE

Whan Kook Chung, M.D., Ph.D.

Benign recurrent intrahepatic cholestasis (BRIC) was first described by Summerskill and Walshe (1). The clinical picture of this disease consists of multiple episodes of cholestatic jaundice without extrahepatic bile duct obstruction. The duration of an episode of jaundice varies from weeks to months. In the anicteric period, liver function tests are normal, and the histology of the liver is also normal or shows only minimal reactive changes and/or mild fibrosis. Familial and nonfamilial forms of BRIC have been described (2). The mechanisms by which episodes of cholestasis are initiated and the factors involved in the maintenance of cholestasis are not known. Altered bile acid metabolism has been claimed to play a role in the pathophysiology of this disease (3,4).

BRIC has no characteristic geographical distribution (5). It is occasionally encountered in Korea also. Cholestatic cases, as described in this chapter, are often mistaken in Korea for cases of primary biliary cirrhosis or sclerosing cholangitis.

The author presents the morphological and biochemical findings of one typical example from among the cases with BRIC. To provide better understanding of the significance of observations on BRIC of undetermined origin, the findings were compared with those of two cases with persistent cholestatic jaundice of unknown etiology, and of another two HBsAg carriers with BRIC.

I. Benign recurrent intrahepatic cholestasis of undetermined origin

Case. A 27-year-old male patient had been suffering from jaundice, itching, fatigue and mild fever for a month preceding his admission to St. Mary's Hospital. (Table 11-1). This episode of jaundice was his third.

Ten years before the admission, he had had an operation for gastric ulcer perforation and, five years before the admission (first episode), he had had the first bout of icterus and itching which lasted for almost three months but disappeared spontaneously. Two years before the admission (second episode), the patient had suffered from jaundice with itching which disappeared spontaneously two months later. There was no history of liver disease or jaundice among his family members. The patient had no history of toxic drug ingestion.

Physical examination revealed deep jaundice and there were scratch wounds resulting from severe itching. The liver was palpable one finger breadth under the right costal margin, showing soft consistency and a smooth surface. There was no pressure tenderness of the liver and the spleen was not palpable. The other findings of physical examinations were normal.

The serum total bilirubin was 28.1 mg/100ml (direct bilirubin 12.0 mg/100ml), the total cholesterol 163 mg/100ml, the serum aspartate aminotransferase (SAST) level 104 units and the serum alanine aminotransferase (SALT) level 99 units (Table 11-1). The serum alkaline phosphatase activity showed 39.9 King-Armstrong (KA) units. HBsAg was negative.

On the seventh day of admission, endoscopic retrograde cholangio-pancreatography (ERCP) was done. No obstruction was seen in the main bile duct. A liver scintigram was normal except for slight enlargement of the liver. No bile duct enlargement was evidenced by liver sonography.

The conspicuously elevated serum bilirubin level at the time of admission on Sept. 23, 1985, (third episode) declined to the normal range at the end of the third month of hospitalization. However, since then, it slowly rose again and reached a peak on May 11, 1986 (fourth episode). The serum bilirubin level again fell to the normal range two months after the peak but, thereafter, there were two mild and short episodes (fifth and sixth)—five months (Oct. 1987) and 13 months (June 1988) respectively, after the fourth peak. The direct bilirubin levels were usually high but they were lower than half of the total bilirubin levels.

Concomitant peak elevation of serum alkaline phosphatase activity occurred. Peaks of the aminotransferase activity appeared before and after the peaks of the bilirubin level but aminotransferase ranges were slightly low considering the high levels of bilirubin.

A needle liver biopsy was performed on Oct. 2, 1985, during the third episode of cholestasis. The principal histologic changes observed during the acute attack were predominantly centrilobular necrosis and cholestasis (Fig.

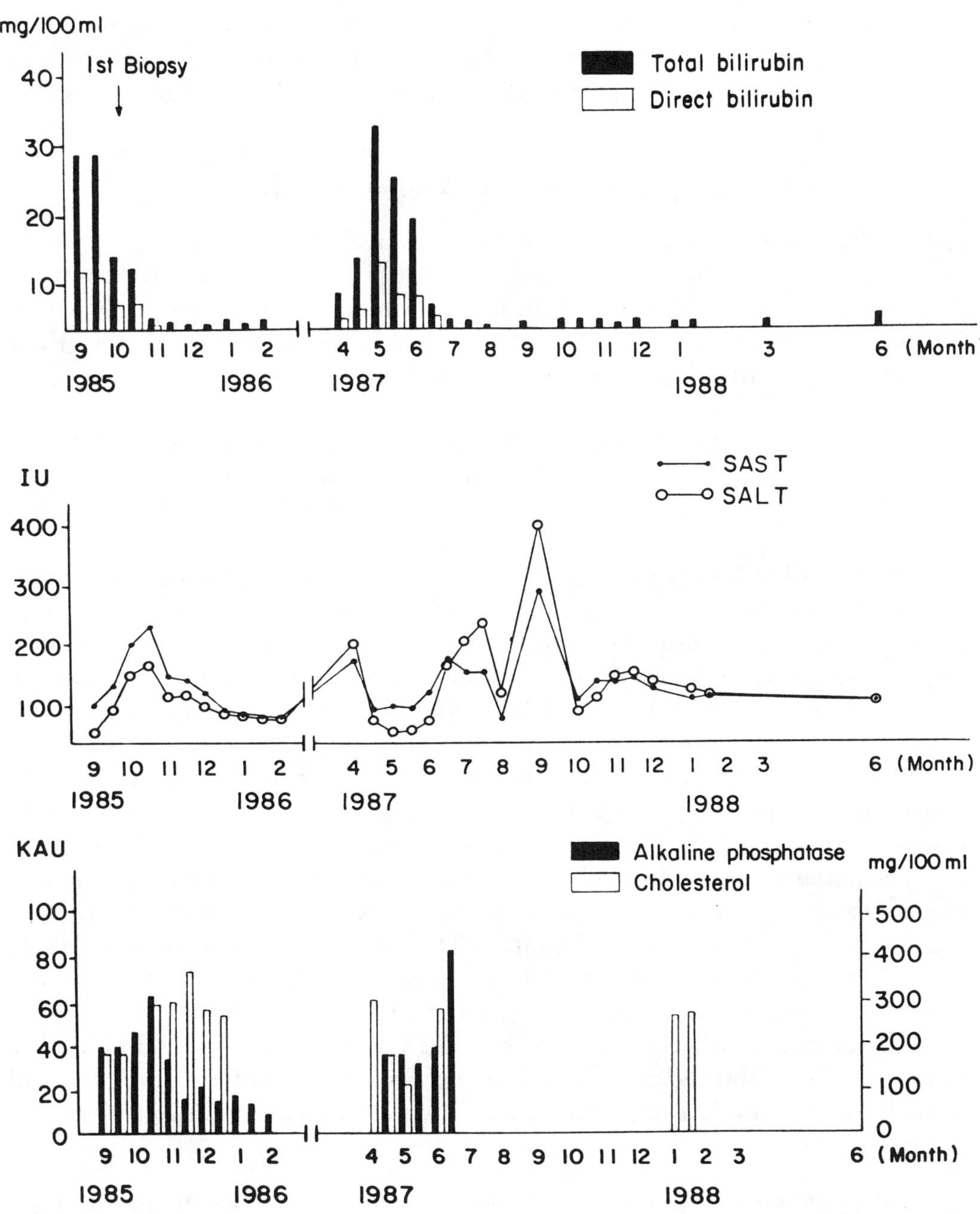

Table 11-1. Biochemical Follow-up Studies of a Case with Benign Recurrent Intrahepatic Cholestasis

143, see page 117). The outstanding cholestatic feature was accumulation of bile pigment in hepatocytes, Kupffer cells and bile plugs in the bile canaliculi. Inflammatory infiltrate with mononuclear cells and neutrophil granulocytes and a few eosinophiles were observed in the edematous portal tracts. Cholangioles were destroyed and bile ductules were hardly seen in the portal tracts.

II. Persistent intrahepatic cholestasis of undetermined origin

In the case of BRIC presented above, episodes of cholestasis lasting for two to three months followed by a process of recovery were repeated. By contrast, there were instances of severe cholestasis of undetermined origin persisting for more than six months, even for several years. In order to document their biochemical and histologic entities, two cases are described below.

Reversible case. A 47-year-old male was admitted because of deep jaundice and severe itching. He had complained of easy fatigue, persistent jaundice with itching that lasted for 45 days preceding the admission. He had clay-colored stool.

The bilirubin level was high during the two-month period of hospitalization fluctuating between 17 mg—32 mg/100ml. The direct bilirubin level was usually more than half the total bilirubin. By comparison, the aminotransferase activities were always low, not exceeding 100 units. However, the serum alkaline phosphatase activities were always higher than 20 KA, paralleling the bilirubin level.

Mild diffuse narrowing of intra- and extra-hepatic bile ducts without disturbance of the bile passage was evidenced by ERCP. No drugs which could possibly induce cholestasis had been taken before the onset of the illness.

The patient was discharged from the hospital two months after the admission, with no sign of recovery from jaundice. Thereafter, he was treated with ursodeoxycholic acid for two months. The jaundice gradually reversed to normal and the bilirubin level declined to the normal range. Thus, the cholestatic jaundice persisted for six months and finally subsided.

A liver needle biopsy was performed 22 days after the admission. The biopsy specimen showed conspicuous cholestasis in the centrilobular area and some inflammation in the portal space. Bile duct proliferation was absent in the portal tract.

Intractable case. A 29-year-old woman was first seen at Wonju Presbyterian Hospital in July 1988 with jaundice, deep but without pruritus (Table 11-2). The disease had begun in May 1988. The patient had no history of allergy, drug exposure, hepatitis or transfusion. Physical examination revealed icterus in the skin and sclerae. The edge of the liver was blunted, smooth and a little tender. The biochemical data were: serum bilirubin, total 12.9 mg/100ml and direct 8.0 mg/100ml; serum alkaline phosphatase 104 KA units; serum total cholesterol 244 mg/100ml; serum albumin 3.6 gm/100ml and globulin 4.4 gm/100ml; SAST 244 units and SALT 250 units. There was no antimitochondrial antibody. Large bile duct obstruction was not seen in ERCP. Splenomegaly was revealed by sonography.

A liver needle biopsy was done on Aug. 9, 1988. The biopsy specimen was referred for consultation to the Armed Forces Institute of Pathology in Washington D.C., which reported that the histologic features were suggestive of a type of primary biliary cirrhosis (Figs. 144, 145, 146, 147, see page 117).

Thereafter, she had herbal medicine for two months, but the disease progressed.

In January of 1989, she was admitted again, this time to Koryo University's Kuro Hospital, because of jaundice. Physical examination revealed hepatosplenomegaly but spider, edema, ascites and xanthomatous change were not seen.

The blood picture indicated slight anemia with the level of hemoglobin standing at 11.2 gm/100ml. There were occasional target erythrocytes. HBsAg and anti-HCV were negative. Antimitochondrial antibody tests were repeated but were always negative.

The biochemical data were: serum bilirubin, total 17 mg/100ml, direct 12 mg/100ml; serum alkaline phosphatase 54.1 KA units; total serum cholesterol 808 mg/100ml; SAST 147 units and SALT 96 units; serum albumin 3.2 gm/100ml and globulin 4.3 gm/100ml; serum copper 200 ug/100ml and serum ceruloplasmin 61 mg/100ml.

ERCP was performed again but no abnormality was noted in the main bile duct. No esophageal varices were found by gastroscopy.

The second liver biopsy was performed on Feb. 1990. The histologic findings were almost similar to those of the first, with only the inflammatory cells showing more sparse infiltration (Fig. 148, see page 117).

As shown in Table 11-2, the biochemical abnormalities persisted without significant interval changes until Jan. 1990, despite treatment with prednisolone or ursodeoxycholic acid.

She was hospitalized for the third time in July 1990, this time at Severance Hospital, because of multiple cranial nerve palsy in addition to jaundice. The abnormal levels of blood chemistries, including bilirubin, transferases, cholesterol, alkaline phosphatase, γ-glutamyl transpeptidase and serum proteins, remained unchanged during the follow-up period. HBsAg, anti-HCV and antimitochondrial antibody were negative but the immunoglobulin M increased a little above the upper border of normal.

An abdominal sonogram revealed gallstone and ascites. A computerized tomogram of the brain showed no abnormality. There was no definite elec-

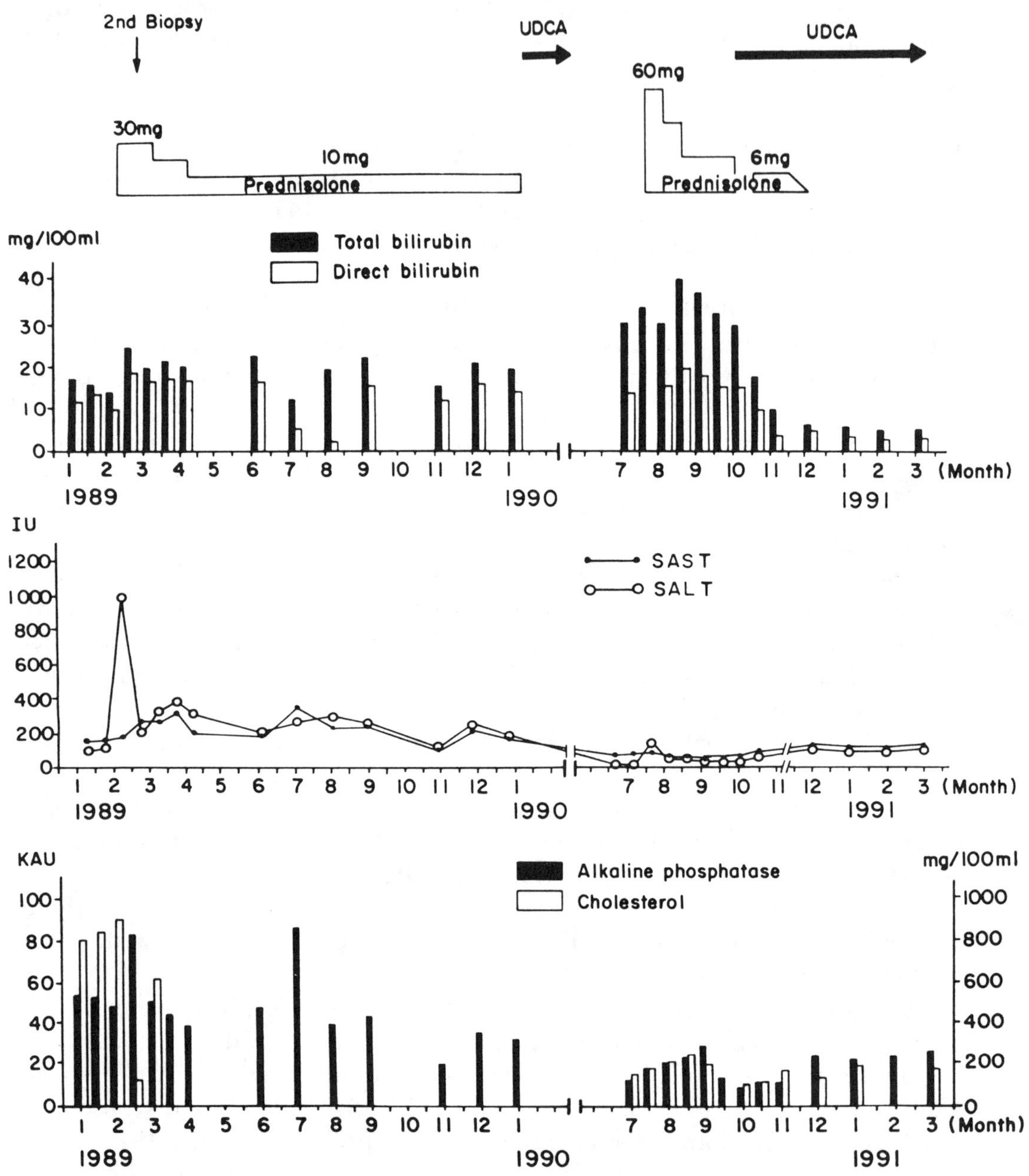

Table 11-2. Biochemical Follow-up Studies of a Case with Intractable Persistent Intrahepatic Cholestasis

trophysiologic evidence of peripheral neuropathy. She was then subjected to prednisolone and ursodeoxycholic acid therapy until early December, 1990. Thereafter, the serum bilirubin declined to 4.3 mg/100ml. The serum cholesterol level and the serum alkaline phosphatase activity declined to the normal ranges. The cranial nerve palsy improved also but there was still mild dysarthria persisting at the time of discharge. (This case was provided by Dr. C. H. Lee, Kuro Hospital and Dr. J. B. Chung, Severance Hospital).

From the biopsy findings, she was suspected of having primary biliary cirrhosis. However, in primary biliary cirrhosis, the absence of mitochondrial antibody and high bilirubinemia with central cholestasis persisting for more than two years following the onset are unusual.

Whether the idiopathic multiple cranial nerve palsy syndrome is related to such a cholestatic syndrome or not is not clear.

The cholestatic syndrome of undetermined origin, regardless of its course being recurrent or persistent, is characterized as follows: 1. Jaundice is pronounced with biochemical signs of cholestasis. 2. Bile pigments in hepatocytes, Kupffer cells and bile plugs in the bile canaliculi occur usually in the centrilobular area. 3. Ducts and ductules are usually absent in needle biopsy. 4. No obstruction is seen in the main bile duct on ERCP. 5. Factors known to produce intrahepatic cholestasis, such as drugs, pregnancy or hepatitis B virus infection or positivity of antimitochondrial antibody, are absent.

Thus, these three types suggest that the spectrum of cholestasis syndrome of undetermined origin in Korea ranges from benign recurrent to intractable persistent. Further investigation may be needed to clarify whether these three types of cholestasis are of the same origin or of different etiologies.

III. Recurrent intrahepatic cholestasis in HBsAg carriers

In Korea, HBsAg carriers are quite common and hepatitis B is superimposed on with other illnesses. Accordingly, when recurrent jaundice occurs in HBsAg-positive cases, whether it is BRIC of undetermined origin or the result of reactivation of hepatitis B, it is sometimes difficult to define. Two cases of type-B chronic hepatitis with recurrent jaundice resembling BRIC are introduced below in an attempt to present an analysis of differences between the former and the latter.

Case 1. A 24-year-old man was hospitalized because of the presence of HBsAg and HBeAg in his blood and elevated serum aminotransferases on screening. Two successive peaks of serum bilirubin levels associated with increased serum aminotransferase activities occurred during the two years and six months after the first admission—the first peak one month after the first admission and the second 17 months after the first (Table 11-3). The serum bilirubin elevations were mild while the serum aminotransferase activities were quite high.

Two biopsies were done 16 months apart. The first biopsy was performed one month after the recovery from the first episode and the second during the second peak. The first biopsy specimen showed nonspecific reactive hepatitis, and the second exhibited very active cholestatic hepatitis showing hepatic cell degeneration and pericellular infiltration with acute and chronic inflammatory cells (Fig. 149, see page 118). When last seen 15 years after the second biopsy, the patient appeared healthy with no sequelae.

Case 2. A 19-year-old man was admitted to St. Mary's Hospital because of dark urine and jaundice. He had been healthy up until ten days prior to the admission. He denied previous jaundice. He had mildly icteric sclerae. The liver edge was palpable two cm under the right costal margin and minimally tender. At the time of the admission, the serum bilirubin was 4 mg/100ml with 1.6 mg/100ml of direct bilirubin. The SAST was 1500 units, the SALT 1320 units, the serum alkaline phosphatase 5 KA units and the serum total cholesterol 132 mg/100ml. HBsAg and HBeAg were positive. The serum bilirubin declined to the normal range one month after the hospitalization, but then rose and reached a peak just one year after the first episode.

After the admission, the SAST activity rose sharply, reaching as high as 1500u, and later returned to near normal. Thereafter, it rose slowly again and in parallel with the second peak of the bilirubin level. After the second peak, the bilirubin level and the aminotransferase activity slowly declined to the normal range. However, the alkaline phosphatase and the cholesterol level steadily remained in the normal range from the beginning.

Two liver biopsies were performed, the first two months after the first bout and the second during the second bout. The first biopsy specimen showed nonspecific reactive hepatitis, and the second revealed cholestatic hepatitis in association with degeneration of hepatic cells and pericellular infiltration of acute and chronic inflammatory cells (active cholestatic pericellular hepatitis) (Fig. 150, see page 118).

When the patient was last seen 14 years after the second biopsy, it appeared that complete healing occurred and no sequelae developed.

The two cases mentioned above are HBsAg carriers with benign recurrent intrahepatic cholestasis. Comparison of the clinical and biological findings of these two cases with those of the three cases of recurrent or persistent intrahepatic cholestasis of unknown origin, described earlier in this chapter, re-

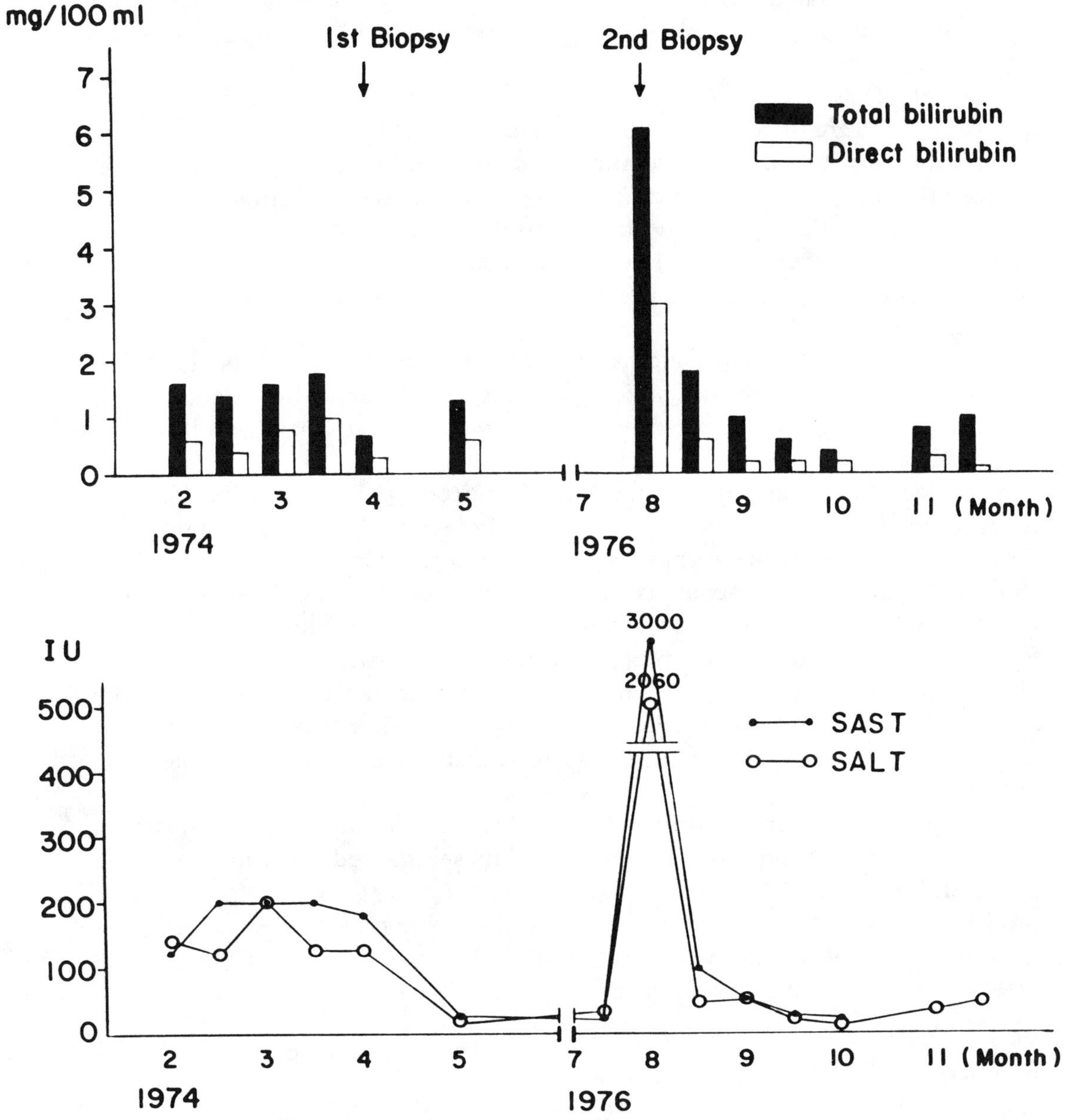

Table 11-3. Biochemical Follow-up Studies of a Case with Recurrent Intrahepatic Cholestasis in a HBsAg Carrier

vealed that the former had a lower bilirubin level, a higher serum aminotransferase level, a shorter duration of hyperbilirubinemia and a longer anicteric phase. Even at its peak, the bilirubin level did not exceed 6.5 mg/100ml, but the serum aminotransferase activity was extremely high, exceeding 2,000 units.

In both HBsAg carriers, serum alkaline phosphatase and the total cholesterol levels remained in the normal range. When hyperbilirubinemia was absent, the biopsy findings were almost normal and, when the bilirubin level reached its peak, the biopsy findings of these two cases were very similar, both showing cholestatic hepatitis with pericellular inflammatory cell infiltration. Thus, the episodic elevation of serum bilirubin is presumed to result from acute bouts of parenchymal necroinflammation, probably due to hepatitis B virus infection.

In presenting the histologic features of these cases, the author feels that convincing evaluation of this histologic evolution is somewhat weakened by the absence of histologic pictures of the first acute attack, as well as the convalescent stage of the second episode.

The reason is that the author failed to produce histologic evidence of recovery at the anicteric phase from acute cholestatic intercellular hepatitis. Fortunately, however, the author recently encountered an HBsAg carrier with cholestatic intercellular hepatitis that showed reversible histologic evolution.

The HBsAg carrier recovered after an episode of cholestasis lasting four months. A liver needle biopsy was performed on the patient at the cholestatic phase, and another biopsy was conducted at the anicteric phase following the cholestasis. The first biopsy revealed active cholestatic pericellular hepatitis. In the second biopsy, the greater part of the specimen was nearly normal, indicating recovery.

The primary finding of active cholestatic intercellular (pericellular) hepatitis was acute inflammation, predominated by segmented neutrophiles in the intercellular space.

Thus, these findings are clear evidence that the irregularities of the histologic pattern, due to intercellular inflammation at the stage of cholestasis, cease to exist at the anicteric phase.

Summary

Morphological and biochemical findings of a case with benign recurrent intrahepatic cholestasis (BRIC) of undetermined origin were described. In addition, to help the reader understand better the significance of observations on BRIC, the findings were compared with those of two cases of persistent cholestasis and two HBsAg carriers with BRIC.

1. The pathological changes, observed during an attack in the liver of a

patient with benign recurrent intrahepatic cholestasis and in the liver of two patients with persistent cholestasis of undetermined origin were similar, with centrilobular bile stasis and portal mononuclear cell infiltration. The ducts or ductules in the portal tracts were destroyed and usually absent in needle biopsy specimens. In the persistent forms, particularly long-standing and intractable kind, chronic sequelae, such as portal fibrosis, were observed.

Thus, the three cases of cholestasis of unknown origin were presumed to represent a spectrum of cholestasis, ranging from a mild recurrent to a long-standing persistent form.

2. By comparison, HBsAg carrier patients with recurrent cholestasis showed a lower bilirubin level, higher aminotransferase activity, a shorter duration of hyperbilirubinemia and a longer interval between episodes than cases with BRIC of unknown origin.

In HBsAg carriers, the serum alkaline phosphatase activities and the total serum cholesterol levels remained in the normal range, while the levels were extremely high in cases with cholestasis of undetermined origin.

3. The pathologic features of recurrent cholestasis in HBsAg carriers, observed during attack, included acute episodic parenchymal degeneration and pericellular infiltration with acute and chronic inflammatory cells. The biopsy findings during silent intervals between cholestatic episodes appeared nearly normal.

4. These limited observations suggest that ursodeoxycholic acid may be effective in therapy for the cholestatic syndrome of unknown origin.

References

1. Summerskill, W.H.J and Walshe, J.M. Benign recurrent intrahepatic "obstructive" jaundice. Lancet 1: 1171–1172, 1960.

2. Van Berge Henegouwen, G.P., Ferguson, D.R., Hofmann, A.F. and De Pagter, A.G.F. Familial and nonfamilial benign recurrent cholestasis distinguished by plasma disappearance of indocyanine green but not cholyglycine. Gut 19: 345–349, 1978.

3. Van Berge Henegouwen, G.P., Brandt, K.H. and De Pagter, A.G.F. Is an acute disturbance in hepatic transport of bile acids the primary cause of cholestasis in benign recurrent intrahepatic cholestasis? Lancet 1: 1249–1251, 1974.

4. Summerfield, J.A., Kirk, A.P., Chitranukroh, A. and Billing, B.H. A distinctive pattern of serum bile acid and bilirubin concentrations in benign recurrent intrahepatic cholestasis. Hepatogastroenterology 28: 139–142, 1981.

5. Beaudoin, M., Feldman, G., Erlinger, S. and Benhamou, J.P. Benign recurrent cholestasis. Digestion 9: 49–65, 1973.

Legends

Fig. 143. A liver needle biopsy was performed during the icteric phase in a case with benign recurrent intrahepatic cholestasis (BRIC) of undetermined origin.

A higher magnification of the central zone (CV) shows centrizonal parenchymal degeneration and necrosis and accumulation of bile pigment in ballooned liver cells (arrows) and activated Kupffer cells. Needle biopsy, HE, ×200.

Fig. 144. A biopsy specimen obtained from a case with intractable persistent cholestasis of undetermined origin.

The first liver biopsy specimen, obtained three months after the onset of jaundice, shows central vein (CV) phlebitis and perivenular zonal necrosis and mild collapse with a little inflammation. Conspicuous cholestasis is noted. Needle biopsy, HE, ×100.

Fig. 145.

Mononuclear cells are accumulated in the expanded and somewhat sclerotic portal tracts (PS). Well-preserved proximal biliary trees are not seen in the two enlarged portal tracts. Needle biopsy, HE, ×100.

Fig. 146.

An enlarged portal space with accumulation of acute and chronic inflammatory cells is demonstrated. Young inflammatory septal fibrosis extends from the portal tract into the parenchyma. There are no bile ductules or ducts. Needle biopsy, trichrome, ×200.

Fig. 147.

There are intralobular accumulation of foamy histiocytes and irregularly arranged cuboidal cells(arrows) that look like proliferated bile duct epithelial cells. Needle biopsy, trichrome, ×400.

Fig. 148.

The second biopsy specimen shows intralobular accumulation of xanthomatous histiocytes. Needle biopsy, HE, ×400.

Fig. 149. Liver biopsy specimens obtained from an HBsAg carrier with BRIC.

The second biopsy was done during the second attack. The hepatocytes are swollen, degenerated and isolated by intercellular acute and chronic inflammatory cell infiltration and hemorrhage. Some hepatocytes are imbibed with bile pigments (arrows). Needle biopsy, HE, ×200.

Fig. 150. Liver biopsies were performed on an HBsAg carrier with BRIC.

The second biopsy was done during the second episode of jaundice. The biopsy findings are almost similar to those shown in Fig. 149. Needle biopsy, HE, ×200.

12 MILIARY TUBERCULOSIS OF THE LIVER

Whan Kook Chung, M.D., Ph.D.

Before the wide use of biopsy, the liver had seldom been considered to be a site of tuberculous involvement, except in cases of acute secondary miliary tuberculosis or terminal hematogenous dissemination in far advanced pulmonary tuberculosis (1,2,3). The primary involvement of tuberculosis in the liver had been considered rare and had usually been regarded as undiagnosable except by laparotomy or postmortem examination. However, the popular use of the needle biopsy procedure has changed this concept.

Furthermore, the use of liver biopsy procedure has broadened the knowledge of the histologic appearance of the liver with miliary tuberculosis.

Clinical significance of liver biopsy

In miliary tuberculosis, with or without pulmonary involvement, clinical evidence of hepatic injury is slight except for occasional hepatomegaly (4). Abnormal serum aminotransferase activity complicates or dominates the picture in rare instances of miliary tuberculosis. In such instances, with hepatomegaly or abnormal aminotransferase activity, liver biopsy is very helpful for the diagnosis of miliary tuberculosis. In some cases, miliary dissemination involves only the liver, spleen and portal lymph nodes in association with fever (4). In these forms, liver biopsy is of particular advantage and may provide the only clue to undiagnosed febrile conditions, leading to immediate and life-saving specific antituberculosis therapy.

Over many decades, the author performed needle biopsies on Korean patients who had undiagnosed hepatomegaly, continuation of fever of undetermined origin and abnormal serum aminotransferase activity of unknown origin (anicteric hepatitis of unknown origin), in order to establish the disease entities. Needle biopsy was also conducted on cases suspected of miliary tuberculosis through chest X-ray findings to discover hepatic dissemination and, if found, to see the histologic pattern.

Among the cases, 11 were thought to be cases of miliary tuberculosis: three of undiagnosed hepatomegaly, two of fever of undetermined origin, two of unknown origin of anicteric hepatitis, and four associated with pulmonary miliary tuberculosis.

In the cases of tuberculosis, histologic alterations of the liver resulted either from tuberculosis in other organs (5) or from tuberculous granulation tissue within the liver. Of the 11 patients, ten had extrahepatic organ tuberculosis before biopsy; four had miliary tuberculosis in the lung (one had miliary tuberculosis combined with bone tuberculosis), one minimal pulmonary tuberculosis, one far advanced pulmonary tuberculosis and four tuberculous pleurisy and/or peritonitis (Table 12-1). Extrahepatic involvement of tuberculosis was not identified in one patient with hepatosplenomegaly.

Laboratory findings

Results of hepatic tests were erratic (Table 12-2).

No abnormality was found in the serum bilirubin level. Serum protein contents and alkaline phosphatase activities were often abnormal but showed slight elevation. Serum aminotransferase activities slightly increased in four cases.

Histologic analysis of biopsy specimens

Histologic analysis was made of biopsy specimens obtained from the liver of 11 patients with miliary tuberculosis and the results recorded (Table 12-3).

Nonspecific reactive hepatitis was frequently accompanied by irregular hepatocellular damage, small areas of focal necrosis, diffuse Kupffer cell activation and portal inflammation. This alteration was observed in all the patients studied. However, hepatic lesion was sometimes characteristic even in the absence of tubercles in the specimen. Focal Kupffer cell proliferation was noted, which occluded the lumens of the sinusoids, leading to compression and disappearance of hepatic cells between two sinusoids (Fig. 151, see page 118). Small nodules containing histiocytic elements (retothelial nodules) were

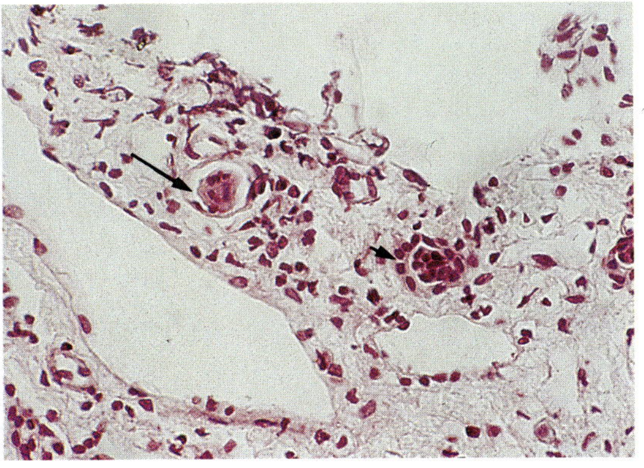

Fig. 167 See Legend page 175.

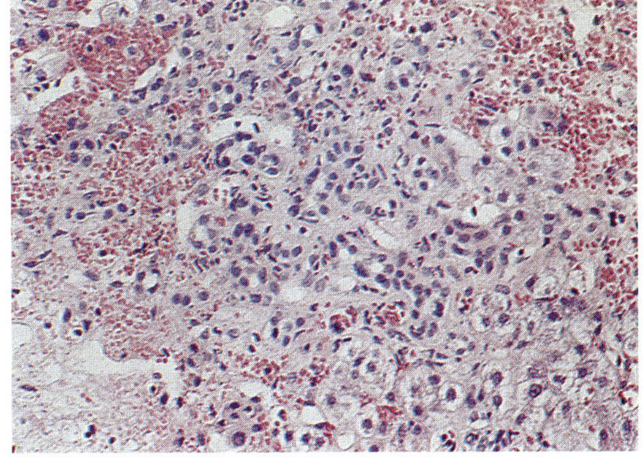

Fig. 168 See Legend page 184.

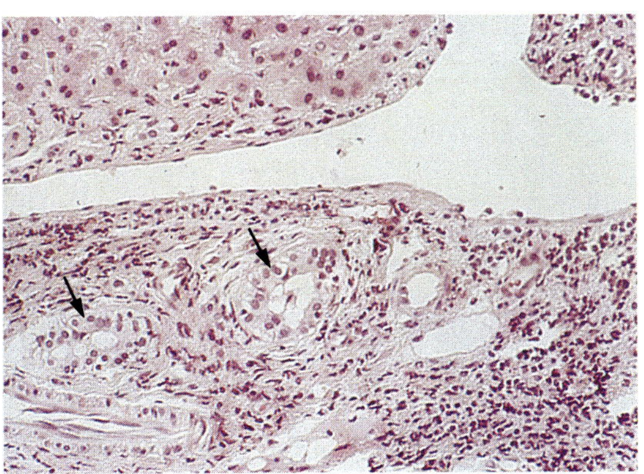

Fig. 169 See Legend page 184.

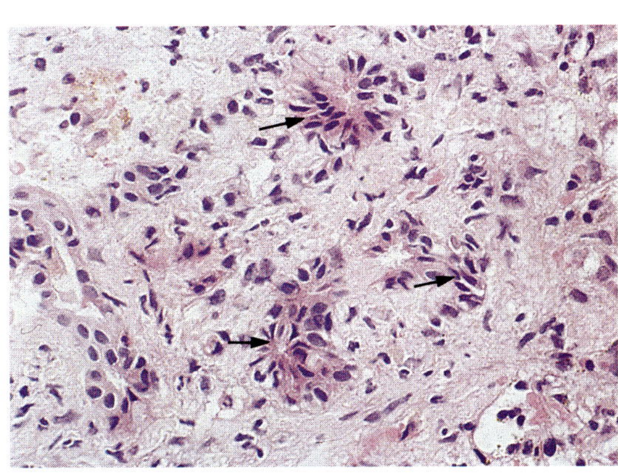

Fig. 170 See Legend page 184.

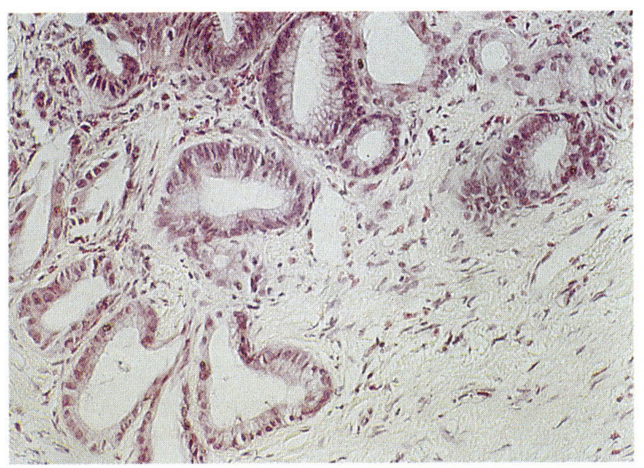

Fig. 171 See Legend page 184.

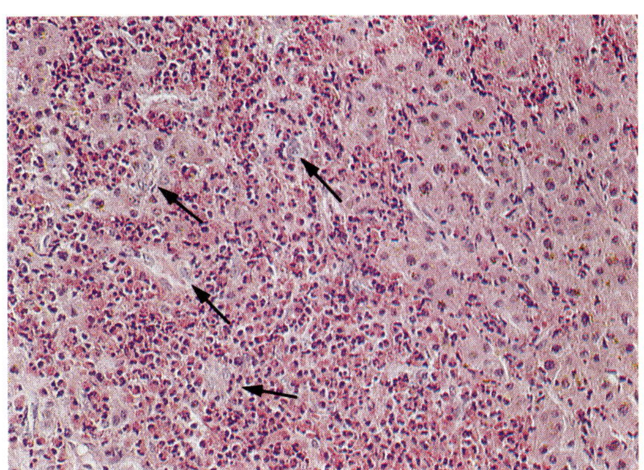

Fig. 172 See Legend page 185.

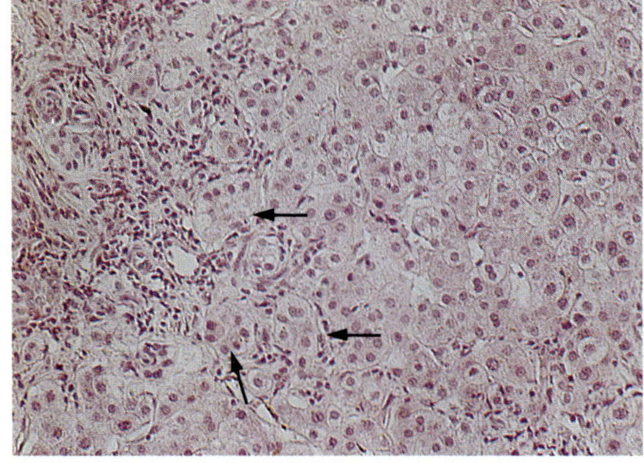

Fig. 173 See Legend page 185.

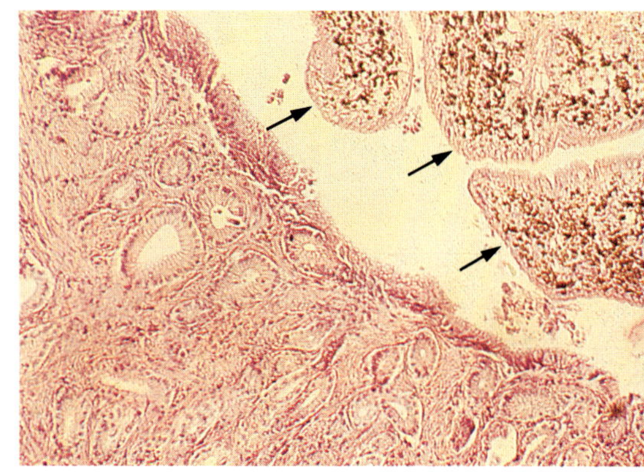

Fig. 174 See Legend page 185.

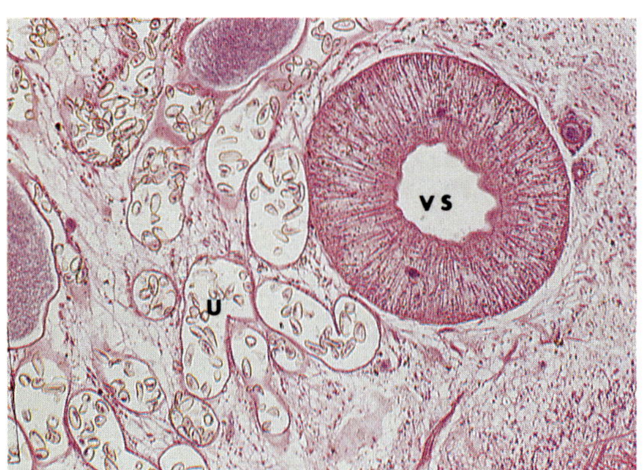

Fig. 175 See Legend page 185.

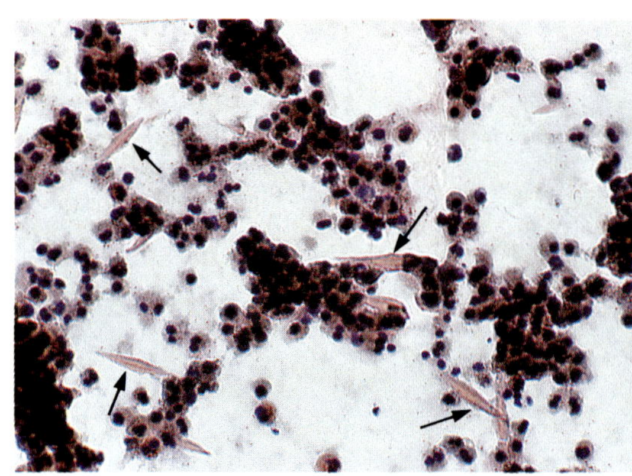

Fig. 176 See Legend page 185.

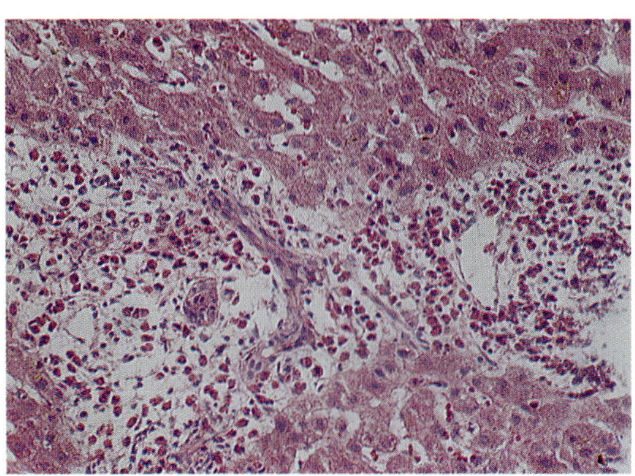

Fig. 177 See Legend page 185.

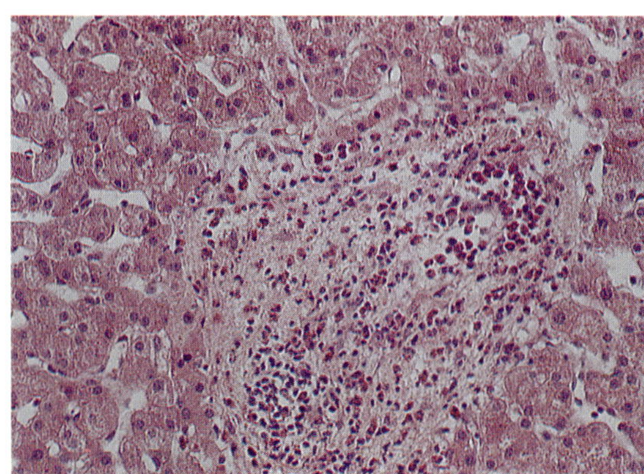

Fig. 178 See Legend page 185.

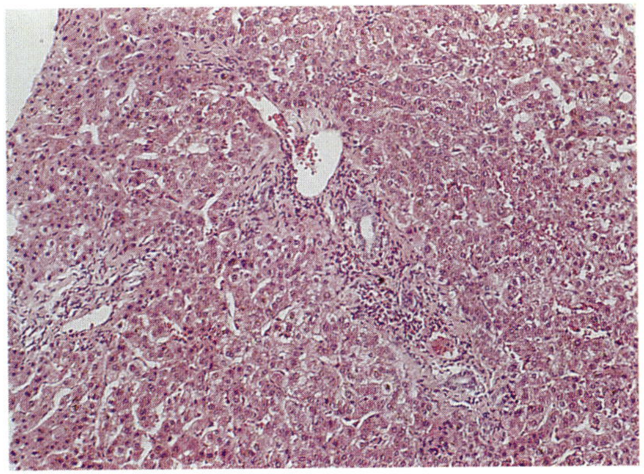

Fig. 179 See Legend page 185.

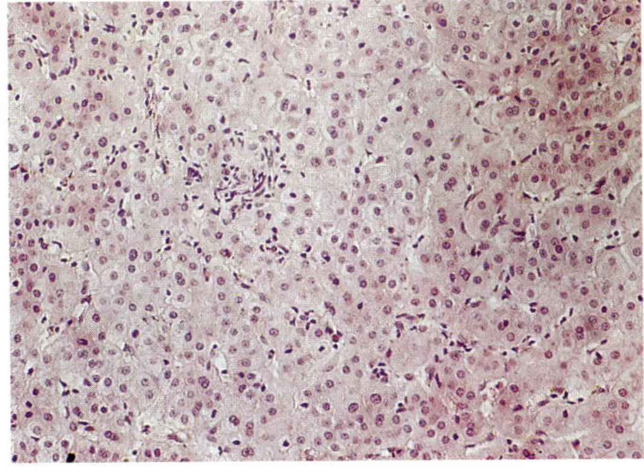

Fig. 180 See Legend page 185.

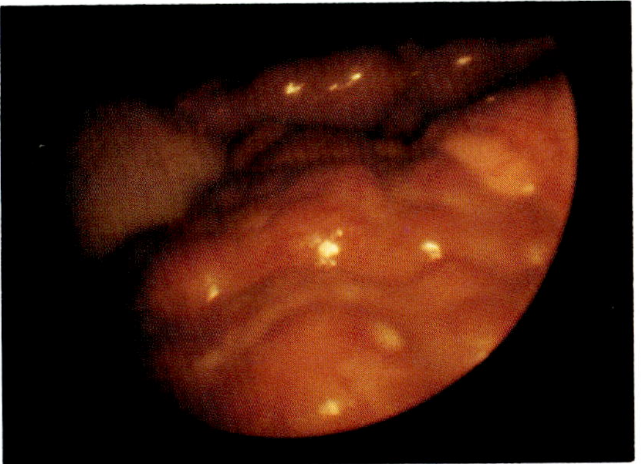

Fig. 181 See Legend page 185.

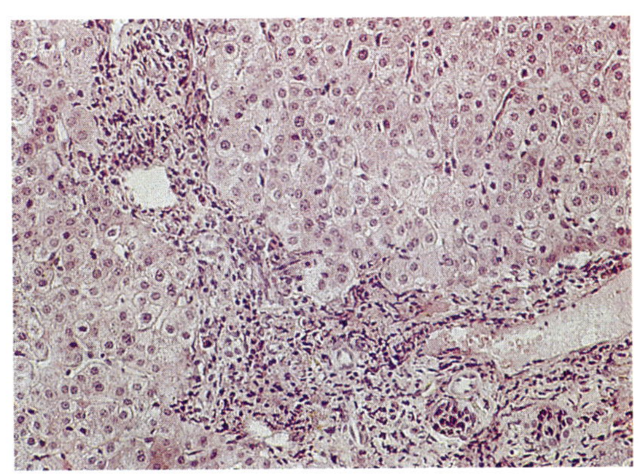

Fig. 182 See Legend page 185.

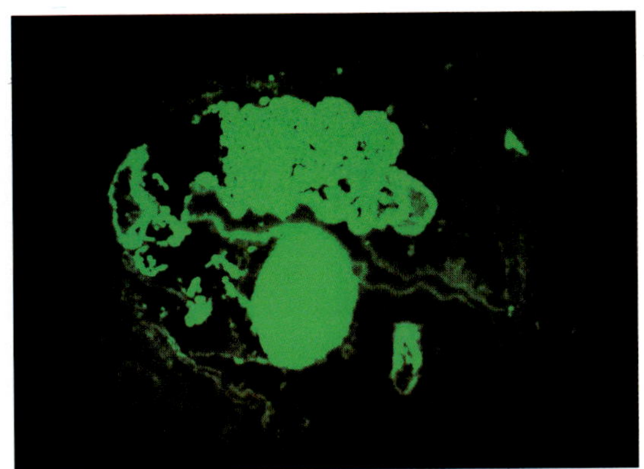

Fig. 183 See Legend page 186.

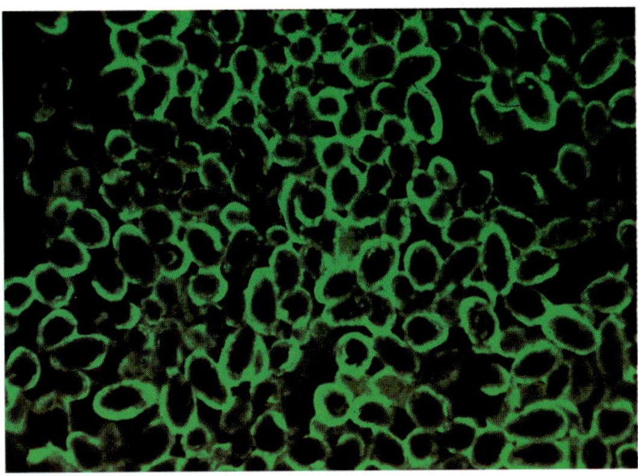

Fig. 184 See Legend page 186.

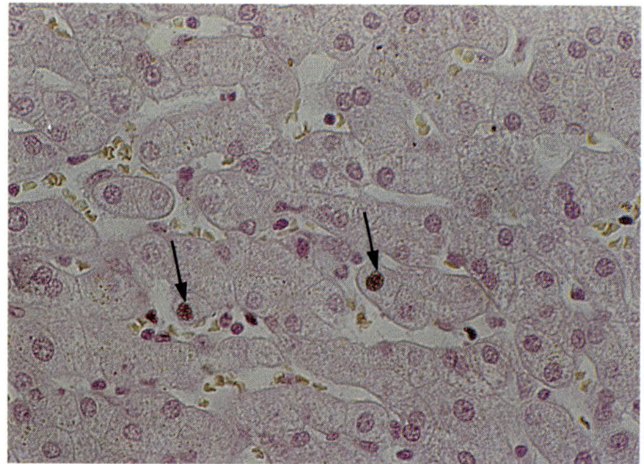

Fig. 185 See Legend page 190.

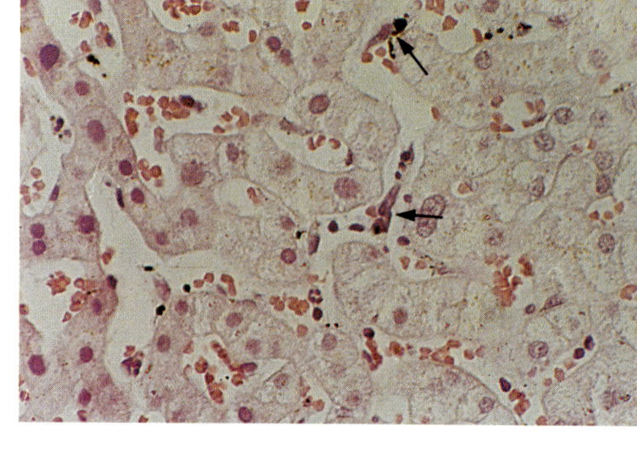

Fig. 186 See Legend page 191.

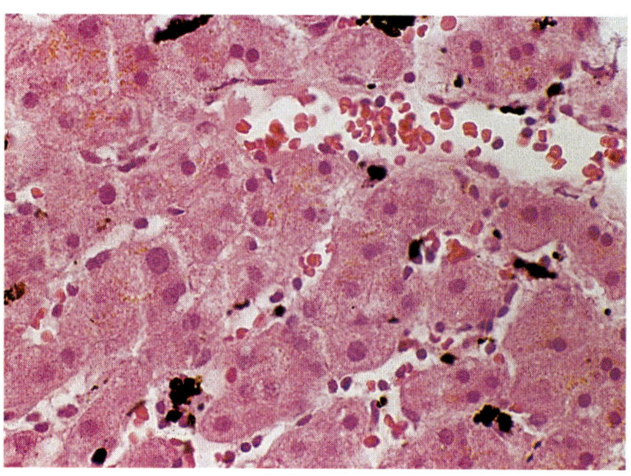

Fig. 187 See Legend page 191.

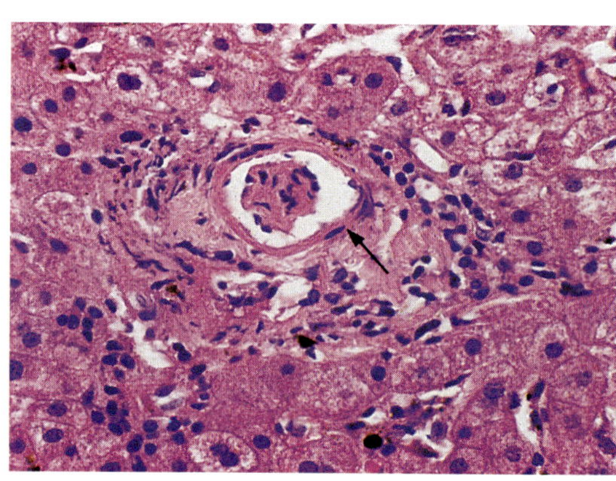

Fig. 188 See Legend page 191.

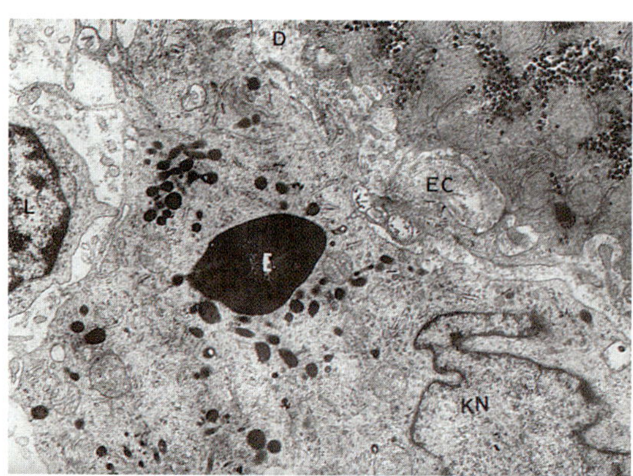

Fig. 189 See Legend page 191.

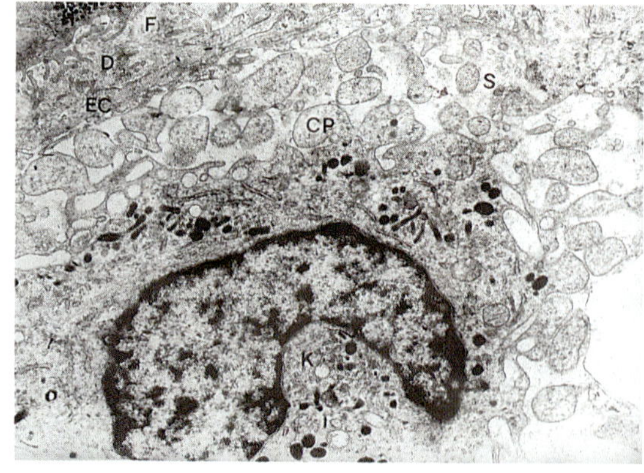

Fig. 190 See Legend page 191.

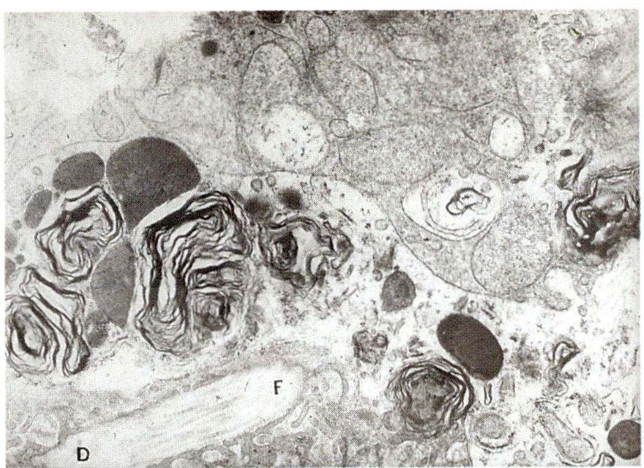

Fig. 191 See Legend page 191.

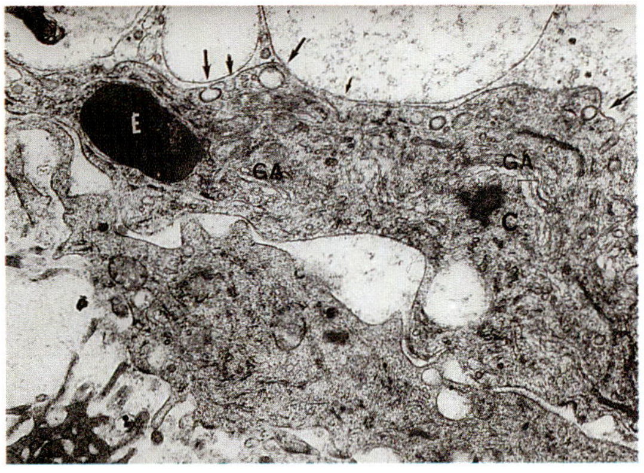

Fig. 192 See Legend page 191.

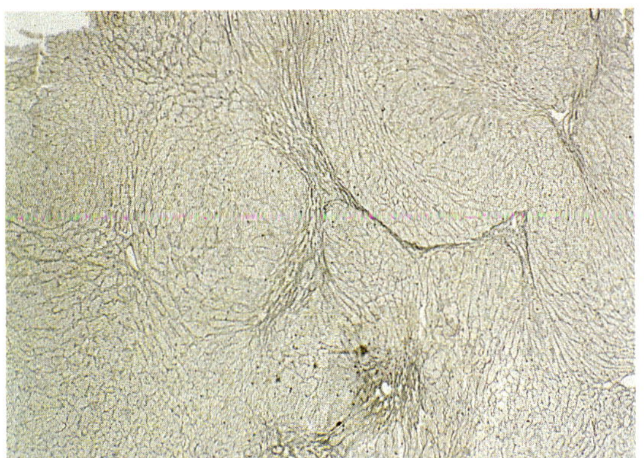

Fig. 193 See Legend page 198.

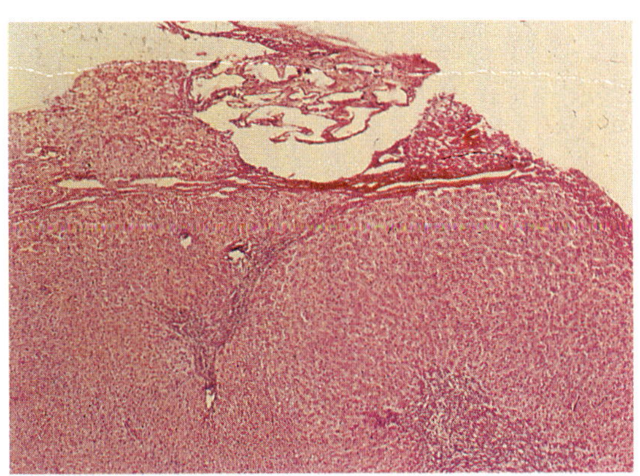

Fig. 194 See Legend page 198.

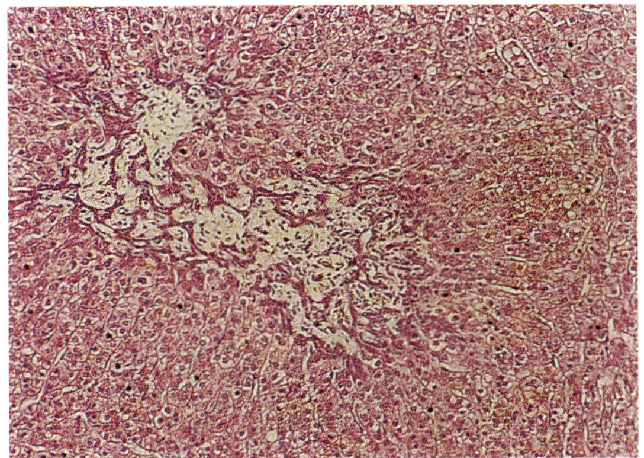

Fig. 195 See Legend page 198.

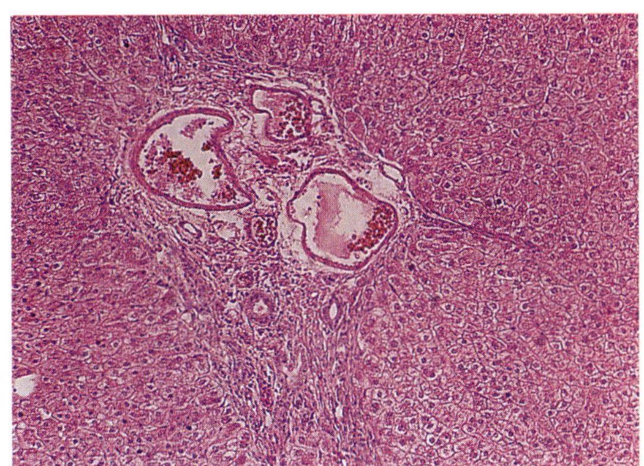

Fig. 196 See Legend page 198.

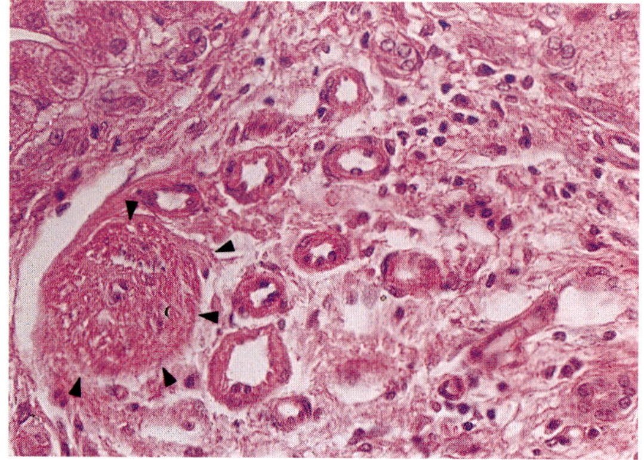

Fig. 197 See Legend page 199.

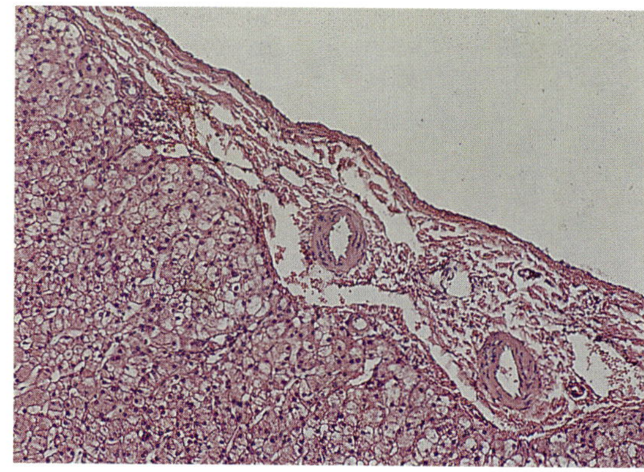

Fig. 198 See Legend page 199.

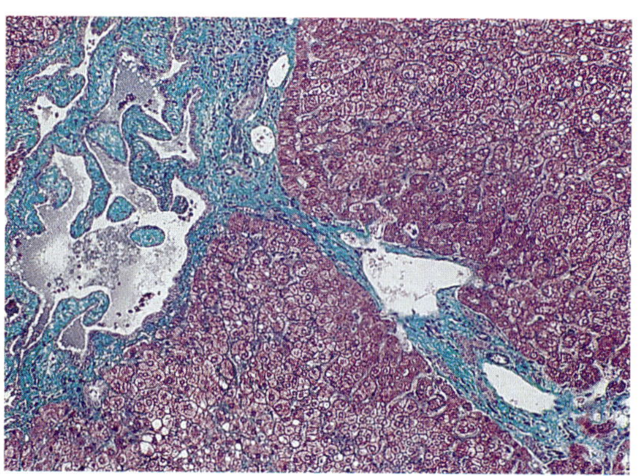

Fig. 199 See Legend page 199.

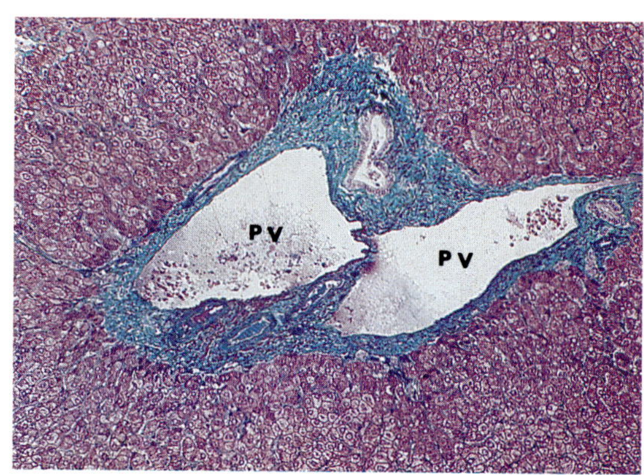

Fig. 200 See Legend page 199.

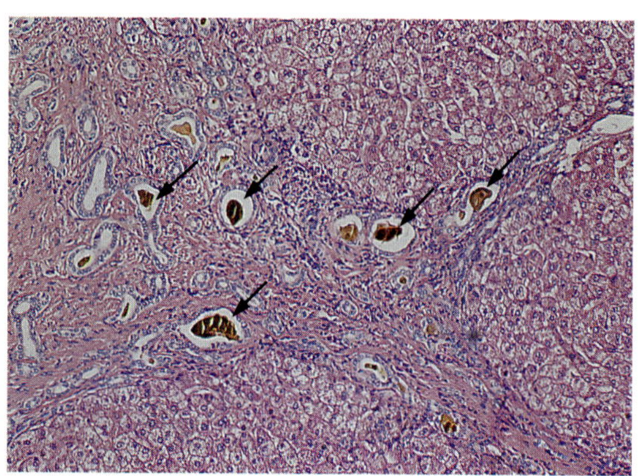

Fig. 201 See Legend page 199.

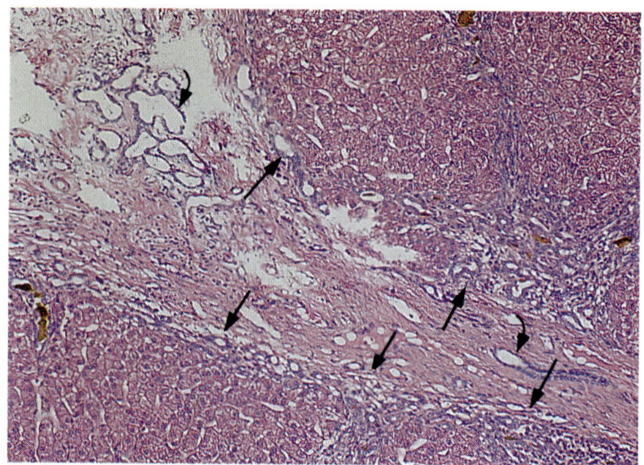

Fig. 202 See Legend page 199.

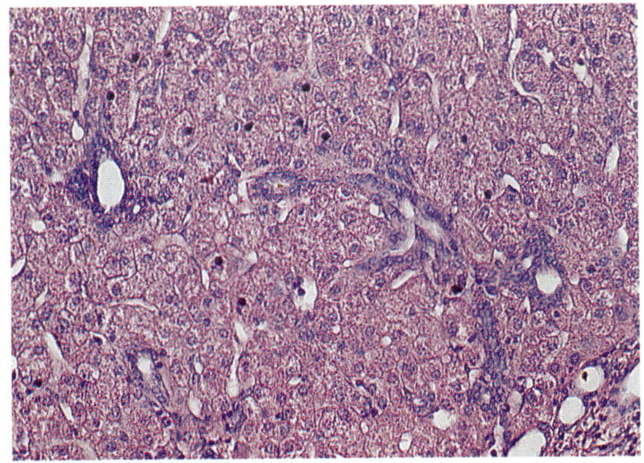

Fig. 203 See Legend page 199.

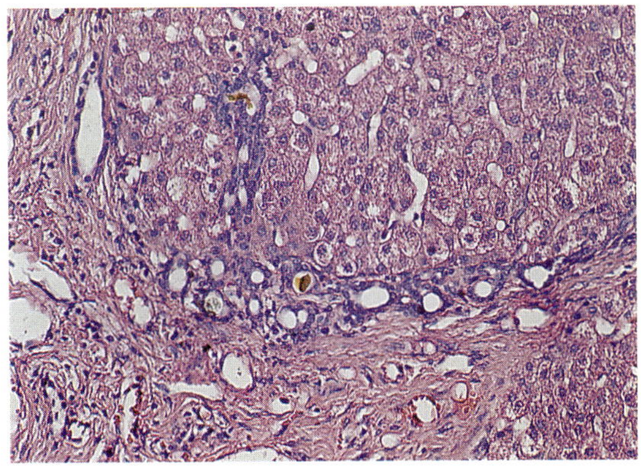

Fig. 204 See Legend page 199.

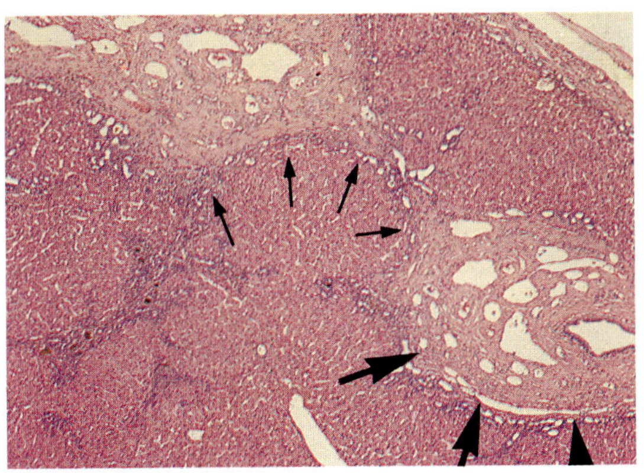

Fig. 205 See Legend page 199.

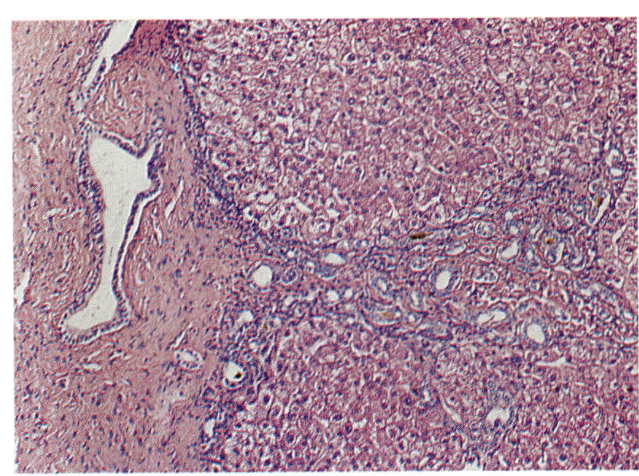

Fig. 206 See Legend page 199.

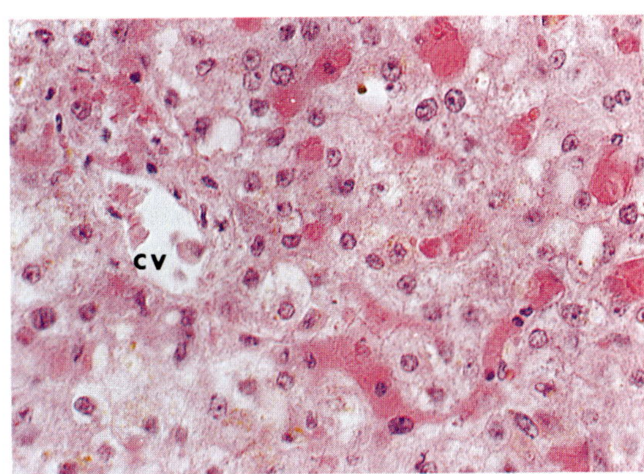

Fig. 207 See Legend page 206.

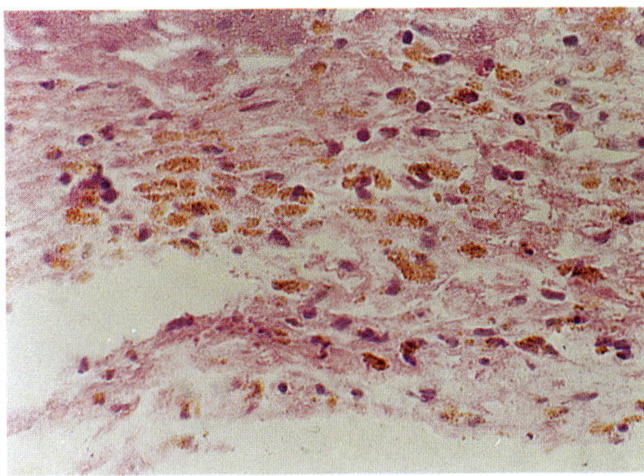

Fig. 208 See Legend page 206.

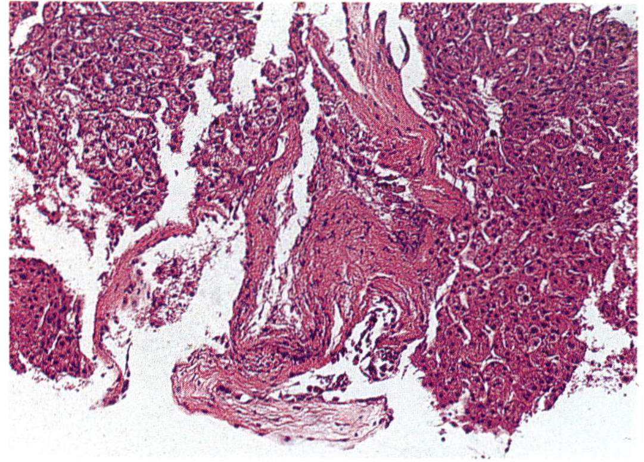

Fig. 209 See Legend page 206.

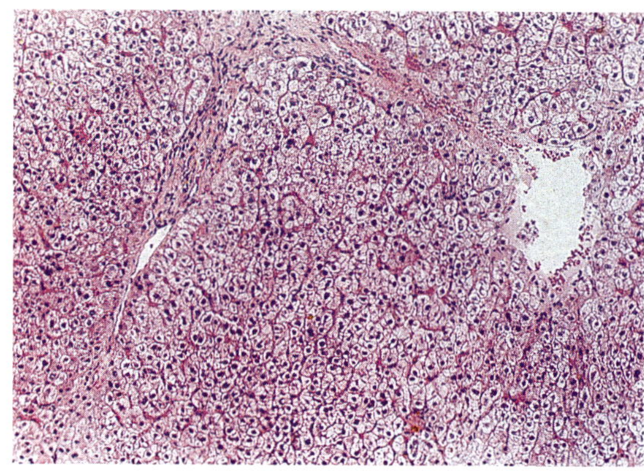

Fig. 210 See Legend page 206.

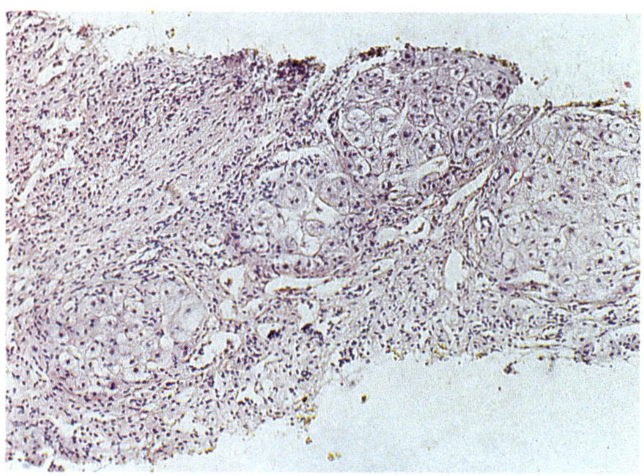

Fig. 211 See Legend page 207.

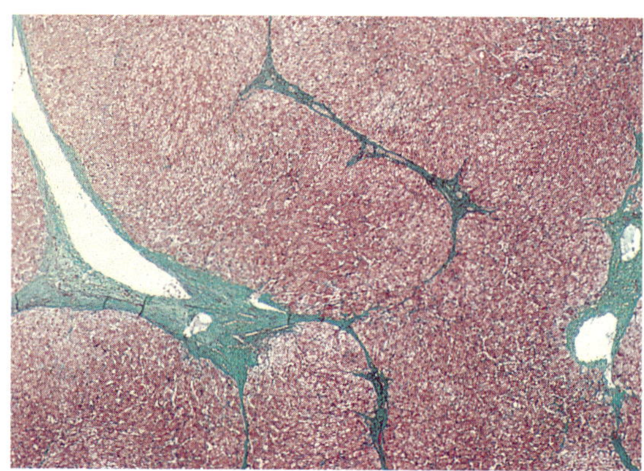

Fig. 212 See Legend page 207.

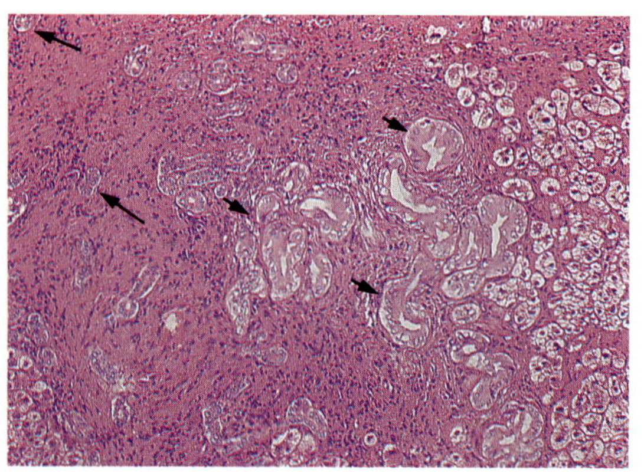

Fig. 213 See Legend page 207.

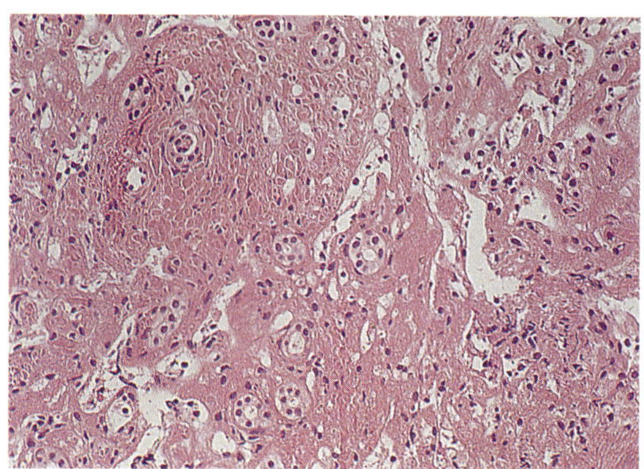

Fig. 214 See Legend page 207.

TABLE 12–1.

Differences Between Clinical Diagnosis Before Biopsies and Biopsy Diagnosis

Case number	*Clinical diagnosis before biopsy*	*Indications for biopsy*	*Histological diagnosis*
1	Tuberculous pleurisy and peritonitis	Undiagnosed hepatomegaly	Nonspecific reactive hepatitis with small histiocytic accumulation in a focal liver cell necrosis
2	Minimal pulmonary tuberculosis	Undiagnosed hepatosplenomegaly	Miliary tuberculosis, mild
3	Far advanced pulmonary tuberculosis and intestinal tuberculosis	Undiagnosed hepatomegaly	Miliary tuberculosis, moderate
4	Tuberculous peritonitis and nephrotic syndrome	Unknown origin of fever and undiagnosed abdominal mass	Miliary tuberculosis, mild
5	Tuberculous peritonitis	Unknown origin of fever	Miliary tuberculosis, mild
6	Chronic anicteric hepatitis	Histologic confirmation of anicteric hepatitis	Miliary tuberculosis, moderate
7	Interstitial pneumonia, tuberculous pleurisy and chronic anicteric hepatitis	Histologic confirmation of anicteric hepatitis	Miliary tuberculosis, severe
8	Miliary tuberculosis in lung	Histologic confirmation of miliary tuberculosis diagnosed by chest X-ray	Miliary tuberculosis, mild
9	Miliary tuberculosis in lung and bone tuberculosis	"	Military tuberculosis, mild
10	Miliary tuberculosis in lung	"	Miliary tuberculosis, moderate
11	Miliary tuberculosis in lung	"	Miliary tuberculosis, severe

Key: Mild, < 4 granulomas; Moderate, 4–10 granulomas; Severe, > 10 granulomas in a biopsy specimen

TABLE 12–2.

Clinical and Laboratory Findings in 11 Cases of Miliary Tuberculosis of Liver

Case number	Age/Sex	Fever	Hepatomegaly	Splenomegaly	Chest X-ray	WBC (/mm³)	Hepatic test results: Serum Protein Albumin/Globulin (gm/100ml)	SAST (units)	SALT (units)	Alkaline phosphatase (KA units)	Total bilirubin (mg/100ml)	Antituberculosis therapy	Clinical diagnosis
1	27/M	–	+	–	Right pleural effusion	5,900	3.9/3.9	17	16	7.6	0.4	+	Tuberculous pleurisy and peritonitis
2	43/M	–	+	+	Minimal tuberculosis	5,300	4.3/3.7	17	16		0.8	–	Minimal pulmonary tuberculosis
3	42/M	–	+		Far advanced tuberculosis	12,500	1.3/3.3	29	8	1.2	0.8	+	Advanced pulmonary tuberculosis and intestinal tuberculosis
4	23/M	+	–		Normal	5,450	4.2/3.2	40	26	2.9	1.2		Tuberculous peritonitis, Nephrotic syndrome
5	25/M	+	+	–	Miliary tuberculosis appeared 2 months after the biopsy	6,500	3.3/4.0	22	15	4.9	0.5	–	Tuberculous peritonitis
6	48/M		+	–	Normal		3.1/3.7	115	70	9.8	1.0	–	Anicteric hepatitis
7	20/M	–	–	+	Interstitial pneumonia, pleural effusion	6,000	4.0/3.9	170	277	21.0	1.0	–	Interstitial pneumonia, Tuberculous pleurisy, Anicteric hepatitis
8	30/M	+	+	–	Miliary tuberculosis	6,500	3.6/3.5	150	53	1.9	0.4	+	Miliary tuberculosis in lung, Chronic anicteric hepatitis
9	43/F	+		–	Miliary tuberculosis, bone tuberculosis	5,600	3.3/3.0	32	25		0.8	+	Miliary tuberculosis in lung, Bone tuberculosis
10	35/F	+			Miliary tuberculosis	5,900	2.1/3.1	112	56	1.9		+	Miliary tuberculosis in lung
11	64/F	+	+		Miliary tuberculosis	9,300	1.8/3.6	26	48	8.7	0.8	+	Miliary tuberculosis in lung

TABLE 12–3.

Histologic Analysis of 11 Cases of Miliary Tuberculosis of Liver

Histologic finding	*Number*
Focal necrosis of hepatic cells	6
Sinusoidal cellular activation	10
Steatosis	6
Portal inflammation	5
Small accumulation of histiocytic elements	6
Expanding histiocytic granuloma before caseation	5
Caseous necrotizing granuloma	
with shell of histiocytic elements	6
without the shell	5
Fibrosed tubercle	5
Conglomeration of granuloma	4
Various stage of granuloma	5

sometimes observed (Figs. 151, 152, 153, see page 118). Small foci of caseation necrosis, in which Kupffer cells and hepatic cells were necrotic, were surrounded by lymphoid and histiocytic elements. This change was seen in nine of the eleven cases. Epitheloid tubercles, usually was caseated necrosis and with a variable rim of lymphoid and histiocytic elements, were observed in six of the eleven cases (Fig. 154, see page 118) (Table 12-3). Large foci of caseous necrosis occasionally showed fibrosis without such cellular shells. Five of the eleven cases had such granulomas. In the center of larger tubercles, a core of a fine granular acidophilic tissue was intermixed with a few fine basophilic nuclear fragments (caseation necrosis). With reticulum fiber stains, the fibers appeared broken in the areas of caseation and the developing epitheloid cells pushed aside the original fiber framework.

Histiocytic nodules, the foci of caseation, and tubercles were irregularly distributed throughout the lobule without reference to lobular topography. Accordingly, they were also found in the vicinity of the central vein (Fig. 155, see page 119). Fully developed and larger tubercles were located more often near or within the portal tracts (Fig. 156, see page 119). Conglomerated tubercles were seen usually in protracted cases, but sometimes in association with severe cases (Fig. 157, see page 119). Five cases with fibrosed tubercles were observed in their healing stage.

In less acute forms, especially those under adequate control with antituberculous treatment, tubercles of various stages were intermixed and conglomerated with the development of fibrosis of the tubercles. Five patients were in the multiple stage of granulomas. Three of these patients were intensively treated with antituberculous drugs.

The process of full development of tubercles, which has been speculated as going through several stages (6), was evidenced by this observation. Initiation of a tubercle seems to be accumulation of histiocytic elements around a small necrotic foci, in response to preexisting tissue injury or accumulation of histiocytic elements without preceding hepatocellular necrosis. Subsequently, the histiocytic elements become transformed into epitheloid cells and eventually some epitheloid cells develop into Langhans' giant cells (Fig. 154, see page 118). Lymphoid elements appear very early around the tubercle, forming a shell. Tubercles near the portal tracts produce inflammatory changes in the tract, sometimes with ductular proliferation (Fig. 156, see page 119). In the center of large tubercles, necrosis of epithelial cells occurs, producing a core of fine granular acidophilic tissue (caseation necrosis) (Fig. 154, see page 118).

Histologic differentiation

In interpreting a granuloma in a liver biopsy, elucidation of the etiology is often difficult and sometimes impossible. In Korea, granulomas, due to tuberculosis and typhoid fever (see Chapter 13), are more frequent than in Western countries, and other types of granuloma, such as sarcoidosis, fungal granuloma, etc., are rare (7).

For the diagnosis of the tuberculous granuloma, the demonstration of acid-fast bacilli, either in section or by culture, although this is rarely possible (5), is the only reliable evidence. Localization of tubercles within the lobular parenchyma, independently of the portal tract, especially in the vicinity of the central vein, seldom occurs in conditions other than tuberculosis, and almost never in sarcoidosis (6). The pattern of caseation is also somewhat helpful in differentiating tuberculous granuloma from typhoid and sarcoidosis, but not from other granulomatous diseases. Usually, the etiology of the hepatic tuberculous granuloma, seen in liver biopsy specimens, has to be established by extrahepatic lesions of tuberculosis. It is necessary for the patient to show a good and apparently specific response to antituberculosis therapy.

In 10 cases studied in this chapter, hepatic granuloma coexisted with various types of tuberculosis of extrahepatic organ, including pulmonary, pleural, peritoneal or osseous tuberculosis. Eight cases revealed a granuloma with the pattern of caseation. In many of the cases, the granulomas were scattered in the lobular parenchyma and portal area. All of the cases had good response to antituberculosis treatment. Therefore, involvement of tuberculosis is strongly suggested in the cause of granulomas in these cases, although acid-fast bacilli were not demonstrated in the biopsy specimens.

Summary

To establish the disease entities, the author performed liver needle biopsies on Korean patients who had undiagnosed hepatomegaly, continuation of fever of undetermined origin and abnormal serum transferase activity of unknown origin (anicteric hepatitis of unknown origin). He did the same on cases suspected of miliary tuberculosis through chest X-ray findings, in order to determine whether there was hepatic dissemination and, if there was any, to find out what was the histologic pattern. Of the cases, 11 were thought to be of miliary tuberculosis.

Of the 11 patients, the number of cases of extrahepatic organ tuberculosis before biopsy was ten; four had miliary tuberculosis in the lung (one of the four had miliary tuberculosis combined with bone tuberculosis), two pulmonary tuberculosis and four tuberculous pleurisy and/or peritonitis. In the remaining one, extrahepatic involvement could not be proved.

Histologic analysis of biopsy specimens is described and discussed. Granulomas ranged from histiocytic micronodules to large caseous necrotizing granulomas. Histiocytic micronodules were present in six cases (56%) and caseous necrotizing granulomas appeared in eight cases (73%). Focal Kupffer cell hyperplasia and diffuse sinusoidal inflammatory reaction were sufficiently frequent to be characteristic of hepatic involvement in tuberculosis.

Liver biopsy has clinical importance in diagnosing hepatic involvement in miliary tuberculosis because it sometimes leads to a correct diagnosis in patients with unexplained fever and sometimes without roentgenologic findings in the lung. In these forms, liver biopsy is of particular advantage and may lead to immediate and life-saving specific antituberculosis therapy.

References

1. Bockus, H.L. Gastroenterology Philadelphia, W.B. Saunders Co., 1946.

2. Lichtman, S.S. Tuberculosis in Diseases of Liver, Gall Bladder and Bile Ducts. Philadelphia, Lea & Febiger, pp. 1068–1075, 1953.

3. Mather, G., Nawson, J. and Hoyle, C. Liver biopsy in sarcoidosis. Quart J Med 24: 331, 1955.

4. Guckian, J.C. and Perry, I.E. Granulomatous hepatitis: An analysis of 63 cases and review of the literature. Ann Intern Med 65: 1081–1100, 1966.

5. Korn, R.J., Kellow, W.F., Heller, P., Chomet, B. and Zimmerman, H.J. Hepatic involvement in extrapulmonary tuberculosis. Am J Med 27: 60–71, 1959.

6. Popper, H. and Schaffner, F. Granulomatosis diseases of the liver: in Liver Structure and Function, McGraw-Hill Book Co., Inc., pp. 507–508, 1957.

7. Neville, E., Piyasena, K.H.G. and James, D.G. Granulomas of the liver. Postgraduate Medical Journal 51: 361–365, 1975.

Legends

Fig. 151. Sinusoidal cell activation and small nodules of histiocytic elements.
Focal Kupffer cell and histiocyte proliferation, which occludes the lumens of sinusoids, leading to compression and disappearance of hepatic cells between two sinusoids. Case #1, needle biopsy, HE, ×400.

Fig. 152. A small histiocytic nodule below the intima of the central vein (CV).
Case #10, needle biopsy, HE, ×200.

Figs. 153. Expanding histiocytic granuloma before caseation.
Intralobular focal necrosis and the beginning of caseation which is surrounded by histiocytic elements. Case #11, needle biopsy, HE, ×200.

Fig. 154. Caseous necrotizing granulomas.
Two large granulomas with extensive caseous necrosis, producing a core of fine granular acidophilic tissue intermixed with a few fine basophilic nuclear fragments, are illustrated. Some epitheloid cells appear to develop into Langhans' giant cells (arrows). Case #7, needle biopsy, HE, ×200.

Figs. 155. Location of granulomas.
A large tubercle is located in the vicinity of the central vein (CV). Case #7, needle biopsy, HE, ×200.

Fig. 156.
A fully developed large epitheloid tubercle is located within the portal tract. Case #7, needle biopsy, HE, ×200.

Figs. 157. Conglomerated tubercles.
This liver biopsy specimen shows a conglomeration of several caseous necrotizing nodules. Case #11, needle biopsy, HE, ×200.

13

HISTOLOGIC STUDY OF TYPHOID LIVER

Whan Kook Chung, M.D., Ph.D. and
Jae Young Yoo, M.D., Ph.D.

Although its incidence has declined remarkably in Korea, typhoid fever still continues to occur sporadically because of inadequate treatment and the existence of longtime carriers. As a result, we have been able to observe many cases with various complications resulting from typhoid fever (1,2). However, reviews regarding complications of typhoid fever, particularly hepatic lesions are scarce (3,4,5). This study, which gives a detailed description of the histologic changes of typhoid liver observed recently, is an extension of our previous study (2). This study was conducted with 22 typhoid fever patients. Of the 22 patients, nine (Group A) were proved bacteriologically, seven (Group B) serologically and, in the remaining six (Group C), neither bacteriologically nor serologically proved. The clinical suggestion was that the patients of Group C had typhoid fever.

There were 11 male and 11 female patients, whose ages ranged from 25 years to 58 years, with an average of 39 years. None of the patients had a history of any previous liver disease or tuberculosis, and none had ever been exposed to hepatotoxic drugs.

Immediately after the performance of biochemical liver studies, liver needle biopsies were performed. These biopsies were conducted with a Menghini needle via the intercostal approach three to 98 days (a mean of 29 days) after the onset of fever, and one to 14 days (a mean of seven days) after the administration of chloramphenicol alone or with steroids.

Case Presentation

Case 1. A 31-year-old man was admitted to St. Mary's Hospital, Seoul. His chief complaints at the time of admission were 15 days of high fever, five days of diarrhea and four days of jaundice. Physical examination revealed obvious jaundice and a body temperature reaching 39.4°C. Hepatosplenomegaly and ascites were observed. Blood culture revealed Salmonella group D. A Widal test proved positive for typhoid fever. Liver chemistries, including serum bilirubin, serum alkaline phosphatase (SALT) and serum aspartate aminotransferase (SAST), showed abnormalities. Hypoalbuminemia and hyperglobulinemia were also noted.

Treatment for typhoid fever began with oral administration of chloramphenicol three grams per day and continued for 10 days. Liver function improved but still showed abnormalities. For the determination of possible hepatic lesion, a liver needle biopsy was performed 25 days after the onset of fever.

The histologic features of the biopsy specimen are shown in Fig. 158 (see page 119). The sinusoid was filled with numerous sinusoidal cells, including proliferated Kupffer cells, macrophages and lymphocytes and micronodules. Necrosis of a group of hepatic cells attracted scavenger cells including lymphocytes, plasma cells, histiocytes and segmented leucocytes (Fig. 158, see page 119). A dark hepatic cell with a pyknotic nucleus, expelled from the liver cell plate, was lying in the center of the hepatic necrosis (Fig. 159, see page 119). Fat metamorphosis was demonstrated at the periphery of the granuloma. A higher magnification of a large granuloma showed accumulation of histiocytes, lymphoid cells and plasma cells in the area from which the group of hepatic cells disappeared.

Widening of the portal tract and inflammation with lymphocytes, plasma cells, histiocytes, segmented leukocytes and proliferated cholangioles with cholangiolar inflammation were seen. Histiocytes and inflammatory cells were wedged into the cholangiolar wall.

Case 2. A 26-year-old housewife, suffering from high fever for 12 days and complaints of tarry stool with anemia for 2 days, was admitted. Her blood culture showed Salmonella group D, and the Widal reaction for typhoid fever proved strongly positive. Two grams of chloramphenicol were given per day for seven days, but the high fever persisted and the liver test results showed abnormalities. A needle biopsy was carried out 18 days after the onset of the fever.

Biopsy findings revealed zonal (confluent) necrosis in the hepatic lobule with typhoid granulomas, fat metamorphosis, congestion and hemorrhage. The lesion was involved from the portal tract to the central area. An acidophilic body was also seen.

Comments

Typhoid granulomas, which are considered to be a characteristic histologic feature of typhoid hepatitis, were observed in eight of the nine cases whose diagnosis was proved by bacterial culture (Table 13-1). Of these eight patients, four had submassive confluent necrosis. All remaining four exhibited focal necrotic types of granulomas, one showing the type of predominant portal reaction. Marked sinusoidal Kupffer cell mobilization was observed in all the patients. Portal reaction was mild, but inflammatory reaction with mononuclear cells, sometimes with segmented leucocytes, was observed. Only one patient showed central vein reaction. Histologic comparison of these three groups showed no significant differences either in severity or incidence. Hyperbilirubinemia is a relatively rare complication of typhoid fever. It was so even during the pre-antibiotic era. Nonetheless, abnormal liver function was rather frequent. Of the culture-proven nine cases, six showed modest hyperbilirubinemia but there was SAST elevation in all the cases (Table 13-2). Mild serum hyperglobulinemia was also observed in eight patients. Comparison of liver function among the three groups showed no significant differences.

TABLE 13–1.

Histologic Analysis of Liver in Typhoid Fever

Histologic changes	*Group A (n=9)* *Bacteriologically proved* *(%)*	*Group B (n=7)* *Serologically proved* *(%)*	*Group C (n=6)* *Clinically suggested* *(%)*	*Total (n=22)* *(%)*
Histologic findings:				
Intralobular reaction				
Typhoid granuloma	88.9	57.1	100.0	81.8
Acidophilic body	11.1	14.3	16.6	13.6
Focal necrosis	44.4	28.5	66.7	45.5
Confluent necrosis	44.4	28.5	16.6	31.8
Sinusoidal Scavenger cell mobilization	100.0	85.7	100.0	95.5
Congestion	88.9	85.7	100.0	90.9
Hemorrhage	11.1	28.5	16.6	18.2
Fat infiltration	33.3	42.8	33.3	45.0
Portal reaction				
Inflammation	66.7	42.9	66.7	59.1
Periductular reaction	55.6	14.3	33.3	36.4
Vascular reaction				
Central vein	11.1	28.5	16.6	18.2
Portal vein	0.0	28.0	0.0	9.1
Hepatic artery	0.0	14.3	16.6	9.1
Histologic types*	I,3; II,2; III,4	I,4; II,1; III,2	I,5; III,1	I,12; II,3; III,7

*According to text

TABLE 13–2.

Clinical and Laboratory Findings of Typhoid Fever

	Group A (n = 9) Bacteriologically proved		*Group B (n = 7) Serologically suspected*		*Group C (n = 6) Clinically suggested*		*Total (n = 22)*	
	Mean (Range)	*% Abnormal*	*Mean (Range)*	*% Abnormal*	*Mean (Range)*	*% Abnormal*	*Mean (Range)*	*% Abnormal*
Age	39.1 (25–47)		37.9 (26–58)		38.7 (26–55)		38.6 (25–58)	
Sex (M:F)	5:4		4:4		2:4		11:11	
Febrile period (days)	25.2 (7–60)		20.3 (5–90)		90.6 (2–90)		25.1 (2–90)	
Days between biopsy and onset of fever	31.1 (14–70)		23.2 (9–98)		33.2 (3–80)		29.1 (3–98)	
Days of treatment with antibiotics before biopsy	8.0 (1–14)		6.7 (1–8)		5.5 (3–8)		7.1 (1–14)	
Liver test results:								
Serum bilirubin, Total (mg/100ml)	4.3 (0.4–10.4)	(66.7)	3.0 (0.7–8.7)	(22.2)	1.3 (0.3–3.4)	(40.0)	3.1 (0.4–10.4)	(47.6)
Direct (mg/100ml)	2.3 (0.1–6.0)	(44.4)	1.6 (0.2–5.1)	(44.4)	0.6 (0.1–2.3)	(40.0)	1.7 (0.1–6.0)	(66.7)
Serum alkaline phosphatase (Bodansky u)	4.9 (1.2–10.0)	(44.4)	3.4 (1.7–10.1)	(11.1)	4.3 (1.2–11.0)	(40.0)	4.3 (1.2–11.0)	(42.9)
Serum albumin (gm/100ml)	2.9 (1.8–3.9)	(44.4)	2.5 (1.8–3.6)	(22.2)	2.8 (2.5–3.4)	(50.0)	2.7 (1.8–3.6)	(42.9)
globulin (gm/100ml)	3.7 (2.2–5.7)	(88.9)	3.6 (3.2–4.2)	(100.0)	3.4 (2.9–4.2)	(50.0)	3.6 (2.2–5.7)	(85.7)
SAST (Sigma u)	161.0 (43–441)	(100.0)	153.6 (27–375)	(85.7)	180.4 (34–321)	(80.0)	163.1 (25–441)	(90.5)

Key: Criteria of abnormalities; Hyperbilirubinemia $\geq$ 2.0 mg/100ml, Serum alkaline phosphatase $\geq$ 5 BU, Hypoalbuminemia $\leq$ 3.0 gm/100ml, Hyperglobulinemia $\geq$ 3.0 gm/100ml, SAST (Serum aspartate aminotransferase) $\geq$ 40 Sigma u/100ml

Jaundice and/or other abnormalities in liver function, occurring during the course of typhoid fever, must be differentiated from viral hepatitis. Differentiation between typhoid fever and viral hepatitis is important since these diseases tend to occur simultaneously or be endemic in Korea.

As shown in this study, the causative agents cannot always be isolated from patients with typhoid fever. The reason is that treatment with antibiotics alone or with steroids and diagnosis by a culture method might be inadequate. In complicated cases, liver needle biopsy is useful for differentiating the two entities and in making a confirmative diagnosis, even when the case is not proved by a culture method.

The histologic features of the biopsy specimens permitted a division of the cases into the following three types (2):

Type I. Typhoid granuloma and/or predominant sinusoidal scavenger cell reaction—12 cases

Type II. Predominant portal reaction in comparison with other histologic features—three cases

Type III. Submassive zonal (confluent) lobulár necrosis and fat metamorphosis with typhoid granulomas—seven cases

The febrile period, the time interval between biopsy and the onset of fever, and the duration of treatment with chloramphenicol before the biopsy were longest in Type III, followed by Type I and Type II (Table 13-3). Abnormal elevation of the serum bilirubin level, SAST activity and serum alkaline phosphatase activity with hypoalbuminemia and hyperglobulinemia were found most frequently in the patients of Type III.

The *pathogenesis* of the lesion has not been completely clarified yet, but it appears to be caused by the endotoxin of organism (6)(7).

Our previous observation in mice showed that injection of Salmonella typhi endotoxin (typhoid vaccine) produces focal areas of liver cell necrosis, infiltration of mononuclear phagocytes in the area of necrosis and hyperplastic Kupffer cells (2). These lesions closely resemble the pathologic findings in patients with a typhoid liver.

The typhoid nodule seems to go through two courses to reach its full-grown stage:

1. Nodules develop without preceding hepatocellular necrosis, resulting from accumulation of proliferated endothelial phagocytes. 2. Histiocytic elements, either of hepatic origin or blood-borne, accumulate in small necrotic foci in response to a pre-existing tissue injury (Figs. 158, 159, see page 119). Furthermore, segmented leukocytes, lymphocytes and plasma cells also participate in this process.

Several factors are presumed to be the cause or causes of hepatic cell necrosis. One is anoxia due to the occlusion of sinusoids and blood capillaries or arterioles by proliferation and embolization caused by aggregated endo-

TABLE 13–3.

Changes of Clinical and Laboratory Findings According to Histologic Type

Findings / Type	Type I (n = 12)			Type II (n = 3)			Type III (n = 7)		
	Mean	*Range*	*% Abnormal*	*Mean*	*Range*	*% Abnormal*	*Mean*	*Range*	*% Abnormal*
Febrile period (days)	25.9	2–90		9.7	7–15		23.0	8–60	
Days between biopsy and onset of fever	27.8	3–98		16.0	9–25		30.0	16–70	
Days of treatment with antibiotics before biopsy	6.7	1–20		5.7	1–9		7.9	4–14	
Widal reaction (typhoid)	Reactive in 6/11			Reactive in 3/3			Reactive in 4/7		
Liver test results:									
Serum bilirubin, Total (mg/100ml)	1.8	0.4–8.7	(16.7)	1.8	0.6–4.0	(33.3)	5.9	0.8–10.4	(85.7)
Direct (mg/100ml)	0.8	0.1–4.8		1.0	0.3–2.3		3.4	0.2–6.0	
Serum alkaline phosphatase (Bodansky u)	3.2	1.2–11.0	(25.0)	3.8	1.2–6.5	(33.3)	6.4	0.4–10.1	(71.4)
Serum albumin (gm/100ml)	3.2	1.8–3.6	(33.3)	3.2	2.9–3.6	(33.3)	2.9	1.9–3.9	(57.1)
globulin (gm/100ml)	3.7	2.9–4.2	(83.3)	4.1	3.2–5.7	(33.3)	3.4	2.2–4.5	(85.7)
SAST (Sigma u)	153	34–441	(91.7)	112	27–265	(66.7)	245	158–375	(80.0)

Key: Criteria of abnormalities; Hyperbilirubinemia $\geq$ 2.0 mg/100ml, Serum alkaline phosphatase $\geq$ 5 BU, Hypoalbuminemia $\leq$ 3.0 gm/100ml, Hyperglobulinemia $\geq$ 3.0 gm/ml, SAST (Serum aspartate aminotransferase) $\geq$ 40 Sigma unit/100ml, Widal reaction $\geq$ 1:160

thelial phagocytes which are stimulated by endotoxin (Fig. 167, see page 153). Another is an endogenous cytolytic agent (lysosomal hydrolase) probably released from Kupffer cells. A third probable cause is immune injury, such as antibody-dependent cell-mediated cytotoxicity or T-cell cytotoxicity.

A recent case, in which intact bacilli were demonstrated within the liver, suggested that liver injury might occur due to local release of cytotoxin or local inflammatory reactions within reticuloendothelial cells (8).

Sinusoidal cell activation varied from lobule to lobule and was usually limited to part of the lobule. Hepatic congestion was frequent and typhoid nodules were randomly and unevenly distributed throughout the lobule (Fig. 160, see page 119). They were seen sometimes in the central or subcapsular area, even in the portal space (Fig. 166, see page 120).

Occasionally, bridging parenchymal necrosis connected the portal and the central zone, or the central and the central zone, we saw:

1. Severe ischemic necrosis with mild inflammatory cell infiltration.
2. Conglomeration of nodules (Figs. 161, 162, see page 120).
3. Submassive confluent necrosis with related massive mononuclear cell reaction.

Such fibrotic changes are followed by confluent necrosis and subsequent passive collapse of reticulin fibers. Thereafter, collagen fibers gradually develop and are overlaid on the reticulin fibers as time passes (Figs. 163, 164, 165, see page 120). However, these alterations are focal and reversible.

Jaundice is said to be a relatively rare complication in typhoid fever. However, in this study, six of the nine cases of Group A showed hyperbilirubinemia. Although it is usually presumed to be due to mild cholangitis, little or no autopsy evidence supports this. In this study through biopsy, the authors could occasionally observe portal expansion and infiltration of macrophages (Fig. 166, see page 120) and, sometimes, cholangiolitis with cholestasis in the later stage (Fig. 167, see page 153).

Summary

Clinical, biochemical, bacterial-serologic and histologic studies by liver needle biopsy were performed on twenty-two patients with typhoid fever. Of the 22 patients, nine (Group A) were proved bacteriologically, seven (Group B) serologically and the remaining six patients (Group C), neither bacteriologically nor serologically proved, were clinically suspected of typhoid fever.

Histologic comparison of these three groups showed no significant differences either in severity or in frequency.

The histologic features in biopsy specimens permitted a division of the cases into the following three types: Type I—twelve cases had predominantly typhoid granulomas and/or sinusoidal scavenger cell reaction. Type II—three cases had predominant portal reaction in comparison with other histologic features. Type III—the remaining seven cases showed the features of submassive zonal (confluent) lobular necrosis and fat metamorphosis with typhoid granulomas, and clinical and biochemical findings were more severe than in the other two types.

Although the liver needle biopsy is not considered a routine method for the diagnosis of typhoid fever, it seems to be useful when other diagnostical methods, including bacteriologic tests, fail to produce a definite outcome.

References

1. Chung, W.K. Liver biopsy findings of icteric typhoid hepatitis. Korean J Intern Med 19: 88–94, 1976.

2. Yoo, J.Y. and Chung, W.K. Histologic studies on typhoid liver: I. Observation of liver tissue obtained from patients, II. Animal experiment. J Catholic Med College 92: 293–318, 1979.

3. Ayhan, A., Gokoz, A., Karacadag, S. and Telatar, H. The liver in typhoid. Am J Gastroenterology 59: 141–145, 1973.

4. Faierman, D., Ross, F.A. and Seckler, S.G. Typhoid fever complicated by hepatitis, nephritis and thrombocytopenia. JAMA 221: 60–61, 1972.

5. Ramachandran, S., Godfrey, J.J. and Perera, M.V.F. Typhoid hepatitis. JAMA 230: 235–240, 1974.

6. Hornick, R. B. and Greisman, S. On the pathogenesis of typhoid fever. Arch Intern Med 138: 357–359, 1978.

7. Allison, A.C., Davis, P. and Page, R.C. Effect of endotoxin on macrophages and other lymphoreticular cells. J Infec Dis 128: s212-s219, 1973.

8. Schwartz, A., Robinstein, H.S. and Coons, A.H. Electron microscopy of cellular responses following immunization with endotoxin. Am J Path 19: 135, 1968.

Legends

Fig. 158. A biopsy specimen obtained from Case 1.

Destruction of liver cells surrounded by histiocytic elements is seen at the periphery of a granuloma. Needle biopsy, HE, ×400.

Fig. 159.

Necrosis of a group of hepatic cells attract scavenger cells (lymphocytes, plasma cells, histiocytes and segmented leucocytes) which take the place of disappearing hepatic cells. A dark eosinophlic hepatic cell (arrow) with a pyknotic nucleus is expelled from the liver cell plate and lies in the center of the focal necrosis. Fat metamorphosis is demonstrated at the periphery of a granuloma. Needle biopsy, HE, ×400. (Reproduced from Yoo, J.Y. and Chung, W.K. J Catholic Medical College 32: 293–306, 1979, with permission).

Figs. 160. Varied intralobular changes (typhoid hepatitis).

Scattered typhoid micronodules (arrows) and an accumulation of red blood cells in the sinusoid (congestion). Needle biopsy, HE, ×100.

Fig. 161. Conglomeration of granulomas.

A conglomeration of many small granulomas with lymphoid and histiocytic elements. Needle biopsy, HE, ×200.

Fig. 162.

A conglomeration of three nodules. The left upper nodule is more cellular than the lower two. This is presumed to represent the state of ischemic necrosis. These three nodules put together appear to be precursors of confluent necrosis. Needle biopsy, HE, ×200.

Fig. 163. Collapse and fibrosis.

A fibrous granuloma with infiltration of numerous lymphoid cells and histiocytic elements is located in the lobular parenchyma. Fat metamorphosis is seen. Needle biopsy, HE, ×400.

Fig. 164.

The lobular parenchyma with fatty infiltration is divided into three parts by inflammatory septal fibrosis. This alteration, not diffuse but focal, seems to be passive collapse following confluent necrosis. Needle biopsy, HE, ×100.

Fig. 165.

A higher magnification of a part of inflammatory septal fibrosis, illustrated in Fig. 164, discloses various types of cells including lymphocytes, histiocytes, plasma cells and cholangiolar cells. HE, ×400.

Figs. 166. Changes of the portal tract.

An accumulation of macrophages in the edematous portal tract (PV). Needle biopsy, HE, ×400.

Fig. 167.

Microthrombus in the arteriole (long arrow) and cell debris in the bile ductule (short arrow). Needle biopsy, HE, ×400.

14 HISTOLOGICAL CHANGES IN LIVER WITH CLONORCHIASIS

Whan Kook Chung, M.D., Ph.D.

Clonorchis sinensis (CS) is a common liver fluke found in Korea. Before and after the Korean War, millions of people in Korea were infected with CS (1,2). However, recently, the infection rate is quite low for several reasons: one is the extensive use of agricultural pesticides by farmers, which has led to a reduction in the population of miracidia-carrying snails, the first intermediate host; a second is the nationwide education campaign discouraging the eating of fresh-water fish that contain encysted metacercaria, the second intermediate host, plus better dietary habits thanks to improved socio-economic conditions. A third reason is the popularization of treatment with drugs, like "praziquantel," which are very effective against CS. Nevertheless, severe symptomatic cases are still occasionally found in Korea. During the period of this observation, because no adequate treatment method was available, the disease was left to run its natural course once infection occurred.

Clonorchiasis is regarded by some as a cause of fatal cirrhosis (3,4), but others find no connection with cirrhosis (5). It can lead to cholangiocarcinoma.

Patients

For the purpose of documenting the histologic entities of hepatic involvement of clonorchiasis and its histologic evolution, 105 patients infected with

Clonorchis sinensis were observed by means of liver biopsy. Their conditions varied in severity, ranging from a mild, symptomless form to full-blown cirrhosis. Eighteen of the 105 patients were subjected to serial biopsies at intervals of three months to six years with an average of 12.2 months. Of the 105 patients, 31 had nonspecific reactive hepatitis (Table 14-1). Because hepatic injury due to CS infection is a space-occupying lesion, sampling errors can occur by liver needle biopsy. It was not easy for the needle to approach the focus where the true CS lesion was located, which frequently necessitated a histologic diagnosis of nonspecific reactive hepatitis (29%).

Two cases of acute viral hepatitis were superimposed on clonorchiasis.

In this study, 21 cases (20%) had both CS infection and chronic hepatitis histologically presumed to be of viral origin; it was difficult to determine which was the primary cause. In Korea, chronic hepatitis B is quite common and there are occasions when the disease is superimposed with CS infection. Among these cases, some develop cirrhosis as described below in this chapter. On the contrary, when the CS carrier has cirrhosis, whether the patient carries nonspecific reactive hepatitis or chronic hepatitis caused by virus infection, it can be found through retrograde tracing. Therefore, very few cases of cirrhosis develop from CS infection alone.

TABLE 14–1.

Histologic Classification of Hepatic Lesions due to Infection of Clonorchis sinensis (CS)

Groups	*Histologic characteristics*	*No. patients*
1. Nonspecific reactive hepatitis	Only Kupffer cell mobilization, some single cell necrosis, and a little portal reaction	31
2. Acute viral hepatitis, with or without CS reactions	Diffuse parenchymal spotty necrosis and hepatic cell variation in size and staining quality from one cell to next	2
3. Chronic viral hepatitis, with or without CS reactions	Periportal inflammation (piecemeal necrosis) or subacute hepatic necrosis in association with progression	21
4. Hepatic lesions showing CS reaction alone	Adenomatosis, ductular proliferation and hyperplasia, periductular fibrosis and eosinophilic infiltration in expanding portal space	51
(Cholangiocarcinoma)*		(2)

*Two of the 51 cases of Group 4 had cholangiocarcinoma

Histological Finding

Cases of hepatic lesions with piecemeal necrosis and subacute hepatic necrosis thought to have resulted from CS infection alone were very few but these can be frequently observed in chronic viral hepatitis (see Chapter 6). Hepatic lesions resulting from CS reaction include bile ductular proliferation (Fig. 168, see page 153) and hyperplasia (Figs. 169, 170, see page 153) and adenomatous alterations (Fig. 171, see page 153). Periductular fibrosis (Figs. 169, 170, see page 153) and eosinophilic cell infiltration (Fig. 172, see page 153) were usually present. Subcapsular edema and inflammation were sometimes distinct.

In the presence of CS infection, 51 cases (49%) had such conditions (Group 4). Histologic analysis of the biopsy specimens taken from the 51 cases is shown in Table 14-2.

TABLE 14–2.

Histologic Findings of Liver Biopsy Specimens Obtained from 51 Cases with CS Reaction Alone

Histologic findings	*No. cases*	*Positivity (%)*
Lobular architecture		
Distorted	6	(11.7)
Hepatic cell damage		
Degeneration		
Acidophilic body	0	(0.0)
Fatty	7	(13.7)
Excessive lipofuscin pigmentation	3	(5.9)
Cholestasis	3	(5.9)
Necrosis		
Single cell or focal	24	(47.1)
Confluent	0	(0.0)
Regeneration		
Multiple cell thick plate	16	(31.4)
Regenerative nodule	2	(3.9)
Intralobular mesenchymal reaction		
Sinusoidal cell mobilization	27	(52.9)
Central vein reaction	6	(11.8)
Portal reaction		
Widening	48	(94.1)
Mononuclear cell	46	(90.2)
Polymorphonuclear cell	43	(84.3)
Eosinophilic cell	37	(72.5)
Bile ductule proliferation	47	(92.2)
Periductular fibrosis	38	(74.5)
Piecemeal necrosis	6	(11.8)
Fibrosis		
Portal	35	(68.6)
Septal		
Focal	12	(23.5)
Diffuse	0	(0.0)
Pericellular	1	(2.0)
Adult worm of Clonorchis sinensis	3	(5.9)

Because patients who had the characteristic findings of acute or chronic hepatitis of viral origin (see Chapter 6) were not included in the 51 cases, none of them (51 cases) had acidophilic bodies or subacute hepatic necrosis. Central vein reactions (six cases) and periportal piecemeal necrosis (six cases) were rare and mild. One case with bile ductular proliferation showed the characteristic periductular inflammatory fibrosis, and acinus formation of ductular cells, both of which are looked like the circumscribed hepatic necrosis (Fig. 173, see page 154). However, the changes were very focal and mild. Diffuse septal fibrosis or regenerative nodules, usually observed in cirrhosis, could not be seen. The lobular architecture was well preserved in most of the cases.

An interesting factor was that CS adult worms (Figs. 174, 175, see page 154) were found in three cases and, in one case, Charcot-Leyden crystals were detected through aspiration needle biopsy (Fig. 176, see page 154).

In most of the cases, prominent microscopical findings were that the portal tracts had been infiltrated with mononuclear cells, polymorphonuclear cells and abundant eosinophilic cells, and that the portal space was expanded (Fig. 177, see page 154).

Bile ductule proliferation occurred in 47 cases of the 51, and the proliferation was still continuing (Fig. 168, see page 153). Many cases (38 cases) were complicated with periductular fibrosis (Figs. 169, 170, see page 153). Portal fibrosis also developed. The fibrosis that developed in the portal tracts was limited to the portal space (Fig. 178, see page 154), sometimes extending into the parenchyma, forming fibrotic septum, but it was not diffuse and did not develop to cirrhosis (Fig. 179, see page 155). Frequently, intralobular histologic changes included sinusoidal cell mobilization (27 cases), mild hepatic cell regeneration patterns (two-cell-thick plates) (16 cases), focal necrosis, portal inflammation and fat metamorphosis of a mild degree and excessive lipofuscin pigmentation in liver cells, which are usually seen in nonspecific reactive hepatitis (Fig. 180, see page 155) (see Chapter 3). Of the 51 cases, two developed cholangiocarcinoma (see Chapter 8).

Laboratory findings

Hyperbilirubinemia was found in about a half of the cases belonging to Group 4 (Table 14-3), reaching as high as 18 mg/100ml. The serum alkaline phosphatase activity and the serum total cholesterol level were abnormal in 55% and 23%, respectively, in cases that were available for tests. Thus, cases showing cholestasis were frequently observed in Group 4.

Serum aminotransferase activity was frequently increased. Hypoalbuminemia and hyperglobulinemia were mild. Hematologic examination frequently showed slight anemia and eosinophilia. In a severe case, eosinophilic cells amounted to 87% of the leucocytes of 31,700/mm3.

TABLE 14–3.

Laboratory Test Results in Patients Showing Clonorchis sinensis Reaction Alone in the Liver

Tests	*No. tested*	*Abnormal*	*%*	*Mean (Range)*
Serum bilirubin (mg/100ml)				
Direct	50	>0.2	42%	111 (0.1–9.6)
Indirect	50	>1.0	56%	1.3 (0.1–18.0)
SAST	51	>45u	68%	106.1 (20–850)
SALT	48	>40u	77%	120.6 (10–640)
Alkaline phosphatase (Bodansky u)	45	>5u	55%	9.7 (1.0–61.5)
Serum cholesterol (mg/100ml)	43	>200mg	23%	215.7 (113–345)
Serum protein (gm/100ml)				
Albumin	45	<30gm	31%	3.7 (1.9–4.5)
Globulin	45	>3.0gm	57%	3.8 (2.7–5.7)

Histological progression

Seven cases were followed-up by sequential liver biopsy. Histological progression in Cases 1–5 was apparent during a six-month follow-up period. This was thought to be due to the fact that the results were different according to the region of a liver needle biopsy sampling rather than to the fact that progression had occurred during that period. Among the cases, septal fibrosis already appeared from the time of the first biopsy, though Cases 4 and 5 seemed to develop early cirrhosis four months and three months later, respectively. Probably the origin is hepatitis virus infection rather than CS infection.

Case 6 and Case 7 were HBsAg carriers in addition to being CS carriers. Of the two cases, Case 7 is described below in detail.

Case report

Case 7. A 23-year-old man was admitted to St. Mary's Hospital because of easy fatigability, intermittent epistaxis and indigestion. He had been suffering for seven years from the above complaints when his illness was diagnosed as type B viral hepatitis.

He had no history of alcohol abuse or exposure to toxic drugs. On physical examination, he was found to be chronically ill. No conjunctival icterus and collateral vessels on the body surface were noted. The liver was felt two-finger breadth under the right costal margin and the spleen was palpable 5 cm below the left costal margin. The lower legs showed mild pitting edema.

His stool contained CS ova and a skin test for CS was positive. The total serum bilirubin level was 1.4 mg per 100 ml, and the serum total protein 6.8 gm (the albumin 4.1 gm and the globulin 2.7 gm) per 100 ml. The serum aspartate aminotransferase (SAST) and the serum alanine aminotransferase

(SALT) were 74 and 87 units, respectively. The prothrombin time was 100% of normal. The alkaline phosphatase activity was 21.0 BU units. The serum HBsAg and the HBeAg were positive. An abdominal ultrasonogram showed a coarse parenchymal echogenic pattern with splenomegaly. Laparoscopic examination showed a micronodular liver surface with splenomegaly. A liver needle biopsy specimen showed minute portal fibrosis but no definite cirrhosis.

After discharge, he was followed-up at the outpatient clinic. He was admitted again to St. Mary's Hospital six years after the first admission. He had been well until 20 days earlier, when he had hematemesis and tarry stool.

On physical examination, he was pale and chronically ill. His skin was clammy and dark, and multiple vascular spiders were found on the upper chest but he had neither conjunctival icterus nor collateral veins on the abdominal wall. The liver was felt two-finger breadth under the right costal margin and the spleen was palpated one palm width under the left costal margin. No ascites was noted.

The hematocrit was 26.9 percent and the white cell count 2,200/mm3. The serum bilirubin level was 0.9 mg per 100 ml, and the serum total protein 5.8 gm (the albumin 3.1 gm and the globulin 2.7 gm) per 100 ml. The SAST and the SALT were 55 units and 4 units, respectively. The alkaline phosphatase activity was 6.3 BU units. Alpha-fetoprotein was not detected. CS ova were found in his stool.

An emergency gastroscopic examination disclosed grade III esophageal variceal engorgement with a red color sign and emergency sclerotherapy with ethanolamine was performed.

A laparoscopic examination showed extensive macronodular cirrhosis (Fig. 181, see page 155) and a liver biopsy specimen revealed cirrhosis. Lobular parenchymal cells were highly regenerative and dysplastic, and Orcein-stain-positive hepatic cells were scattered throughout the lobule. He was transferred to the surgical department and had portal-caval shunt, and surgical wedge liver biopsy was performed. The biopsy specimen showed multilobular cirrhosis with incomplete strand septal fibrosis.

It was concluded that this patient had suffered from Type B chronic viral hepatitis 13 years before and had CS infection for at least six years prior to the last admission. During that period of six years, this case developed from early cirrhosis to advanced macronodular cirrhosis with complication of esophageal variceal bleeding. Such progression seems to be caused by hepatitis B virus infection rather than by CS infection (see Chapter 5).

Pathogenesis

The pathogenesis of histologic progression of liver injury in CS infection remains problematic. Fibrosis in a CS liver occurs in the portal tracts around proliferated bile ductules. In this process, proliferated bile duct epithelial cells penetrate into and anchor in the lobular parenchyma, and then basement membrane is created around the epithelial cells. Thereafter, fiber bundles get attached to the basement membrane and several types of mesenchymal cells surround the ductules (6) and, finally, development of periductular fibrosis occurs. Thus, ductular proliferation extends into the periportal area and forms an invasion pattern resembling piecemeal necrosis (Fig. 173, see page 154), sometimes connecting two portal tracts (Fig. 182, see page 155).

Bile duct proliferation is believed by some to result from mechanical or chemical stimulation caused by adult worms or ova of CS parasite on the bile duct (4), and by some others to be a kind of immune response (Figs. 183, 184, see page 155) (7).

Characteristically, primary biliary cirrhosis (PBC), like CS infection, shows bile ductular proliferation in its early stage. However, in PBC, the etiologic factor that causes the disease is still unknown. Furthermore, in PBC, subsequent bile ductular destruction occurs and its course is chronically progressive and perpetuating. However, in clonorchiasis, unlike in PBC, the new formation of bile ductules is more lasting and its disease course depends on the biological state of CS, and there are fewer progressive cases in clonorochiasis than in PBC. Cases are very few in which cirrhosis develops from CS infection alone.

Summary

For the purpose of documenting the histologic entities of hepatic involvement of clonorchiasis and its histologic evolution, 105 patients infected with CS were observed by means of liver biopsy. Their conditions varied in severity, ranging from a mild, symptomless form to full-blown cirrhosis. Eighteen patients out of the 105 were subjected to serial biopsies at intervals of three months to six years with an average of 12.2 months.

Of the 105 patients, 31 were cases of nonspecific reactive hepatitis, two cases of acute viral hepatitis superimposed with CS infection, and 21 cases with chronic hepatitis appearing in histologic patterns to be of viral origin in association with CS infection. The remaining 51 cases had the characteristic histologic features of CS reaction alone. Of the 51 cases, two developed cholangiocarcinoma.

Cases of hepatic lesions, thought to have resulted from CS infection, showed marked portal reaction, including bile ductular proliferation and hyperplasia, periductular fibrosis and inflammation, biliary adenomatosis and, sometimes, abundant infiltration of eosinophils intermingled with lymphoid and segmented leucocytes.

In the cases of CS infection, the fibrosis which developed in the portal tracts was usually limited to the portal space, and sometimes extended into the parenchyma, forming fibrotic septum, but it was not diffuse and did not develop into cirrhosis. In most CS carriers who develop cirrhosis, the disease (CS) is histologically in association with chronic hepatitis that appears to be of viral origin. Therefore, the cause of cirrhosis in such cases is probably hepatitis virus infection rather than CS.

References

1. Chung, W.K. A case with common bile duct obstruction due to adult worms of Clonorchis sinensis. Korean Armed Forces Med J 6: 3, 1956.
2. Chung, W.K. Distribution of Clonorchis sinensis carrier in residents living around the Kum River. Korean Armed Forces Med J 6: 25, 1956.
3. Germer, W.D., Mah, H.Y. and Shulze, W. Die Klinik der Clonorchiasis. Z Hyg u Infektionskrht 141: 132–139, 1955.
4. Lee, J.K. Clinical, laboratory and histologic studies on clonorchiasis. J Catholic Med Coll 19: 107–127, 1970.
5. Hou, P. C. The pathology of Clonorchis sinensis infestation of the liver. J Path Bact 19: 53–64, 1955.
6. Popper, H. and Schaffner, F. The problem of chronicity in liver disease. Progress in Liver Diseases, eds: Popper and Schaffner, Grune & Stratton, New York and London, vol II. pp. 519–538, 1965.
7. Kee, C.S. and Chung, W.K. Immunocytochemical studies on guinea pig liver infested with Clonorchis sinensis. J Catholic Med Coll 25: 177–189, 1973.

Legends

Fig. 168. Changes in bile ductules.

Bile ductules have proliferated and there are neutrophils in the wall of ductules and the surrounding tissue. Needle biopsy, HE, ×200.

Fig. 169.

A widened large portal tract shows acute and chronic inflammatory cell infiltration. The epithelial cells of the small interlobular bile ducts are apparently hyperplastic cells (arrows). Needle biopsy, HE, ×200.

Fig. 170.

Some of the proliferated bile ductules in scar tissue show flattened and elongated hyperplasia (arrows) of epithelial cells. Needle biopsy, HE, ×400.

Fig. 171. Biliary adenomatous change. Needle biopsy, HE, ×400.

Fig. 172. Abundant eosinophilic cells surround the proliferated bile ductules (arrows) and infiltrate into the sinusoids. Needle biopsy, HE, ×200.

Fig. 173. Chronic inflammatory cell infiltration around the proliferated small bile ducts extends from the portal tract into the parenchyma. Periductular inflammation and acinus formation (arrows) of ductular cells are noted. Needle biopsy, HE, ×200.

Fig. 174. An adult worm of CS in liver.
An adult worm (arrows) of Clonorchis sinensis is seen in the bile duct. The bile duct wall shows adenomatosis. Wedge biopsy, HE, ×200.

Fig. 175.
An aspirated adult worm of CS shows its ventral sucker (VS) and numerous ova in its uterus (U). Needle biopsy, HE, ×400.

Fig. 176. A liver needle-aspirated specimen obtained from a case with CS infection shows Charcot-Leyden crystals (arrows) among liver cells. Needle aspiration, HE, ×400.

Figs. 177. Portal inflammation.
Two edematous and expanded portal tracts with marked infiltration of eosinophils mixed with some mononuclear cells are connected with each other. Needle biopsy, HE, ×200.

Fig. 178. Widened sclerotic portal tracts.
Eosinophilic leucocytes and lymphoid cells infiltrate into the edematous and sclerotic portal space. A few ductular cells are seen.
The limiting plate is intact. Needle biopsy, HE, ×200.

Fig. 179. Minute portal fibrosis.
Bile ductules have proliferated and periductular inflammation and fibrosis have developed in the bridge which connects the portal tracts. Needle biopsy, HE, ×100.

Fig. 180. Nonspecific reactive hepatitis.
Increased sinusoidal cell reaction and a focal necrosis of hepatic cells. Needle biopsy, HE, ×200.

Fig. 181. A case of hepatitis B carrier in whom macronodular cirrhosis developed later.
Hobnail patterns in the liver surface are seen in laparoscopic observation six years after the initial observation.

Fig. 182. Patterns of progressive parenchymal invasion.
Inflammatory bridging between portal tracts.
In the bridge, there are numerous proliferations of bile ductules which are surrounded by inflammatory cells and fibrosis. Needle biopsy, HE, ×200.

Fig. 183. Immunocytochemical study of a guinea pig liver infected with Clonorchis sinensis.

Sections from a guinea pig liver, four weeks after the infection of Clonorchis sinensis. The sections are treated with mixed serum obtained from four rabbits with clonorchiasis, and then with fluoresceinated anti-rabbit gammaglobulin antiserum. An adult worm is stained brightly. Periductal fiber is also stained but to a lesser degree. ×100.

Fig. 184.

A section from a guinea pig liver, eight weeks after the infestation of Clonorchis sinensis. The section is treated with a serum from a patient with clonorchiasis, and then with fluoresceinated anti-human gammaglobulin antiserum. The capsule of ova are stained. ×400.

15 HEPATIC INJURY IN PATIENTS WITH FALCIPARUM MALARIA

When Kook Chung, M.D., Ph.D. and
Ahn Ki Lee, M.D., Ph.D.

The prevalence of vivax malaria had been endemic in Korea until the end of the Korean War. Since then, it has been difficult to find patients with that disease in this country. However, in a period of several years after 1965, we encountered, among Korean military personnel who had served in the Vietnam War, many with falciparum malaria, an illness which had never been found in Korea before 1965. Thereafter, falciparum malaria continued to be detected among Korean workers who returned from service in Middle East countries.

The liver has been believed to be the main organ for the destruction of the malarial parasite (1), but reports on studies of the function and histologic changes of the liver in patients with malaria are scarce (2).

For the purpose of clarifying the causes of fever and/or hepatomegaly of unknown origin and of evaluating the persisting abnormal liver test results shown by patients who later turned out to have falciparum malaria, liver biopsies were performed on 35 cases of falciparum malaria (Table 15-1). All the patients were males and their ages ranged from 21 to 38 years, averaging 25 years.

Clinical, biochemical and histologic studies by means of liver needle biopsy were carried out on these 35 cases. In all instances, the diagnosis was confirmed by identification of malaria parasites in the peripheral blood. In order to elucidate the ultrastructural changes in infected livers, transmission electron microscopic examination was also performed.

Light microscopic and electron microscopic study of liver biopsy tissue

The period from the onset of the disease to biopsy was 10–134 days (average 44.4 days) (Table 15-1). Among 33 cases, six had liver needle biopsy at the time of the first attack, of which only one had a biopsy performed at the recovery stage after the first attack. In the remaining 27 cases, biopsy was carried out at the recrudescent stage. In 25 cases, chloroquine was administered for the purpose of preventing malarial infection before attack and, in 20 cases, chloro-

TABLE 15–1.

Histologic Features and Some Clinical Conditions at the Time of Liver Biopsy in 35 Men with Malaria

	No. cases observed	*Mean*	*Range*
Age	35	25	21–38
Days from onset to biopsy (days)	34	44.4	10–134
Attacks at biopsy (days)	33		
Bouts of recrudescence before biopsy	33		0–10
Mean time interval between recrudescences (days)	25	24.5	6–50
Malaria plasmodium contained erythrocytes (/million RBC)	25		0–13581
		Positivity	
		No. cases	*(%)*
Histologic features			
Parenchymal cells			
Anisocytosis	35	14	40.0
Acidophilic body	35	1	2.9
Lipofuscin pigment	35	9	25.7
Bile pigmentation	35	2	5.7
Histiocytic nodule	35	7	20.0
Focal necrosis	35	9	25.7
Mitosis	35	14	40.0
Fatty metamorphosis	35	3	8.6
Sinusoidal reaction			
Widening and/or congestion	35	33	94.3
Mononuclear cells	35	25	70.1
Kupffer cell, endothelical cell activation with malaria pigment	35	35	100.0
Kupffer cell mitosis	35	5	14.3
Central vein reaction	35	11	31.4
Portal reaction	35	26	74.3
Thromboarteritis	35	6	17.1

(Some of these cases are from Lee, A. K. and Chung, W. K., J Catholic Med. College 34: 801–812, 1981, with permission)

quine, quinine and pyrimethamine were administered, either alone or in combination, for the treatment of malarial attack.

I. Light microscopic findings

Biopsy findings showed that parenchymal cell alterations were less severe in degree and rarer in frequency than sinusoidal cellular changes. Anisocytosis, lipofuscin pigmentation, focal necrosis and fat metamorphosis of liver cells, as seen in nonspecific reactive hepatitis, were frequent. In one case, acidophilic bodies were scattered throughout the lobule, despite mild damage to other hepatic cells. Occasionally, mitotic figures of nuclei of liver cells (Fig. 185, see page 156) and sinusoidal cells appeared. On the contrary, sinusoidal cell reaction was severe in all the cases. The sinusoids were congested and dilated (Fig. 186, see page 156). Characteristic and prominent histologic changes included active mobilization of Kupffer cells and perisinusoidal endothelial cells (Figs. 186, 187, see page 156), some in the active febrile stage and some others in the recovery stage. Both of these cells engulfed erythrocytes containing malarial pigment (Fig. 187, see page 156). The pigmentation was pronounced in the centrilobular area.

Erythrocytes, infected with malarial parasites, significantly accumulated in the sinusoids and the central vein. More than 80% of the erythrocytes in the sinusoids were infected with malarial parasites and, on the contrary, the infected red blood cells in the peripheral blood of the same patient were only 0.2%. In Cases 24 and 26, infected erythrocytes could not be found in the peripheral blood (Table 15-1), but many infected erythrocytes could be seen in the sinusoid and the central vein. The situation was the same in Case 10, even though the patient had recovered from fever. Many lymphocytes often accumulated in the sinusoids.

The central vein was severely congested in about 30% of the patients and, sometimes, a pattern due to bleeding from a ruptured central vein wall could be observed. Occasionally, the vascular wall was thickened.

The portal tracts were widened and infiltrated with mononuclear cells and phagocytes, which engulfed the malarial pigment. This type of portal tract involvement was observed in about 74% of the cases but the degree was mild. The arterioles in the portal tract sometimes showed thromboangitis (Fig. 188, see page 156).

II. Electron microscopic findings

The most characteristic and prominent electron microscopic change in the liver, infected with plasmodia of falciparum malaria, was the appearance of hyperplastic and hypertrophic Kupffer cells and perisinusoidal endothelial cells. Phagocytotic phenomena of Kupffer cells and endothelial cells (Figs. 189, 190, see page 156), occurring during the removal process of erythrocytes containing malarial parasites from the blood, were observed by electron microscopic examination of liver biopsy tissue.

Voluminous hypertrophy of Kupffer cells and endothelial cells with large irregular nuclei were observed (Figs. 189, 192, see pages 156, 157). Kupffer cells had pinocytotic vesicles and numerous fusiform or slender cytoplasmic projections extending into the lumen of the sinusoid. Numerous osmiophilic dense bodies of varying sizes and shapes, which were presumed to be malarial pigments, erythrocytes, lipofuscin pigment and lamellated myeloid bodies, were seen in Kupffer cells (Figs. 189, 191, 192, see pages 156, 157).

Perisinusoidal endothelial cells had a prominent Golgi apparatus and a centriole (Fig. 192, see page 157). Several pinocytotic vesicles and invaginations of the cell membrane were observed on the surface of perisinusoidal endothelial cells, among which some bristle-coated ones were detectable (Fig. 192, see page 157). Endothelial cells also contained malarial pigments and erythrocytes.

Summary

The primary injury of the liver in patients with infection of falciparum malaria seems to be a diffuse involvement of the reticuloendothelial system, which is produced by malarial parasites. The hepatocellular abnormalities noted in this study are presumed to have resulted from anoxia, due probably to anemia and mechanical vascular damage. Liver needle biopsy is a useful diagnostic procedure for malaria.

References

1. Dockrell, H.M., Souza, J.B. and Playfair, J.H.L. The role of the liver in immunity to blood-stage murine malaria. Immunology 41: 421–430, 1980.

2. White, L.G. and Doerner, A.A. Functional and needle biopsy study of the liver in malaria. JAMA 155: 637–639, 1954.

3. Lee, A.K. and Chung, W.K. Histologic and ultrastructural studies on liver infested with falciparum malaria. J Catholic Med Coll 34: 801–822, 1981.

{This is an extension and revision of a study which was carried out formerly by Lee, A.K. & Chung, W.K. (1981) (3).}

Legends

Fig. 185. Hepatic cell alterations.

Two mitotic figures (arrows) of liver-cell nucleus are seen. Case 11, needle biopsy, HE, ×400.

Fig. 186. Sinusoidal reaction.

Activated Kupffer cells (arrows) containing malarial pigment and numerous erythrocytes in the dilated sinusoid. Case 33, needle biopsy, HE, ×400.

Fig. 187.

Activated Kupffer cells engulf malarial pigment. Case 19, needle biopsy, HE, ×400.

Fig. 188. Portal reaction.

An arteriole in a portal tract shows the thickening of the wall and an intravascular thrombus (arrow). Perivascular inflammation and fibrosis are noted. Needle biopsy, HE, ×400.

Fig. 189. Electron microscopic findings.

(Reproduced from Lee, A.K. and Chung, W.K. J. Catholic Medical College 34: 801–822, 1981, with permission).

An electron micrograph of a Kupffer cell and two lymphocytes in the sinusoid. The voluminous cytoplasm of the Kupffer cell contains multiple osmiophilic dense bodies, vacuoles, a large irregularly shaped nucleus (KN) and an erythrocyte (E). The free surface of the Kupffer cell bounds the space of Disse (D) and comes into contact with the edge of the endothelial sheet (EC).

A lymphocyte (L) is closely applied to the Kupffer cell by several cytoplasmic processes from the lymphocyte. ×12,500.

Fig. 190.

A hypertrophied Kupffer cell (K) extends numerous cytoplasmic projections (CP) into the lumen of the sinusoid (S).

Numerous osmiophilic dense bodies varying in shape and size, an abundance of rough endoplasmic reticulum and several mitochondria are seen in the cytoplasm of a Kupffer cell. The space of Disse (D) is widened and contains a large quantity of collagen fiber (F) beneath the endothelial cell (EC). H: hepatocyte. ×8,332.

Fig. 191.

In the sinusoid, lamellated and fibrillar materials and osmiophilic electron-dense bodies are surrounded by several cytoplasmic processes (pseudopod) from the Kupffer cell. Bundles of collagen fiber (F) are seen among the microvilli of the hepatocyte in the space of Disse (D). ×25,000.

Fig. 192.

An electron micrograph of part of a perisinusoidal cell (endothelial cell). Several pinocytotic vesicles and invaginations (long arrows) of the cell membrane are observed on the surface of the perisinusoidal cell, among which some bristle-coated ones (short arrows) are detectable. This cell has a prominent Golgi apparatus (GA), several mitochondria, smooth endoplasmic reticulum and an erythrocyte (E).

C: centriole. ×29,900.

16 NONCIRRHOTIC PORTAL HYPERTENSION

Whan Kook Chung, M.D., Ph.D. and
Jin Wu Jeong, M.D., Ph.D.

Portal hypertension is most often associated with cirrhosis, but some other types of portal hypertension are not. In this chapter, we treat two types of portal hypertension, not associated with cirrhosis, whose causes are unknown and whose entities have not been established yet. One is called "regenerative nodular hyperplasia" (Group 1) (Fig. 193, see page 157), and the other is a type variously called "idiopathic (primary) portal hypertension" (1), "hepatoportal sclerosis" (2) or "noncirrhotic portal fibrosis" (3) (Group 2).

Microhamartomas (von Meyenberg complexes) rarely give rise to cirrhosis, but multiple lesions are associated with portal hypertension, and the lesions tend to merge imperceptibly with congenital hepatic fibrosis (4). Patients with congenital hepatic fibrosis are liable to portal hypertension without hepatic parenchymal disease or obstruction of the main portal vein (5). Both of these cystic diseases belong to another group of noncirrhotic portal hypertension (Group 3).

Patients

For the purpose of clarifying the histologic patterns of noncirrhotic portal hypertension of unknown etiology in Korea, histologic and clinical changes were examined in three cases from Group 1, six cases from Group 2 and three cases from Group 3 (Table 16-1). In nine out of 12 cases, surgical hepatic wedge

TABLE 16–1.

Clinical Summary of Noncirrhotic Portal Hypertension

Case No.	1	2	3	4	5	6	7	8	9	10	11	12
Age and Sex	45/F	34/F	21/F	54/M	17/F	51/F	16/F	46/F	65/F	30/M	34/F	17/F
Vascular spiders	–	–	–	–	–	–	–	+	–	–	–	–
Hepatomegaly	+	+	–	–	–	+	–	–	+	+	+	+
Splenomegaly	+	+	+	+	+	+	+	+	+	+		
Abdominal wall veins	+ + + +	+	–	–	–	–	±	?	–	–	–	–
Ascites	+ +	±	–	–	–	+ +	+	–	–	–	–	–
Bleeding varices	+	–	–	+	+	–	+	+	+	+	+	+
Liver scan												
Size of liver	Shrunken rt. lobe	Slightly enlarged		Moderately collapsed	Slightly decreased	Slightly enlarged	Normal	Normal	Normal	Normal	Slightly enlarged	Slightly enlarged
Mottling	±	–		–	±	±	±	±	+	+	+	+
Portal vein venography	Markedly dilated	Moderately dilated	Portal thrombosis				Moderately dilated	Markedly dilated			Markedly dilated	Markedly dilated
Mesenteric arteriography						Portal V. dilation					Portal V. dilation	Portal V. dilation
Esophageal varices	Moderate	Mild		Moderate	Moderate		Moderate	Moderate	Severe	Moderate	Severe	Severe
Portal venous pressure (during surgery)	280mmH_2O	32OmmH_2O			350mmH_2O	270mmH_2O	365mmH_2O	380mmH_2O			300mmH_2O	
Liver surface												
Laparoscopy	Small multiple nodules		Normal liver	Normal liver		Fibrin deposit			Area of umbilica-tion	Normal	Irregular	Irregular
Laparotomy	Slightly nodular	Slightly nodular			Not cirrhotic					Normal surface	Fibrotic surface	Fibrotic surface
Histologic diagnosis	Regenera-tive nodular hyperplasia	Regenera-tive nodular hyperplasia	Regenera-tive nodular hyperplasia with portal vein throm-bosis	Portal sclero-sis	Portal sclero-sis	Portal sclero-sis	Portal sclero-sis	Portal sclero-sis	Portal sclero-sis	Portal sclero-sis	Congenital hepatic fibrosis	Congenital hepatic fibrosis

Some cases are from Jeong, J. W. and W. K. Chung, J Catholic Medical College, 35:537–546, 1982, with permission.

biopsy was possible. In the remaining three cases, needle biopsy specimens were used. No cause was proved in the 10 cases of portal hypertension, except in those with congenital hepatic fibrosis.

Ten of the 12 patients were females. The remaining two were males belonging to Group 2. Their ages ranged from 16 to 65 years, averaging 38 years. Usually, the liver was not enlarged and sometimes was shrunken. Intraoperative measurement of portal vein pressure was done in seven cases, with 270–380mm H_2O, averaging 328mm H_2O. Liver test results remained fairly good (Table 16-2). Only one of six cases tested for HBsAg was positive. The liver surface was not cirrhotic and slightly diffuse nodules were noted in two cases from Group 1, focal undulation and umbilication were seen in one case from Group 2, and slight irregularity with fibrosis was observed in two cases from Group 3. Splenomegaly with pancytopenia (Table 16-3) of peripheral blood and esophageal varicosities were found in all cases. While one case from Group 1 showed extra-hepatic portal vein thrombosis by splenoportovenography, the remaining cases had patent but dilated extra-hepatic portal veins.

TABLE 16–2.

Biochemical Findings (Before Shunt Operation)

	Mean
Total bilirubin (mg/100ml)	1.1
S A S T (Sigma U)	43.9
S A L T (Sigma U)	21.6
Alk. phosphatase (B.U)	3.6
Total protein (gm/100ml)	7.1
Albumin	4.0
Globulin	3.2

TABLE 16–3.

Hematologic Findings (Before Shunt Operation)

	Mean
WBC (/mm^3)	2892
Hemoglobin (gm/100ml)	9.0
Hematocrit (%)	27.6
Platelet (1000)	93
Reticulocyte (%)	2.0
Prothrombin time (sec/% of normal)	11.4/82.7
Bleeding time (min)	1.7
Coagulation time (min)	4.8

Histological Findings

In all the cases from Group 1, regenerative nodules of varied size abutting on one another compressed the normal hepatic parenchyma between them. This resulted in stromal collapse and reticulin condensation (Fig. 193, see page 157). In the center of the nodule, seemingly located in the intralobular area, a group of duct-like structures, perhaps resulting from compressed hepatic cells by exudate of the lymph between the plates, gave an appearance of "reversed lobulation" (Figs. 194, 195, see page 157). It seemed to have been induced as the result of outflow block from the lobular parenchyma, perhaps due to the compression of the parenchyma by regenerative nodules.

There were multiple dilated vessels in a single nodule. Markedly dilated and proliferated sclerotic portal veins and arterioles were observed in a widened and edematous portal tract (Figs. 196, 197, see pages 157, 158). Vascular thrombi were occasionally seen in portal tracts (Fig. 197, see page 158).

In Group 2, the histologic changes were characterized by periductal fibrosis, phlebosclerosis and perivascular fibrosis of the portal vein system. Several dilated vessels in and around a fibrosed portal tract and multiple sinusoidal cystic dilatation were observed. Bleb-like abnormal spaces were in the immediate subcapsular area (Fig. 198, see page 158).

In a case with a change resembling primary biliary cirrhosis, the liver surface observed by laparoscopy showed focal undulation and an umbilication. Approximation of portal tracts resulting from parenchymal atrophy occurred probably as a result of a secondary reaction to portal circulatory insufficiency. In the portal tracts, portal vein radicles and proximal bile ducts had disappeared or were unrecognizable. Old thick fibrosis with a sharp outer border was observed in the expanded portal space.

In one case, a von Meyenberg complex was connected with a portal tract which had sclerosis very similar to that seen in Group 2 (Figs. 199, 200, see page 158). In a case of congenital hepatic fibrosis (Case 11), the liver surface observed by laparoscopy showed multiple gray-whitish scars that were triangular or stellate in shape. Microscopically, there were ductular proliferation and portal fibrosis of varying degrees (Figs. 201, 202, see page 158). The cholangioles were generally dilated and showed varying degrees of atrophy of epithelial lining cells (Fig. 202, see page 158). These ducts sometimes formed microcysts, showing a close resemblance to microhamartomas (Fig. 203, see page 159). The patient had no jaundice but had bile-containing dilated ducts (Figs. 201, 204, see pages 158, 159). There was little or no inflammatory infiltration in the fibrotic septa, and the junction of septa and parenchyma was sharply defined (Figs. 201, 202, 205, see pages 158, 159), except where the abnormal ducts abutted on liver cells (Fig. 204, see page 159).

Proliferated bile ductules extended into the parenchyma and a group of hepatic lobules was entrapped and encircled by the proliferated ductules (Fig. 205, see page 159). We presumed that atrophy of the intervening parenchyma and eventual development of a large portal sclerosis with thick fibrosis occur (Fig. 205, see page 159). The liver parenchyma was intersected by serpinginous septa of mature fibrous tissue, between which the lobular structure remained more or less intact (Figs. 202, 205, see pages 158, 159). A few islands of parenchyma appeared isolated by fibrosis, but hyperplastic nodules were nearly always absent (Figs. 205, 206, see page 159). The scar tissue contained multiple cystic dilations (Figs. 202, 205, 206, see pages 158, 159).

Multiple dilated vessels or cystic sinusoids, as were noted in a single lobule, and thinly walled bypass channels in and around the portal tracts (Figs. 197, 199, see page 158), dilated portal veins (Figs. 196, 199, 200, 201, 205, see pages 157, 158, 159) and proliferated and sclerotic arterioles (Figs. 197, 198, see page 158) were seen in all three groups. The changes were presumed to have resulted from compensatory phenomena due to lack of blood perfusion into the parenchyma.

Sometimes, portal vein radicles and proximal bile ducts were unrecognizable in the fibrotic portal space. The outer border of sclerotic portal tracts was usually sharp.

Whether or not the different histologic features shown in Groups 1 and 2 are due to the same causative factors, and whether or not the microhamartoma is associated with idiopathic portal hypertension as in Case 10 are not clear. The portal hypertension due to congenital hepatic fibrosis does not come within the category of so-called "idiopathic portal hypertension". However, congenital hepatic fibrosis does not exist in combination with true cirrhosis but frequently causes esophageal variceal bleeding due to portal hypertension. For this reason, we have evaluated congenital hepatic fibrosis in this chapter which is assigned to the description of noncirrhotic portal hypertension.

Summary

Noncirrhotic portal hypertension does not seem to be rare in Korea. This disease cannot be ruled out even when needle liver biopsy is normal, and changes are likely to be more effectively detected by operative wedge biopsy. Accordingly, more attention should be paid in the future to the availability of more credible and accurate tests than the surgical wedge biopsy. This focus will ultimately lead to more extensive detection of this disease and the establishment of its clinical and pathologic identity. Such efforts will eventually result in the clarification of its cause.

References

1. Boyer, J.L., Hales, M.R. and Klatskin, G. Idiopathic portal hypertension due to occlusion of intrahepatic portal veins by organized thrombi. Medicine, Baltimore 53: 77–91, 1974.

2. Mikkelson, W.P., Edmondson, H.A., Peters, R.L., Redeker, A.G. and Reynolds, T.B. Extra- and intrahepatic portal hypertension without cirrhosis (hepatoportal sclerosis). Ann Surg 162: 602–620, 1965.

3. Ramalingaswami, V., Wig, K.L. and Sama, S.K. Cirrhosis of the liver in Northern India. A clinicopathologic study. Arch Intern Med 110: 350–358, 1962.

4. Scheuer, P.J. Liver Biopsy Interpretation. Second edition, Williams & Wilkins, Baltimore, page 116, 1977.

5. Kerr, D.N.S., Harrison, C.V., Sherlock, S. and Milnes Walker, R. Congenital hepatic fibrosis. Q J Med 30: 91–117, 1961.

6. Jeong, J.W. and Chung, W.K. Noncirrhotic nodular transformation of the liver with portal hypertension. J Catholic Med Coll 35: 537–548, 1982.

{This is an extension and revision of a study which was carried out formerly by Jeong and Chung (1982)(6).}

Legends

Fig. 193. Regenerative nodular hyperplasia (Case 1) (Group 1).

Regenerative nodules of varied size, abutting one another, compressing the normal hepatic parenchyma between them, resulting in stromal collapse and reticulin fiber condensation. Wedge biopsy, reticulin stain, ×40.

Fig. 194.

Note a regenerative nodule (right lower) which compresses the normal parenchyma of terminal acinus resulting in elongated slender perinodular parenchymal collapse. In the center of the nodule, located apparently in the intralobular area, a group of duct-like structures, perhaps due to hepatic cells compressed by exudate of the lymph between the plates, has an appearance of "reversed lobulation". A hamartoma vascular change is seen at the top of the figure. Wedge biopsy, HE, ×40.

Fig. 195.

In the center of the nodule, two-cell-thick hepatic cell plates are seen compressed by edematous exudate of the lymph between the plates, representing perhaps the result of compression and the blockage of hepatic venous outflow by nodules. Wedge biopsy, HE, ×100.

Fig. 196.

Four markedly dilated thin-walled portal veins are seen in a widened portal tract, resulting probably from a long-standing blockage of outflow of portal blood. Part of the portal tract is compressed by regenerative nodules. Wedge biopsy, HE, ×100.

Fig. 197.

A high magnification of the edematous portal space shows proliferation of arterioles and a thrombus (outlined by arrowheads) filling a portal vein branch. Note a thin-walled vascular channel adjacent to the thrombus. Wedge biopsy, HE, ×400.

Fig. 198. Noncirrhotic portal sclerosis (Case 5) (Group 2).

Two sclerotic arterioles are seen in the bleb-like subcapsular space. Wedge biopsy, HE, ×100.

Fig. 199. Noncirrhotic portal sclerosis associated with von Meyenberg complex (Case 10) (Group 3).

A microhamartoma (left) and portal sclerosis. Wedge biopsy, trichrome, ×100.

Fig. 200.

Two dilated portal veins (PV) are seen in the fibrosed portal tract representing perhaps a compensatory phenomenon resulting from the lack of portal blood perfusion into the parenchyma. Wedge biopsy, trichrome, ×100.

Fig. 201. Noncirrhotic portal sclerosis with congenital hepatic fibrosis (Cases 11 and 12) (Group 3).

There are various types of ductular proliferation in the fibrous portal tract. Bile thrombi are seen in the dilated bile ducts (arrows). Wedge biopsy, HE, ×100.

Fig. 202.

There is no inflammatory infiltration in the fibrotic septum, and the junction of the septum and the parenchyma is sharply defined, except where the abnormal ducts abut on the liver cells (arrows). The cholangioles are dilated and show atrophy of the epithelial lining cells of varying degrees (curved arrows). Wedge biopsy, HE, ×100.

Fig. 203.

Bile ducts form microcysts which show close resemblance to microhamartoma. Wedge biopsy, HE, ×200.

Fig. 204.

Abnormal ducts abut on liver cells. Wedge biopsy, HE, ×200.

Fig. 205.

Proliferated bile ductules extend into the parenchyma and a group of hepatic lobules are entrapped and encircled by the proliferated ductules (thin arrows). They are presumed to be caused by the atrophy of the intervening parenchyma and finally develop to a large portal sclerosis with thick fibrosis (thick arrows). There are multiple cystic dilatations in the scar tissue. Several islands of parenchyma appear isolated by fibrosis, but hyperplastic nodules are absent. Wedge biopsy, HE, ×40.

Fig. 206.

Proliferated bile ductules with fibrosis, which seem to have originated from a sclerotic portal tract extend into the parenchyma to isolate it. The lobular structure remains more or less intact. Wedge biopsy, HE, ×100.

17 HEPATIC VENOUS CONGESTION AND OUTFLOW BLOCK

Whan Kook Chung, M.D., Ph.D., Byung Min Ahn, M.D., Jae Kwang Kim, M.D., Chang Don Lee, M.D., Ph.D., In Sik Chung, M.D., Ph.D., Kyu Won Chung, M.D., Ph.D., Hee Sik Sun, M.D., Ph.D., Boo Sung Kim, M.D., Ph.D., Yong Bok Koh, M.D., Ph.D. and Chang Hong Lee, M.D., Ph.D.

Disturbances in hepatic function and morphologic changes are frequent in patients with heart disease. In acute hepatic congestion, the morphologic changes range from simple passive congestion to extensive centrilobular necrosis and infarction.

Occasionally, in patients with congestive heart failure, the manifestations of liver injury may develop rapidly and dominate the clinical picture, so that the circulatory basis for the liver injury may be obscured. Such patients are often mistakenly diagnosed as having acute viral hepatitis.

Constrictive pericarditis leads to chronic hepatic congestion and, if this begins, portal hypertension develops, splenomegaly and ascites are caused and there are occasional incidents where clinical investigation begins with a clinical impression of cirrhosis.

Among cases of Budd-Chiari syndrome observed in Korea, many are due to inferior vena caval obstruction (1). These are usually diagnosed as cirrhosis accompanying portal hypertension and, since the cause is not evident, the diagnosis can be easily missed.

Biopsy examination of the role of such acute and chronic congestion in the production of hepatic lesion is more reliable than necrospy and is important in guiding management (2).

Patients

The authors had a chance to analyze histologically liver biopsy material obtained from 25 patients in whom acute and chronic hepatic venous congestion and outflow block were produced by cardiovascular origin.

Of the 25 cases, five had congestive heart failure (Group I), five had constrictive pericarditis (Group II) and the remaining 15 Budd-Chiari syndrome (Group III). Suggestive etiologies of congestive heart failure are mentioned in Table 17-1. In most cases, constrictive pericarditis was supposed to be caused by tuberculosis. In all the cases we treated, the Budd-Chiari syndrome was induced by segmental obstruction of inferior vena cava at the level of the diaphragm, which was confirmed by clinical, laboratory and radiologic findings.

In most of the cases of Group I, the symptoms resembled those of acute viral hepatitis (Table 17-2), and the patients of the latter two groups revealed chronic liver diseases.

TABLE 17–1.

Age and Sex Distribution

Group	*Diagnosis*	*Age*	*Sex*
Group I.			
1.	Congestive heart failure with acute renal failure	21	F
2.	Congestive heart failure with rodenticide intoxication	25	F
3.	Congestive heart failure with chronic renal failure	34	M
4.	Congestive heart failure with Graves' disease	46	M
5.	Congestive heart failure with right atrial myxoma	42	M
		Mean (Range)	*M/F*
		33.6 (21–46)	3/2
Group II.	Constrictive pericarditis	37.8 (19–58)	3/2
Group III.	Budd-Chiarl syndrome with inferior vena cava obstruction	37.8 (26–57)	6/9

TABLE 17–2.

Hematologic and Biochemical Findings in Patients with Hepatic Congestion

Group	*Hb/Hct (gm%/%)*	*WBC (/cu mm)*	*Platelet (/cu mm)*	*Alb/Glob (gm/dl)*	*TB/DB (mg/dl)*	*AST/ALT (units)*
I	11.4±1.72/ 35.9±6.29	*9,633 ±3,614	313,000 ±139,000	3.13±0.39/ 2.91±0.95	*3.3±3.6/ 1.5±1.8	*515±640/ 321±571
II	11.7±1.34/ 33.6±1.82	5,800 ±1,542	182,000 ± 79,654	2.46±0.52/ 3.78±0.63	1.0±0.5/ 0.2±0.1	134±132/ 121±102
III	11.5±0.98/ 35.4±2.93	5,253 ±1,128	143,266 ± 38,458	2.93±0.42/ 3.21±0.73	1.4±0.74/ 0.4±0.44	34± 16/ 19± 8

Key: *, $p < 0.05$ as compared to Group III; Alb/Glob, albumin/globulin; TB/DB, total bilirubin/direct bilirubin

Histological Finding

Mild active congestion resulted in the dilatation of central hepatic venules and the compression of hepatic cells in the center of the lobules due to dilated sinusoids filled with blood, sometimes with eosinophilic exudate and sometimes with edematous fluid in the tissue space (Fig. 207, see page 159). In more severe cases, hemorrhage and ischemic centrizonal necrosis or atrophy of liver cells were seen. Such patients often had marked serum aminotransferase increase that suggested viral hepatitis. Correct diagnosis was readily established by liver biopsy.

In severe cases with congestive heart failure, extensive parenchymal cell necrosis, even with confluent necrosis, was seen. Red blood cells extravasated and infiltrated into hepatic cell plates. The intensity of changes decreased toward the portal area. Fatty changes were common, especially in the central zone and on the borders of the congested area. The Kupffer cells showed few changes except for phagocytosis of ceroid pigment (Fig. 208, see page 159). Sometimes cholestasis and a mild degree of portal inflammatory reaction were found. When congestion persisted, the reticulin fiber framework in the center of the lobule collapsed and collagen fibers radiated from the central area into the lobular parenchyma.

Severe acute congestion was also seen in cases with acutely exacerbated chronic forms, including constrictive pericarditis and Budd-Chiari syndrome.

True congestive or cardiac cirrhosis is a rare lesion. When venous congestion is prolonged and severe, fibrosis, in addition to the above changes, is progressive. In such cases among the authors' materials, thrombosis of medium-sized radicles of the hepatic venous tree was seen. Fibrosis due to chronic venous congestion appeared first in the center of the lobule, and sometimes near or complete obstruction by fibrosis of the central vein occurred. Thus, the hepatic venules were often difficult to discern within the fibrous tissue (Fig. 209, see page 160). Thin-walled by-pass channels formed from sinusoids were occasionally mistaken for the original venules. Around the scarred area was a zone of dilated sinusoids.

When hepatic congestion is more prolonged and becomes severe enough, central fibrosis may extend to the portal tracts (Fig. 210, see page 160). This leads to portal-hepatic venous anastomoses and to destruction of the lobular architecture. It seems that the lobule is then dissected, and regenerative nodules form (Fig. 211, see page 160), leading to compression of the hepatic vein and portal hypertension. Under these circumstances, progressive cirrhosis may develop.

Recently, we conducted surgical repair (transcaval finger fracture and thrombectomy) on patients with Budd-Chiari syndrome due to inferior vena caval obstruction. We were able to obtain some hitherto-unknown information through liver wedge biopsy conducted before and after the operation.

Histologic examination revealed fibrotic thickening in most hepatic capsules and the central zone. Occasionally, hematoma was seen in the broad fibrotic scar tissue.

The fibrosis that occurred between the central zone and the portal space formed bridges between them, and the bridges developed into septal fibrosis and dissected the lobule (Fig. 212, see page 160). This enabled us to confirm the changes observed through needle biopsy (Fig. 210, see page 160). Most efferent vein walls had fibrotic thickening, but veins that still had distensibility were dilated (Fig. 212, see page 160). Especially, newly developed efferent veins in the single lobule were markedly dilated. Numerous cystic dilations of sinusoids were observed in the vicinity of proliferated efferent veins.

Many portal tracts showed fibrotic scars and well-developed dilated bypass channels. These phenomena were presumed to be the results of compensatory reaction to the lack of blood perfusion into the parenchyma. Bile ducts and ductules in the portal fibrotic scar were proliferated (Fig. 213, see page 160). The epithelial cell of the ducts was sometimes hyperplastic and swollen.

The major finding from wedge biopsies conducted immediately after the repair of inferior vena caval obstruction, in comparison with the biopsy which was performed before the repair, was the disappearance of dilated intralobular veins, sinusoids and bypass channels in and around the portal tracts. These alterations were presumed to be due to sudden release from the congestion and abrupt collapse of those dilated vascular lumens. However, several days after the operation, confluent ischemic necrosis was observed in the central area and bypass channels began to recur in and around the portal space (Fig. 214, see page 160). Sinusoidal cystic dilation also began to return. These later changes were presumed to have happened as the result of sudden interruption of blood perfusion into the parenchyma.

Hepatocytes had become tolerant to the reduction of sinusoidal circulation up to a point. Further reduction after shut-down of bypass circulation was presumed to accelerate the centrilobular ischemic necrosis. These findings signify that many changes can be found by means of needle biopsy and that important changes not discovered by needle biopsy can be detected through wedge biopsy.

As shown in Table 17-3, cirrhosis with regenerative nodules was much more commonly seen in cases with Budd-Chiari syndrome (93%) than in patients with constrictive pericarditis (20%), while no hepatic cirrhosis was observed in cases with congestive heart failure.

In hepatic congestion, extensive variations of histologic changes throughout the liver partly explain a poor correlation between the structural changes and the clinical and laboratory findings, between the degree and duration of the cardiac failure and between the regions of venous out-flow block on the liver.

TABLE 17–3.

Histologic Analysis of Hepatic Congestion

Histologic findings	*Group I (%)*	*Group II (%)*	*Group III (%)*
1. Lobular architecture			
Distorted	0/5 (0)	1/5 (20)	12/15 (80.0)
Preserved	5/5(100)	4/5 (80)	3/15 (20.0)
Reversed lobulation	4/5 (80)	1/5 (20)	7/15 (46.7)
2. Hemorrhage			
RBC intermingled with hepatocyte	4/5 (80)	3/5 (60)	4/15 (26.7)
Centrizonal	5/5(100)	3/5 (60)	4/15 (26.7)
Over-centrizonal	3/5 (60)	3/5 (60)	1/15 (6.7)
3. Central Vein reaction	5/5(100)	4/5 (80)	9/15 (60.0)
Dilatation	5/5(100)	4/5 (80)	10/15 (66.7)
Fibrous narrowing or obstruction	3/5 (60)	2/5 (40)	9/15 (60.0)
Perivascular edema	4/5 (80)	1/5 (20)	6/15 (40.0)
Perivascular fibrosis	1/5 (20)	2/5 (40)	14/15 (93.3)
Recanalization	0/5 (0)	2/5 (40)	7/15 (46.7)
4. Sinusoidal change			
Dilatation	4/5 (80)	5/5(100)	13/15 (86.7)
Blood	3/5 (60)	4/5 (80)	5/15 (33.3)
Exudate	2/5 (40)	2/5 (40)	4/15 (26.7)
Fibrin thrombi	1/5 (20)	2/5 (40)	5/15 (33.3)
Bile thrombi	0/5 (0)	0/5 (0)	0/15 (0.0)
Kupffer cell activation	5/5(100)	4/5 (80)	11/15 (73.3)
Ceroid pigment	1/5 (20)	0/7 (0)	1/15 (6.7)
Fibrosis and Capillarization	1/5 (20)	3/7 (43)	4/15 (26.7)
5. Parenchymal change			
Compression of hepatic cell plate	2/5 (40)	4/5 (80)	3/15 (20.0)
Hydropic degeneration	2/5 (40)	2/5 (40)	2/15 (13.3)
Centrizonal necrosis	3/5 (60)	1/5 (20)	6/15 (40.0)
Focal necrosis	0/5 (0)	1/5 (20)	1/15 (6.7)
Confluent necrosis	0/5 (0)	2/5 (40)	4/15 (26.7)
Fat	2/5 (40)	2/5 (40)	2/15 (13.3)
Adenomatous hyperplastic nodule	1/5 (20)	1/5 (20)	4/15 (26.7)
Regenerating nodules	0/5 (0)	1/5 (20)	14/15 (93.3)
6. Cholestasis	3/6 (60)	1/5 (20)	1/15 (6.7)
7. Fibrosis			
Centrizonal	3/5 (60)	3/5 (60)	13/15 (86.7)
Bridging	3/5 (60)	2/5 (40)	12/15 (80.0)
8. Portal reaction	5/5(100)	4/5 (80)	11/15 (73.3)
9. Cirrhosis	0/5 (0)	1/5 (20)	14/15 (93.3)

(Some cases are from Ahn B.M. et al. Korean Gastroenterology 21; 947–955, 1989, with permission)

Summary

Of the 25 cases with hepatic congestion, five had congestive heart failure, five had constrictive pericarditis and the remaining 15 had Budd-Chiari syndrome.

In most cases, constrictive pericarditis was supposed to be caused by tuberculosis and, in all the cases we treated, the Budd-Chiari syndrome was induced by segmental obstruction of inferior vena cava at the level of the diaphragm.

In most of the cases of congestive heart failure, the symptoms resembled those of acute viral hepatitis, and the patients of the latter two groups revealed chronic liver diseases.

Cirrhosis was much more commonly seen in patients with Budd-Chiari syndrome (93%) than in patients with constrictive pericarditis (20%), while no hepatic cirrhosis was observed in patients with congestive heart failure.

References

1. Chung, I.S., Won, D.S., Sun, H.S., Kim, B.S., Kim, S.S., Chung, W.K. and Sim, K.S. Budd-Chiari syndrome with obstruction of inferior vena cava. Korea J Int Med 18: 694–704, 1975.

2. Bynum, T.E., Boitnott, J.K. and Maddrey, W.C. Ischemic hepatitis. Digestive Diseases and Sciences 24: 129–135, 1979.

3. Ahn, B,M., Kim, J.K., Chung, I.S., Chung, K.W., Sun, H.S., Kim, B.S. and Chung, W.K. Clinical and morphological findings in acute and chronic hepatic congestion: A retrograde study on 22 patients. Korean J Gastroenterology 21: 947–955, 1989.

(This is an extension and revision of a study which was carried out originally by Ahn, B.M. et al., (3))

Legends

Fig. 207. Congestive heart failure.

Eosinophilic exudate (clumped erythrocytes ?) in the dilated sinusoids around the central vein (CV). Needle biopsy, HE, ×400.

(Reproduced from Ahn, B.M., Kim, J.K., Chung, I.S., et al. Korean J Gastroenterology 21: 947–955, with permission).

Fig. 208.

Phagocytosis of ceroid pigment in macrophages (Kupffer cells) in the area adjacent to the central vein. Needle biopsy, HE, ×400.

(Reproduced from Ahn, B.M., Kim, J.K., Chung, I.S., et al. Korean J Gastroenterology 21: 947–955, with permission).

Fig. 209. Budd-Chiari syndrome.

Thick fibrous scar in the central zone. Needle biopsy, HE, ×100.

(Reproduced from Ahn, B.M., Kim, J.K., Chung, I.S., et al. Korean J Gastroenterology 21: 947–955, with permission).

Fig. 210.

Central-central and central-portal fibrous septa where the dissection of the lobule has begun. Needle biopsy, HE, ×100.

(Reproduced from Ahn, B.M., Kim, J.K., Chung, I.S., et al. Korean J Gastroenterology 21: 947–955, with permission).

Fig. 211.

The hepatic lobule is dissected by fibrotic tissue and several regenerative nodules form. Needle biopsy, HE, ×100.

(Reproduced from Ahn, B.M., Kim, J.K., Chung, I.S., et al. Korean J Gastroenterology 21: 947–955, with permission).

Fig. 212.

Fibrosis occurs around the efferent veins and in the portal tracts, and they extend between efferent veins or between portal tracts or between efferent veins and portal tracts. Regenerative nodules are surrounded by fibrous septa. Dilated efferent veins and bypass channels are seen in the fibrotic scar. Wedge biopsy, trichrome, ×40.

Fig. 213.

There are many ducts and ductules in the portal fibrotic scar tissue. Numerous proliferated ducts in the periphery of the scar consist of enlarged and swollen epithelial cells (short arrows) while those in the inside are not enlarged (long arrows). Wedge biopsy, HE, ×100.

Fig. 214.

A liver biopsy was performed 10 days after surgery for repairment of the obstruction in a patient with Budd-Chiari syndrome due to inferior vena cava obstruction.

Sclerotic portal space containing many bile ductules. Beginning of bypass channels is noted in and around the portal tract. Needle biopsy, HE, ×100.

Addendum

18 THE HISTOLOGIC FINDINGS OF CHRONIC HEPATITIS C AND B: A COMPARATIVE STUDY

Whan Kook Chung, M.D., Ph.D.
Boo Sung Kim, M.D., Ph.D.

The histopathological changes in non-A, non-B (NANB) hepatitis have been studied extensively in several papers over the past decade (1–4). However, they could not be validated because of the lack of confirmatory diagnostic markers and, moreover, in most studies, evidence of infection with a single virus could not be conclusively established. The development of a serological test for antibody to a nonstructural antigen (C100-3) of a parenterally transmitted NANB hepatitis agent, hepatitis C virus (HCV) (5), provided the opportunity to study the pathology of at least one form of this disease. However, first-generation tests gave both false-positive and false-negative results (6–8). Second-generation tests have detected antibodies to both structural and nonstructural components of the virus, and have demonstrated that most patients with parenterally transmitted NANB hepatitis are infected with hepatitis C virus (HCV) (9).

However, whether or not cases, in which the presently available second-generation tests for the detection of HCV-antibody (anti-HCV) are not sensitive enough, or are secondary to other as yet unidentified causes, remains to be seen.

The etiological diagnosis of hepatitis B is confirmed by hepatitis B surface antigen (HBsAg). HBsAg was analysed by solid phase radioimmunoassay, one of the best examination methods which was developed at an early stage. Therefore, the serological and etiological diagnosis of hepatitis B has been possible for a long time before now. Accordingly, the histological characteristics of chronic hepatitis, infected by hepatitis B virus (HBV) have been established early in Korea (10). Through second-generation testing, anti-HCV positive chronic hepatitis C (CH-C) was selected, of which there had been recent reports of histopathologic studies (11, 12). However, there were no established reports on the pathognomonic features of CH-C.

For the purpose of detecting the specific character of the biopsy findings of CH-C and chronic hepatitis B (CH-B), we made a histological comparative examination between these two diseases.

Materials and Methods

Seventy-six consecutive chronic patients with liver diseases, who underwent liver biopsy during a period of 22 years (1970–1992), were studied histopathologically. All patients were HBsAg seronegative and were considered to have NANB hepatitis on the basis of exclusion of other causes of hepatitis by clinical, serological, immunological and biochemical criteria. All patients were positive for anti-HCV by second-generation testing. Among those who underwent second-generation testing, anti-HCV tests were carried out and interpreted following Abbott Co. directions. Fifty-six were men. The mean age of the cohort was 50 (range = 20–67) years (Table 18-1).

Eighty-one consecutive patients, who had undergone a liver biopsy, were randomly selected over a period of 23 months (January, 1988 until November, 1989) and were studied for hepatic histopathology. All patients were HBsAg seropositive and negative for anti-HCV, and had type B chronic hepatitis on the basis of exclusion of other causes of hepatitis by clinical, serological, immunological and biochemical criteria.

All specimens were obtained by the percutaneous needle biopsy, using a Menghini needle. Surgical biopsies were excluded, in order to standardize the amount of tissue examined. None of the liver biopsies were performed in the acute phase of the disease and no patient had immunosuppressive therapy before biopsy.

Hepatitis C markers were measured by second-generation ELISA (Abbott HCV EIA 2nd Generation). These assays were used to detect antibody to the non-structural (NS3 and NS4) region and to the structural core of the HCV. The formalin-fixed-paraffin-embedded section was stained with hematoxylin-eosin and trichrome. Overall histologic diagnosis was made using standard criteria (11–13).

The following features were chosen for this assessment on the basis that they had previously been considered characteristic of or common in NANB hepatitis (2–4, 13, 14): lymphoid aggregates or follicles in the portal tract, infiltration of small bile ducts by inflammatory cells or damaged duct, acidophilic body formation, steatosis and infiltration of sinusoids by lymphoid cells (Table 18-1).

Hepatitis B (control) group of 81 biopsy specimens from 81 HBsAg seropositive patients with CH-B were studied to compare the prevalence of hepa-

TABLE 18–1.

Histopathological Features of Chronic Hepatitis C and B: A Comparative Analysis

Type of chronic hepatitis	*C*	*B*	*p-Value*
No. patients	76	81	
Age: mean (range) yr.	50 (21–67)	34 (15–55)	
Sex: Male to Female ratio	56:20	65:16	
Histological findings			
Portal tract alteration			
Widening with chronic inflammatory cells			
Piecemeal necrosis	46 (60%)	50 (61%)	
dense lymphocyte aggregation (lymphoid follicle)	19 (25%)	13 (16%)	
Without/or mild piecemeal necrosis	32 (42%)	7 (8%)	P<0.01
dense lymphocyte aggregation (lymphoid follicle)	27 (35%)	4 (4%)	P<0.01
Bile duct			
Bile duct proliferation	2 (2%)	2 (2%)	
Bile duct damage and/or loss	45 (59%)	19 (23%)	P<0.01
Intralobular change			
Steatosis			
Microvesicular	1 (1%)	2 (2%)	
Macrovesicular			
Diffuse (massive)	3 (3%)	4 (4%)	
Focal (sublobular)	19 (25%)	5 (6%)	P<0.01
Spotty (mild)	37 (48%)	44 (54%)	
Subtotal	*60 (79%)*	*55 (68%)*	
Dysplastic cells			
Large	5 (6%)	4 (4%)	
Small	5 (6%)	1 (1%)	
Sinusoidal cellular activation (focal)	18 (23%)	9 (11%)	P<0.05
Acidophilic body	9 (19%)	13 (16%)	
Ballooning cell	14 (18%)	15 (18%)	
Focal necrosis replaced by lymphocytic micronodule	55 (72%)	20 (24%)	P<0.01
Spotty necrosis	6 (7%)	6 (7%)	
Subacute hepatic necrosis with/without collapse	6 (7%)	18 (22%)	P<0.05
Circumscribed hepatic necrosis with/without collapse	3 (3%)	9 (11%)	
Cirrhosis			
Strand septal fibrosis	11 (14%)	11 (13%)	
Developing cirrhosis	10 (12%)	19 (23%)	

tohistopathologic features with those in hepatitis C. All patients were seronegative for anti-HCV by second-generation testing as described above.

Serum sampling was done at the time of liver biopsy and stored at −20°C. Statistical analysis was performed using the Chi-squire test.

Results

Over a period of 22 years (from 1971 to 1992), liver biopsy specimens were obtained from 1,445 patients who were considered to have chronic liver dis-

TABLE 18–2.

Serological Diagnosis of Chronic Hepatitis

Tests	*No. of Patients*	*(%)*
anti-HCV (+) & HBsAg (−)	100	(6.9)
anti-HCV (−) & HBsAg (+)	874	(60.5)
anti-HCV (+) & HBsAg (+)	15	(1.0)
anti-HCV (−) & HBsAg (−)	456	(31.5)
Total	1445	

eases before biopsy (Table 18-2). All of the 1,445 cases were submitted to tests for both HBsAg by solid phase radioimmunoassay and anti-HCV by second-generation testing.

Results showed that 100 cases (6.9%) were anti-HCV positive only and 874 cases (60.5%) were HBsAg positive only and, however, 15 cases (1%) were both HBsAg and anti-HCV positive. The remaining 456 cases (31.5%) were both HBsAg and anti-HCV negative. Of the 456 cases, 258 did not enter into the chronic hepatitis category according to the results of the biopsy. The remaining 198 cases had findings of the histological features of chronic hepatitis (10) and it is hoped that further investigation will disclose the cause.

At the time of biopsy, the average age of patients with CH-C was 50 years and the average age of patients with CH-B was 34 years. Of the patients with CH-C, 74% were men and 26% were women and, of the patients with CH-B, 80% were men and 20% were women.

Histopathologic features are summarized in Table 18-1.

Varying degrees of portal tract inflammation were present in almost all biopsy specimens in both groups.

Portal widening with piecemeal necrosis and lymphocytic aggregation were of no significant difference in both groups, whereas patients with mild or without piecemeal necrosis (42%) with dense lymphocytic aggregation (35%) (Fig. 215, see page 217) seen in CH-C patients were more common than those with CH-B combined with dense lymphocytic aggregation (4%) ($P<0.01$). Lymphocytes were the main contributors to the portal inflammatory infiltrates in both groups. The lymphoid lesion seemed to range from loose aggregates of lymphocytes to dense aggregates. Piecemeal necrosis in CH-C was focal, involving part of a portal tract's circumference (Fig. 216, see page 217), patchy and involving some portal tracts and sparing others.

Bile duct injury has been reported to be a feature of NANB hepatitis (4, 15). Of the biopsy specimens from patients with CH-C, 59% had bile duct damage, compared with 23% of those with CH-B. Bile duct injury or loss (Fig. 217, see page 217), or both, involved small-sized bile ducts. Both of these are of different statistical significance ($P<0.01$). Bile duct proliferation was rarely seen both in and around lymphoid aggregation in the portal tract (2% in each group) (Fig. 218, see page 217).

Lobular activity, assessed by inflammation and hepatocellular necrosis, was more severe in patients with CH-B than in patients with CH-C.

Steatosis, especially sublobular focal type and predominantly macrovesicular, was more frequent in CH-C than in CH-B (25% vs. 6%) ($P<0.01$).

Hepatocellular dysplasia was noted in 12% of biopsies from patients with CH-C, whereas it was only shown in 5% of biopsy specimens from patients with CH-B.

Severe sinusoidal cell activations and spotty necrosis in the focal area of biopsy specimens were present in the sinusoids in 23% of patients with CH-C, compared with 11% of patients with CH-B (Fig. 219, see page 217) ($P<0.05$).

The acidophilic bodies were either surrounded by lymphocytes (Fig. 220, see page 217) or "naked" (Fig. 219, see page 217). No specific pattern was noted in either group. Multinucleated ballooning cells were present to some degree in 18% of biopsy specimens in both groups (Fig. 219, see page 217).

Intralobular focal necrosis, replaced by lymphocytic micronodules, was present in more than 70% of the specimens in the CH-C group (Fig. 220, see page 217) (Fig. 221, see page 218), in comparison with the group of CH-B (24%) ($P<0.01$), whereas massive piecemeal necrosis (Fig. 222, see page 218) and subacute hepatic necrosis, (SHN, bridging or multilobular necrosis), was the predominant form in CH-B (22%) (Fig. 223, see page 218) ($P<0.01$). The circumscribed hepatic necrosis (CHN) (10), was more severe in patients with CH-B (11%) (Fig. 224, see page 218) than in patients with CH-C (3%).

SHN (22%) and CHN (11%), which are usually considered as developing collapse and cirrhosis later, were seen more frequently in CH-B than the frequency of SHN (7%) and CHN (3%) in CH-C. Consequently, developing cirrhosis was also seen more frequently in patients with CH-B (23%) than in patients with CH-C (12%).

Discussion

In Korea, B type chronic liver infection is more prevalent than C type while, on the contrary, C type is more prevalent in neighboring Japan. The reason given by some experts is presented as follows.

During and after the Korean War, liver diseases with CH-B were prevalent in Korea. These liver diseases presented a grave health hazard to a population already suffering from the ravages of a long war (10). On the other hand, the high prevalence of CH-C in Japan was caused by previous surgical operations and blood transfusions for patients with lung tuberculosis, aged around 30. Some of them were infected by HCV, and 30 years later they developed CH-C (13).

It is important to find out whether or not these are the only reasons or if there are other causes.

Compared with the CH-B group, the age of CH-C patients is higher.

Also, while CH-B is most probably a primary infection in childhood, CH-C is associated with adulthood, and the histologic features of CH-B are seen as being more aggressive in comparison with CH-C.

Overall, although histological features and prevalence of different markers varied significantly in the two groups, we found no single pathognomonic feature for either disease. We do believe, however, that certain findings may be highly suggestive of a particular diagnosis.

The most striking feature was the presence of lymphoid aggregation or follicles in the portal tract (3). The lymphoid lesion seemed to range from loose aggregates of lymphocytes to well-defined dense structures of lymphoid aggregates. Clearly, follicles are not restricted to CH-C. They are seen, for example, as being confirmed in CH-B in this study. However, in this research, well-defined lymphocytic aggregates were found more less frequently in CH-B (4%) than in CH-C (35%) ($P<0.01$) (Table 1). The reason for the formation of lymphoid follicles remains obscure and deserves further study.

Bile duct injury has been reported to be a feature of NANB hepatitis (4, 14). Of the biopsy specimens from patients with CH-C, 59% had bile duct damage, compared with 23% of those with CH-B. Bile duct injury, loss or both, involved small-sized bile ducts. Both of these differences reached statistical significance ($P<0.01$). Bile duct proliferation was seen to varying degrees.

Steatosis, which has been described as a feature of NANB hepatitis (4), was noted in a more significant number of patients with CH-C than in patients with CH-B ($P<0.01$). A predominant macrovesicular steatosis was found. Whether or not the macrovesicular steatosis is directly related to the HCV infection, or is secondary to other predisposing conditions, is not clear.

Large dysplastic cells, regarded as precursor cells of hepatocellular carcinoma, are not significantly different from both type C and B hepatitis patients. The sinusoidal lymphocyte activation in the focal area is more frequently seen in patients with CH-C (23%) than in patients with CH-B (11%) ($P<0.05$).

Dienes et al. (3) proposed that hepatocellular damage, with "naked" acidophilic bodies or those not being attacked by lymphocytes, was a common feature of NANB hepatitis. It was found that many of the acidophilic bodies, seen in CH-C were accompanied by lymphocytic infiltration and, therefore, the earlier observation could not be confirmed. Ballooning degeneration of hepatocytes was only rarely observed in either group and no diffeent frequency was observed in each group.

Another difference observed was related to varying patterns of the distribution of lobular necroinflammation in the two diseases.

The intralobular focal necrosis, replaced by lymphocytic micronodules in patients with CH-C (72%), was more prominent than in patients with CH-B (24%) (P<0.01), whereas spotty necrosis was rare and of the same frequency in both groups (7%). The lymphocytic micronodules in focal necrosis were presumed to be CH-C-related histologic features, but it remains to be further confirmed in the future.

Diffuse intralobular (confluent) necroinflammation was more frequent in patients with CH-B. These types of confluent necrosis, followed by collapse, usually come from SHN or CHN (10).

SHN was observed in 22% of patients with CH-B and in 7% of patients with CH-C (P<0.05). CHN was also more frequent and with severe lesions in patients with CH-B than in patients with CH-C. These two types of hepatic necrosis induce and probably progress to collapse and cirrhosis (4, 15–17).

Therefore, developing cirrhosis cases are seen more often in CH-B patient groups than in CH-C patient groups.

Conclusion

It has been observed that subacute hepatic necrosis and circumscribed hepatic necrosis present an aggressive picture of frequently causing collapse, after confluent necrosis, more in CH-B type than in CH-C type. Accordingly, it would seem that cirrhosis develops more often in CH-B patients than in CH-C patients.

Differing characteristics of each disease were not revealed. Features more frequently seen in CH-C patients than in CH-B patients are, including dense lymphoid aggregation or follicles in the portal tracts, small-sized bile duct damage and loss, moderately developed macrovesicular steatosis, focal sinusoidal cellular activation and focal necrosis replaced by lymphocytic micronodules.

While a specific pathognomonic feature has not been identified in either disease, we believe that, in combination, certain histological patterns, as mentioned above, may be helpful in differentiating these two diseases.

References

1. Popper, H., Dienstag, J.L., Feinstone, S.M., Alter, H.H. and Purcell, R.H. Pathology of viral hepatitis in chimpanzees. Virchows Arch (A) 387:91–106, 1980.

2. Bamber, M., Murray, A., Arborgh, B.A.H., Scheuer, P.J., Kernoff, P.B.A., Thomas, H.C. and Sherlock, S. Short incubation non-A, non-B hepatitis transmitted by factor VIII concentrates in patients with congenitalcoagulation disorders. Gut 22:854–859, 1981.

3. Dienes, H.P., Popper, H., Arnold, W. and Lobeck, H. Histologic observation in human hepatitis non-A, non-B. Hepatology 2:562–571, 1982.

4. Schmid, M., Pirovino, M., Altorfer, J., Gudut, F. and Bianchi, L. Acute hepatitis non-A, non-B: are there any specific light microscopic features? Liver 2:61–71, 1982.

5. Kuo, G., Choo, Q.L., Alter, H.J., gitnik, G.L., Redecker, A.G., Purcell, R.H., Miyamura, T., Dienstag, J.L., Alter, M.J., Stevens, C.E., Tegtmeier, G.E., Bonino, F., Colombo, M., Lee, W.S., Kuo, C., Berger, K., Shuster, J.R., Overby, L.R., Bradly, D. W. and Houghton, M. An assay for circulating antibodies to a major etiologic virus of human non-A, non-B hepatitis. Science 244:362–364, 1989.

6. Gray, J.J., Wreghitt, T.G., Friend, P.J., Wight, D.G.D., Sundaresan, V. and Calne, R.Y. Differentiation between specific and non-specific hepatitis C antibodies in chronic liver disease. Lancet 335:609–610, 1990.

7. McFarlane, I.G., Smith, H.M., Johnson, P.J., Bray, G.P., Vergani, D. and Williams, R. Hepatitis C virus antibodies in chronic active hepatitis: pathogenetic factor or false-positive result? Lancet 355:754–757, 1990.

8. Weiner, A.J., Kuo, G., Bradley, D.W., Bonino, F., Saracco, G., Lee, C., Rosenblatt, J., Choo, Q.I. and Houghton, M. Detection of hepatitis C viral sequences in non-A, non-B hepatitis. Lancet 335:1–3, 1990.

9. Brown, D., Powell, L., Chrispeels, J., Morris, A., Rassam, S., Sherlock, S., McIntyre, N., Zuckerman, A. and Dusheiko, G. Improved diagnosis of chronic HCV infection by antibody to core epitopes (Abstract). Hepatology 14:69A, 1991.

10. Chung, W. K. Chronic hepatitis in Korea. Popper, H., Schaffner, F., editors. Progress in Liver Diseases, Vol. VIII. Philadelphia: Grune and Stratton, pages, 469–484, 1988.

11. Scheuer, P.J., Ashrafzadeh, P., Sherlock, S., Brown, D. and Dusheiko, G.M. The pathology of hepatitis C. Hepatology 15:567–571, 1992.

12. Bach, N., Thung, S.N. and Schaffner, F. Histological features of chronic hepatitis C and autoimmune chronic hepatitis: A comparison analysis. Hepatology 15:572–577, 1992.

13. Shikada, T. Hepatitis C in Japan. Syllabus of the Plenary Lectures in APASL, April 6–8, 1992, pages 105–107, 1992.

14. Bianchi, L., Desmet, V.J., Popper, H., Scheuer, P.J., Aledort, L.M. and Berk, P. D. Histological patterns of liver disease in hemophiliacs with special reference to morphological characteristics of non-A, non-B hepatitis. Semin Liver Dis 7:203–209, 1987.

15. MacSween, R.N.M. Pathology of viral hepatitis and its sequelae. Clin Gastroenterol 9:23–45, 1980.

16. Carithers, R.L. Jr. and Fallon, H.J. When does acute hepatitis become chronic? Cohen, S., Soloway, R.D., eds. Chronic active liver disease. New York: Churchill Livingstone, pages 189–206, 1983.

17. Cooksley, W.G.E., Bradbear, R.A., Robinson, W., Harrison, M., Halliday, J.W., Powell, L.W., Seah, H.N.G., Okuda, K., Scheuer, P.J. and Sherlock, S. The prognosis of chronic active hepatitis without cirrhosis in relation to bridging necrosis. Hepatology 6:345–348, 1986.

Legends

Fig. 215. Lymphoid aggregation with bile duct damage.

Chronic hepatitis C. A portal area from the liver biopsy specimen shows a lymphoid aggregate with damaged bile duct (arrow). Needle biopsy, HE, × 400.

Fig. 216. Lymphoid aggregation with piecemeal necrosis.

Chronic hepatitis C. Dense aggregate of lymphocytes eccentrically located in a portal tract (lymphoid follicles) and focal areas of circumference show piecemeal necrosis (arrows). Needle biopsy, HE, × 200.

Fig. 217. Lymphoid aggregation with bile duct loss.

Chronic hepatitis C. A portal area shows circular lymphoid aggregate in a portal tract without well-recognized small bile duct. Needle biopsy, HE, × 400.

Fig. 218. Lymphoid aggregation with bile duct proliferation.

Chronic hepatitis C. Multiple bile duct proliferations are seen in a lymphoid aggregate in a portal tract. Needle biopsy, HE, × 200.

Fig. 219 Sinusoidal cell activation and spotty necrosis.

Chronic hepatitis B. Note the marked diffuse spotty necrosis, sinusoidal cell infiltration, ballooning of the liver cells (slender arrow) and naked acidophilic body (thick arrow). The sinusoidal cells consist of mononuclear cells and polymorphonuclear cells. These findings are limited to a part of the specimens. Needle biopsy, HE, × 100.

Fig. 220. Focal necrosis with acidophilic body.

Chronic hepatitis C. Of the two foci of focal necrosis, replaced mainly by lymphocytes, one focus has acidophilic body (arrow) which is surrounded by inflammatory cells. Needle biopsy, HE, × 400.

Fig. 221. Focal necrosis.

Chronic hepatitis C. A large focal necrosis replaced by inflammatory cells is located in the vicnity of a central vein. The inflammatory cells consist predominantly of lymphocytes. Occasional polymorphonuclear leucocytes are present. Needle biopsy, HE, × 400.

Fig. 222. Piecemeal necrosis.

Chronic hepatitis B. Massive piecemeal necrosis involving the entire circumference of a portal tract is noted. Bile duct is absent. Needle biopsy, HE, × 200.

Fig. 223. Subacute hepatic necrosis (bridging necrosis).

Chronic hepatitis B. The portal inflammatory fibrosis links portal to portal tracts and portal tracts to central vein (arrow) and disrupts the normal lobular architecture. Needle biopsy, HE, × 100.

Fig. 224. Circumscribed hepatic necrosis.

Chronic hepatitis B. The biopsy specimen shows circumscribed hepatic necrosis with extensive collapse. Diffuse perihepatocellular fibrosis with acinar arrangement of hepatocytes is noted. Needle biopsy, HE, × 200.

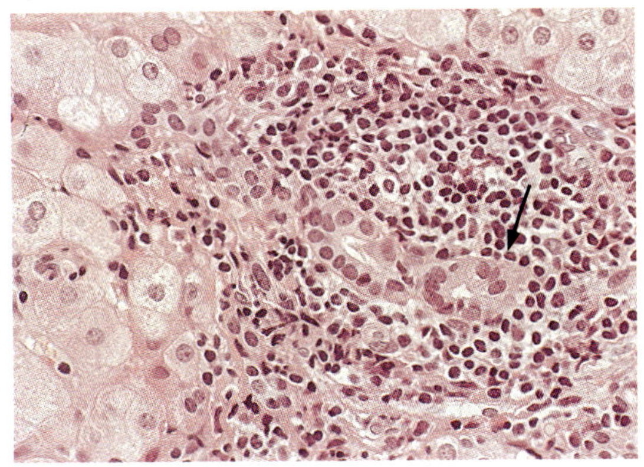

Fig. 215 See Legend page 215.

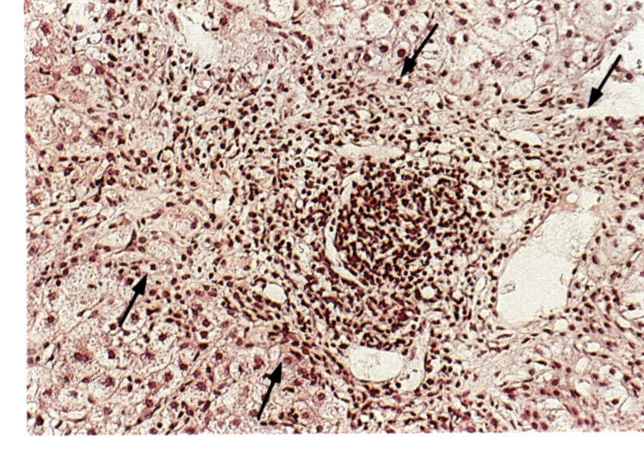

Fig. 216 See Legend page 216.

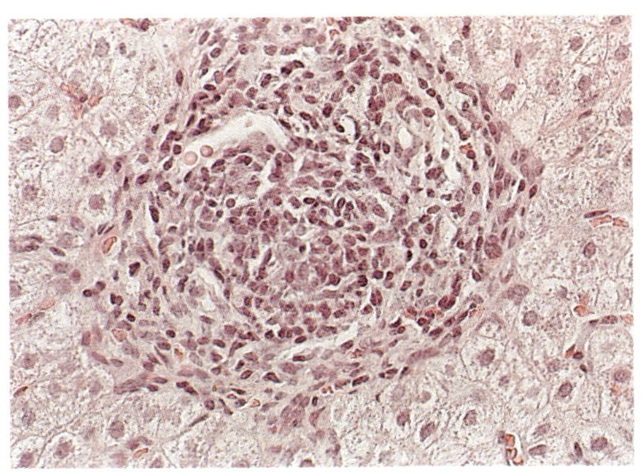

Fig. 217 See Legend page 216.

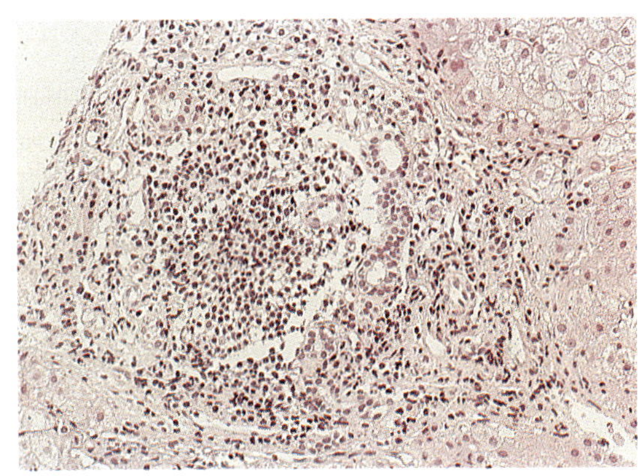

Fig. 218 See Legend page 216.

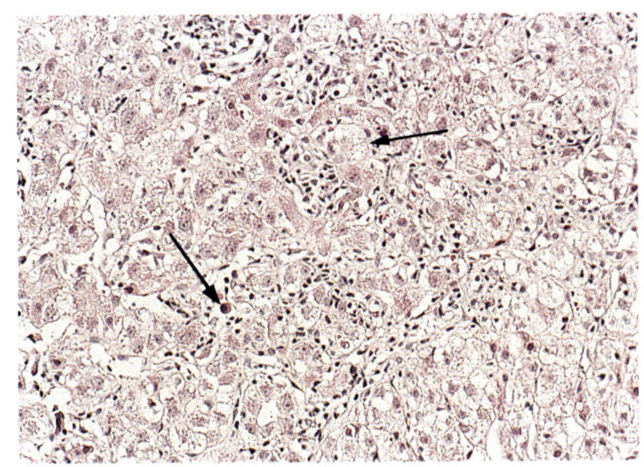

Fig. 219 See Legend page 216.

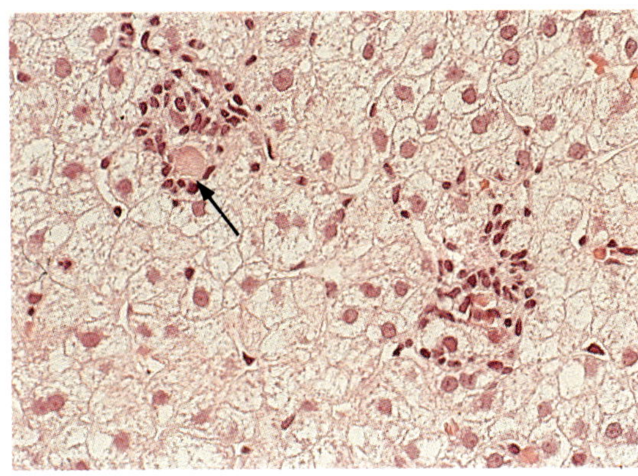

Fig. 220 See Legend page 216.

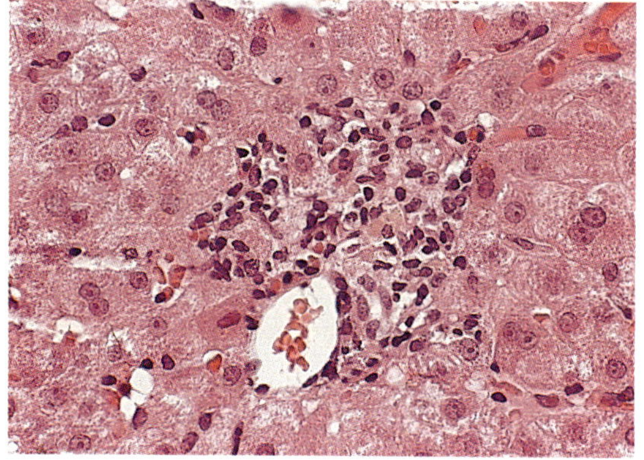

Fig. 221 See Legend page 216.

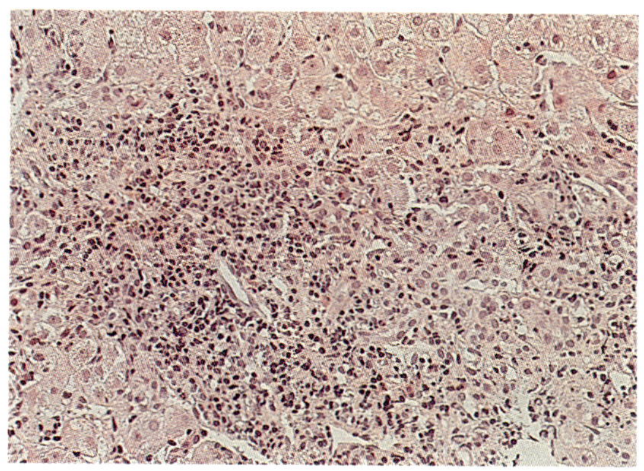

Fig. 222 See Legend page 216.

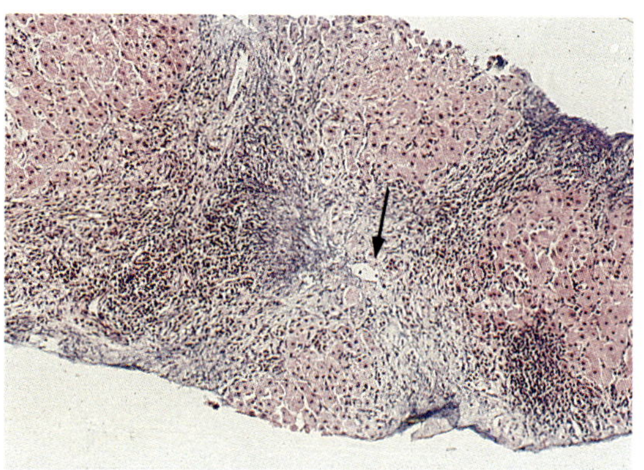

Fig. 223 See Legend page 216.

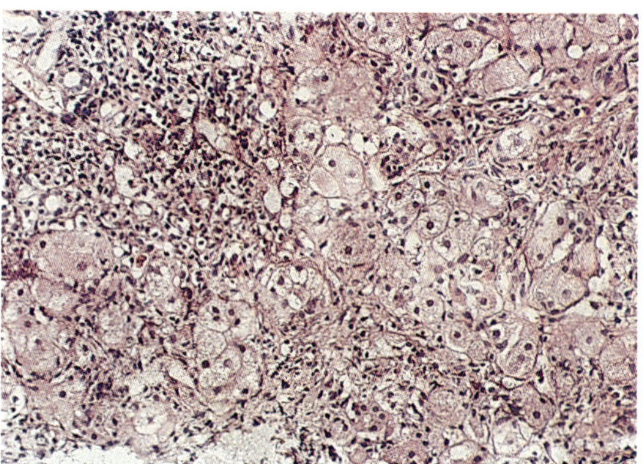

Fig. 224 See Legend page 216.

INDEX

D

E

F

G

H

I

J

K

L

M

N

O

P